THE FETUS AS MEDICAL PATIENT

Moral Dilemmas in Prenatal Diagnosis from a Catholic Perspective

Rev. Dr. Alfred Cioffi, STD

UNIVERSITY PRESS OF AMERICA

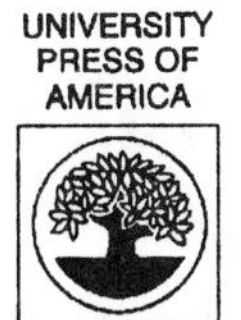

Lanham • New York • London

University Press of America,® Inc.
4720 Boston Way
Lanham, Maryland 20706

3 Henrietta Street
London WC2E 8LU England

Printed in the United States of America
British Cataloging in Publication Information Available

Library of Congress Cataloging-in-Publication Data

Cioffi, Alfred.
The fetus as medical patient : moral dilemmas in prenatal diagnosis from a Catholic perspective / Alfred Cioffi.
p. cm.
Includes bibliographical references.
1. Prenatal diagnosis—Religious aspects—Catholic Church.
I. Title.
RG628.C56 1995 241'.6425—dc20 94–24378 CIP

ISBN 0–8191–9780–7 (cloth : alk. paper)

The paper used in this publication meets the minimum requirements of American National Standard for Information Sciences—Permanence of Paper for Printed Library Materials, ANSI Z39.48–1984.

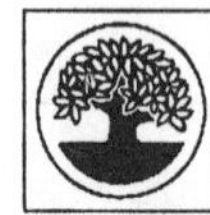

PART TWO

TEN NORTH AMERICAN CATHOLIC MORAL THEOLOGIANS

PART THREE

CRITICAL EVALUATION OF SEVEN RELEVANT THEMES

Abbreviations

AAS: *Acta Apostolicae Sedis*

ACOG: American College of Obstetrics and Gynecology

ACOGTechB: ACOG Technical Bulletin

AGenMedGem: Acta Geneticae Medicae et Gemellologiae

AJHumGen: American Journal of Human Genetics

AJMedGen: American Journal of Medical Genetics

AJObGyn: American Journal of Obstetrics and Gynecology

AmerCathPhilQ: American Catholic Philosophical Quarterly

Ang: Angelicum

Anthr: Anthropotes

BMedJ: British Medical Journal

CanCathHCRev: Canadian Catholic Health Care Review

CathLawyer: Catholic Lawyer

CDF: Congregation for the Doctrine of the Faith

CHA: U.S. Catholic Health Association

ChristCent: Christian Century

CITM: Congresso Internazionale di Teologia Morale

CivCat: La Civiltà Cattolica

ClinGen: Clinical Genetics

ClinObGyn: Clinical Obstetrics and Gynecology

CTSAProceeds: Catholic Theological Society of America Proceedings

CVS: Chorionic villus sampling

DH: *Dignitatis Humanae*

DocCath: La Documentation Catholique

EHumDev: Early Human Development

EscrVedat: Escritos del Vedat

Et: Études

EthMed: Ethics and Medics

EurJObGynReprBiol: European Journal of Obstetrics & Gynaecology and Reproductive Biology

FASEBJ: FASEB Journal

FC: *Familiaris Consortio*

FertSter: Fertility and Sterility

FetalTher: Fetal Therapy

GenCounsel: Genetic Counseling

Genom: Genommics

GMetaf: Giornale di Metafisica

Greg: Gregorianum

GS: *Gaudium et Spes*

HastingsCRep: Hastings Center Report

HealthProgr: Health Progress

HGeneTher: Human Gene Therapy

Hor: Horizons

HospPract: Hospital Practice

HospProgr: Hospital Progress

HumanRepr: Human Reproduction

HV: *Humanae Vitae*

IntJGynOb: International Journal of Gynaecology and Obstetrics

IntJTechAssHealthCare: International Journal of Technological Assessment in Health Care

IssHealthCareW: Issues in Health Care of Women

JAMA: Journal of the American Medical Association

JGenCounsel: Journal of Genetic Counseling

JInherMetabDis: Journal of Inherited Metabolic Disease

JMedEthics: Journal of Medical Ethics

JMedPhil: Journal of Medicine and Philosophy

JRCPhysLondon: Journal of the Royal College of Physicians of London

JReprInfPsy: Journal of Reproductive and Infant Psychology

JReprMed: Journal of Reproductive Medicine

JUltrasMed: Journal of Ultrasound Medicine

KennedyInstEthJ: Kennedy Institute of Ethics Journal

Laurent: Laurentianum

LavalPhilT: Laval Philosophique et Théologique

LG: *Lumen Gentium*

LumVie: Lumière et Vie

MedCare: Medical Care

MedMor: Medicina e Morale

MelScRel: Mélanges de Science Religieuse

MentalRet: Mental Retardation

MilbankMemQ: Milbank Memorial Quarterly; Health and Society

MMNewsletter: Medical-Moral Newsletter

Mor: Moralia

NatApostMentRet: National Apostolate for the Mentally Retarded

NCCB: U.S. National Conference of Catholic Bishops

NEJM: New England Journal of Medicine

NewSchol: New Scholasticism

NRT: Nouvelle Revue Théologique

ObGyn: Obstetrics and Gynecology

ObGynNews: Obstetrics and Gynecology News

Par: Parameters

Ped: Pediatrics

PND: Prenatal Diagnosis (procedure)

Pract: The Practitioner

PrenatDiag: Prenatal Diagnosis (journal)

RasT: Rassegna di Teologia

RazFe: Razón y Fe

RFil: Revista de Filosofía

RH: *Redemptor Hominis*

RIMJ: Rhode Island Medical Journal

RMetaph: Review of Metaphysics

RMetaphMor: Revue de Métaphysique et de Morale

RTLv: Revue Théologique de Louvain

RTMor: Rivista di Teologia Morale

RTPhil: Revue de Théologie et de Philosophie

SalTer: Sal Terrae

Sap: Sapientia

ScandJGastroenter: Scandinavian Journal of Gastroenterology

SecondOp: Second Opinion

SemPer: Seminars in Perinatology

SocBiol: Social Biology

SocIndRes: Social Indicators Research

SocWHealthCare: Social Work in Health Care

Suppl: Le Supplement

Thom: The Thomist

USCath: U.S. Catholic

USCC: U.S. Catholic Conference

VirgLawR: Virginia Law Review

WHealthF: World Health Forum

Preface

Any expectant mother in this day and age is a courageous woman. Consider this: even at the first news of your pregnancy, you will begin to run into what seems to be an endless stream of people, known and unknown to you, who will have a definite opinion about your pregnancy. And they will all be very willing to share their opinions with you! Some will be in favor of your pregnancy and may even be supportive and encouraging. Others will be very critical, or downright rude and insensitive in their comments and suggestions. While the latter must be graciously endured in any civil society, the former are really the ones capable of making a positive contribution at a time when true relationships make a difference.

Yet, among this seemingly endless stream of advice, there is one particular set of opinions that may be of great concern to pregnant women today: medical opinion. Why? Because today, unlike a few short years ago, the medical profession is able to determine many things about the condition of the human embryo even *before* he or she is born.

For example, it is no secret that through prenatal diagnosis the sex of the child in the womb can be known. But way beyond that, through the use of ultrasound, amniocentesis, chorionic villus sampling and various other techniques, a wide range of information about the fetus or embryo can be obtained. In fact, by the proper application of these diagnostic procedures, literally thousands of genetic and developmental abnormalities can now be detected *in utero*. This means that couples who are expecting a child today are also expected to deal with an immense amount of information about their pregnancy that was simply unavailable in former times. Since much of this information is highly technical, expectant couples could find themselves at a loss as to how to interpret the results of such prenatal technologies.

The whole enterprise becomes compounded by the fact that, even if the medical profession is capable of providing a wealth of scientific data about the human fetus or embryo, there is still the issue of what will each particular couple do with the information provided. In other words, given the high impact which some of this information may have, and given also the current legal availability of abortion on demand in the United States, a couple may conclude that a particular abnormality detected in their pre-born may be too much for them to endure (*amelia*, for instance), whereas in reality the condition is totally compatible with life (a missing hand or foot).

This puts the medical doctor in a tremendous predicament, for while in theory he or she is supposed to keep his or her own value system out of the picture, in practice we are talking about human relationships. And in real human life it is impossible to maintain a totally value-neutral stance, especially when dealing with issues which ultimately affect an entire new generation. Therefore, even if the medical doctor wanted to present only the "mere" facts, the very way in which such results are conveyed is already betraying an underlying value judgment.

Then, the expectant couple today is left with no alternative than to "own" their pregnancy, as it were, and take full responsibility for it and for the complex decisions which at times have to be made. But in doing so, it is very important that they realize that they are certainly not alone! And this is why I honestly believe that this book is a definite contribution at this point in time.

Over the years, in researching the topic of human pregnancy from a Catholic perspective, I have found that while there is indeed much ethical and moral material on the subject, there seems to be a lack of sources that are at the same time equally thorough in their bio-medical presentation of prenatal diagnosis. Conversely, there are many references that go into in-depth treatment of the procedures involved in prenatal diagnosis from a bio-medical perspective, but they generally refrain from a deep moral analysis of the issues involved, especially taking in consideration the Catholic perspective.

This is why in this book I have undertaken to write, first, a fairly detailed description of human embryonic development, and also the things that can go wrong along such time of development. Second, I have summarized the opinions of the ten Catholic moral theologians who have written most extensively on the subject of prenatal diagnosis over the past twenty years (the time period when these techniques have been perfected to the point of becoming standard medical practice for all pregnancies). But the third part of the book is truly the one that seeks to apply current Catholic teaching to the multiple issues associated with prenatal diagnosis and conflict situations.

With this in mind, and because of its interdisciplinary scope, this book may seem to the unspecialized reader a bit technical at times, either in its bio-medical part or in its theological one. This notwithstanding, the language in either of these sections is certainly not unaccessible to anyone who is willing to ponder patiently over dilemmas which were non-existent a few years ago simply because the "window" into the womb did not yet exist.

Hence, every Catholic couple who is expecting or planning a child should take the time to read this book. Regardless of how knowledgeable they may be in both the medical and the moral fields, they will undoubtedly find new and relevant information on which to base their decisions about their pregnancy. And I'm sure you'll agree that the quality of our decisions greatly depends on the quality and amount of information we have at the time of such decisions. For non-Catholic couples who consider themselves Christian, I am certain that the conclusions reached in this book are in accordance with your beliefs, for it is the common vision of the human person which unites us. Even for non-Christian couples, I believe that you will find in this book a common grounding in the values and principles which have inspired its writing, namely, the intrinsic dignity and integrity of every human being at each stage of his or her development.

I also recommend this book to those in the medical and theological professions who have to deal with issues of human pregnancy and prenatal diagnosis, either in practice or in theory. You will find that the text is accurate, up to date, and well referenced with an international bibliography. Medical and theological students may find a particular advantage to having the large volume of interdisciplinary information on the subject available in a single book such as this one.

Finally, hospitals, libraries, institutions and organizations seeking to serve in some capacity as support systems and resource centers to expectant couples, or to the medical and ethical professionals involved in the multiple issues which surface as a result of the practice of prenatal diagnosis, should consider adding this book to their reference collections. The claim that the theme is focused from a Catholic perspective is evident even by the very subtitle of the book. However, if it is true that we live in a pluralistic society, the fact that this book seeks to put forward the Catholic perspective should be considered, then, a definite contribution to the ongoing social dialogue on the issues at hand.

It is my sincere hope that this book will help all those presently involved with the pre-born to ponder the complex mystery and perfection of that earliest state of all human life; to realize that technology is available to serve us rather than to dominate and intimidate us; to realize also that, given the proper tools for moral analysis, couples and society at large are capable of arriving at responsible decisions even regarding extremely complicated or emotional issues; and that God indeed provides the concomitant grace to arrive at such sound decisions. Fear is useless, what is needed is information, mature decision-making, and trust.

Acknowledgments

No words on paper would ever suffice to thank the many persons who have helped me in the development of this work. Nonetheless, with words I will now attempt the impossible task of recognizing those who have more directly influenced the maturing of this labor.

First and foremost, to my director, Prof. Dr. Klaus Demmer, msc, I offer my deepest gratitude for guiding me during the discernment of a relevant topic, for his wisdom in helping me identify the most critical issues underlying the main theme, and for his generous disposition during my time of research in Rome.

To Prof. Dr. Angelo Serra, SJ, and the library staff of the Università Cattolica del Sacro Cuore and Gemelli Hospital, Rome, I give thanks for their great availability and access to vital resources.

To Mons. Edwin O'Brien, Mons. Charles W. Elmer, Br. Randal Riede, cfx, Sr. Dorothy Beach, snd, Sr. Beth Wood, ihm, the Piccole Ancelle di Maria Immacolata, my colleagues and staff of the Casa Santa Maria, and to my family and friends living in Rome, I present my gratitude for their prayers and tangible support during my years of residence there.

To Prof. Dr. Edmund Pellegrino, MD, staff and friends of the Kennedy Institute of Ethics, Georgetown University, the library of the Catholic University of America, the Dominican House of Studies, Divine Word College, and Mons. Robert Lynch I remain indebted for all the doors which they opened to me while doing research in Washington, DC.

To Drs. Rolando De Leon, MD, Norman Ruíz Castañeda, MD, and associates of Mercy Hospital and Outpatient Center, and Children's Hospital, Miami, I extend my heartfelt thanks for their critical observations regarding the biomedical part of this work, and for their friendship.

To my ordinary, The Most Reverend Edward A. McCarthy, DD, Archbishop of Miami, for presenting me with the magnificent opportunity to pursue higher studies. To Mons. Jude O'Doherty, staff and parishioners of the Church of the Epiphany, Miami, for their years of sincere friendship and encouragement through times high and low in my priestly ministry.

To the students, faculty and staff of St. Vincent de Paul Regional Seminary, Florida, where I now reside, for their extraordinary assistance and understanding during the final stages of this dissertation, with the many impositions which that required.

To my brother, Prof. Claudio Cioffi, PhD, and to my sister-in-law, Jean N. Cioffi, MMusEd, for their unmitigated support, vigilance and understanding during all moments of the journey.

Finally, to my family and friends in Miami, Florida, to Fr. Felipe Estevez, to Carmen and Alberto Martínez-Ramos, and especially to my mother Gloria and my late father Salvatore, who began loving me by granting me the gift of life, and to whom I dedicate this work as a token of my awareness of the sacred quality of all human life which they sought to instill in me from my earliest beginnings.

Many others have gone unmentioned, but not unforgotten, for your prayers, support and encouragement are ingrained in my heart and in my mind: to all of you many, many thanks.

GENERAL INTRODUCTION

Ever since humans became human, they have lived for the greater part of their first year of existence hidden within the secret recesses of their mother's womb. Now, thanks to the skillful application of advanced biomedical technologies, these first nine months of human life are becoming more visible and better understood. What has been hidden is now being revealed. Prenatal diagnosis (PND) presently allows for the possibility of monitoring human embryonic development and of detecting literally thousands of metabolic, genotypic and phenotypic abnormalities *in utero.*

In 1987, the Vatican's *Instruction on Respect for Human Life* stated that: "If prenatal diagnosis respects the life and integrity of the embryo and the human fetus and is directed towards its safeguarding or healing as an individual, the answer [re. its moral licitness] is affirmative."[1]

With an increased capacity to analyze fetal cells in the laboratory and the present possibility of monitoring human embryonic development using advanced diagnostic techniques such as amniocentesis, chorionic villus sampling, measurement of alpha-fetoprotein levels, ultrasound and fetoscopy, PND has become widely diffused in medical practice. Yet, PND results are not unambiguous: they may either lead to a continuation of the pregnancy, or to a procured abortion. Since a moral evaluation of PND depends to a great extent on biomedical advancements, it seems relevant at this point in time to engage in a comprehensive examination of the state of the question regarding the diagnosis and possible treatment of human illnesses *in utero.* Accordingly, this dissertation examines some moral dilemmas found in PND as viewed by contemporary Catholic thought in the United States of America.

The work is divided into three main parts: biomedical considerations of prenatal human life, a survey of ten American Catholic theologians on the subject at hand, and a critical evaluation thereof. A brief description of each part follows.

PART ONE of this dissertation deals with biomedical considerations in

---

[1] Congregation for the Doctrine of the Faith, *Instruction on Respect for Human Life in its Origin and on the Dignity of Procreation: Replies to Certain Questions of the Day.* (Vatican transl.) Boston: Daughters of St. Paul 1987, 14.

prenatal human life. It is divided into four chapters: prenatal diagnosis (PND), human reproduction, human embryonic disorders, and prenatal interventions. The first chapter is subdivided into: definition, and six indications. The second chapter describes basic contemporary facts about human genetics, fertilization, implantation, embryogenesis, and multifetal gestation. The third chapter covers etiology, genetic defects, common human Mendelian disorders, teratogens, congenital malformations of human organ systems, and the case of very low birth weight. The fourth chapter includes a description of techniques which can be used in detecting human embryonic disorders, such as: amniocentesis, chorionic villus sampling, fetal tissue sampling, percutaneous umbilical blood sampling, maternal serum alpha-fetoprotein assay, analysis of fetal cells within maternal blood, ultrasound, magnetic resonance imaging, and preimplantation diagnosis.

PART TWO of this dissertation is a survey of the literature of ten North American Catholic theologians who have written on the topic of moral dilemmas in PND over the past twenty years. The ten authors are: Benedict M. Ashley, OP, Lisa S. Cahill, Charles E. Curran, William E. May, Donald G. McCarthy, Richard A. McCormick, SJ, Albert S. Moraczewski, OP, Thomas J. O'Donnell, SJ, Kevin D. O'Rourke, OP, and Thomas A. Shannon. Ashley and O'Rourke, McCarthy and Moraczewski, and Shannon and Cahill have been grouped because of the similarity of their views in several of the themes and because of joint authorship of various important works; McCormick and Cahill have also been grouped together because of their similar views. The reason for choosing twenty years is threefold. First, PND techniques were simply not available or too experimental before then, and have been vastly perfected since. Second, abortion has been legal in the United States of America for the past twenty years, providing a perception that, if a fetus is found to be defective, its mother has a right to destroy it. Third, it allows one to note a certain maturing and nuancing over time in various arguments proposed by different authors.

Paramount to all ten authors is seeking to uphold the dignity of human life. In the particular setting of PND, it involves a constellation of issues which touch on prenatal life and conflict situations. Because PND is not without risk, both to the mother and to the fetus, there must be corresponding justification for undergoing the procedure. This, in turn, is related to the possibility of benefits to both, such as: *in utero* surgery, a better pregnancy management, and reassurance to the mother of normal fetal development. On the other hand, these techniques also lend themselves to a host of morally unacceptable practices, such as: "therapeutic" abortion, selective reduction of multifetal gestation, and even fetal sex selection. Hence, each author's views of eugenics and of cooperation in PND by Catholic healthcare professionals and facilities are closely examined.

Standard PND is done during the second trimester of pregnancy (or, with greater risk, late in the first trimester), a time when the human fetus is well along the way of development. However, because there is now the technological possibility of pre-implantation diagnosis, the present discussion on immediate versus delayed hominization is of special importance. Here the different authors examined part ways, as will be seen below. At play is their particular interpretation of current biological data regarding fertilization and early embryonic development. Accordingly, some of the authors speak of a preembryo before implantation, while others reject the validity of such terminology.

PART THREE of this dissertation is a critical analysis of the writings of these ten authors on the subject at hand. In the interest of clarity, this analysis is arranged into seven key issues which emerge from the survey. The seven issues are: basic value systems, philosophical and anthropological presuppositions, theories of hominization and personhood, the analysis of the moral act, the moral dilemmas in PND proper, the current shift in the self-understanding of medicine, and the possibility of dialogue with the magisterium.

1. *Basic Value Systems*

A preliminary question is the shared structural principle from which the various basic value systems examined emerge. As stated above, a basic value common to all ten authors is the intrinsic dignity of human life. Regarding prenatal life and conflict situations, this intuition also necessarily extends to the life of the mother, of the father, of the healthcare professional, and of society at large in the specific cultural ethos of our historical instance.

In addition, all authors seek to engage this pluralistic society in the hope of approximating an eventual consensus concerning the application of this structural principle, another basic value which is at least implicit in their publishing. With this in mind, manifest variances are not necessarily found at the level of basic values, rather at subsequent levels of their interpretation and moral evaluation. Hence, it is proper to delve into the various authors' epistemological and hermeneutical presuppositions.

2. *Philosophical and Anthropological Presuppositions*

The various authors examined rally to one or another of two main streams of the theory of the foundation of moral norms, and consequently, of the rightness of moral action: deontological, or teleological theory. B. Ashley, W. May, D. McCarthy, A. Moraczewski, T. O'Donnell, and K. O'Rourke all espouse a fundamentally deductive conceptual structure where pre-moral goodness is determined by the underlying moral value. Hence, the principle here resides in the goodness of duty as binding, circumstances notwithstanding. Contrastingly, L. Cahill, C. Curran, R. McCormick, and T. Shannon, all move in the direction of a more inductive conceptual system where the good conditions the form under which the value appears. Thus, the direction of thought here is from the pre-moral good to the moral value, with the principle residing in the correctness of acting. It is from here that the goodness of duty is vindicated. It is likewise understood that each author exhibits further subtleties and nuances within these two main confluences. Such become more evident in their proposed theories of hominization.

3. *Hominization and Personhood*

The deontologists advance immediate hominization, while the teleologists mediate. Immediate hominization proposes a processural plan commencing with completed fusion, followed by continuous epigenetic polarity and bilaterality from first cleavage. This implies the presence of a succession of primary organizers such that no qualitative leaps are necessary. The teleologists counter that such system is naturalistic and thus reductionistic. Yet in advancing delayed hominization, a similar naturalism seems to occur by grounding the claim in the possibilities of twinning and recombination before nidation. Without doubt individuality and irrepeatability are constituents of the human person. It still needs to be seen how genetic uniqueness substantially differs from developmental individuality, no longer at the level of a biological given but at that of its theological interpretation. Similarly, totipotentiality expends no univocal claim.

4. *Analysis of the Moral Act*

If one is to adequately assess these evaluations of PND, one must also ask what is the structure at the base of the moral action: what is the grounding of the hermeneutics of the moral decision. Here, whether deontological or teleological, intentionality is also at the root of a proper interpretation of the action. Likewise, such action must be understood within the context of a medical practice with its own presuppositions, objectives, and limits. Regarding the cogent application of the principle of double effect, the deontologists must adequately respond to the inquiry: in what sense is the evil effect not willed by the agent if the action is not to be unrealistically split or hopelessly atomized? More importantly: how and in what manner is the fetus living and growing according to the order and dignity of its stage of development, especially given a true positive PND? The teleologists, on the other hand, must guard from a radical chasm between existential and formal logic, which would render the moral norm ungeneralizable. Further, linguistic and propositional medical and theological presuppositions need to be clarified in as much as this is possible interdisciplinarily.

5. *Moral Dilemmas in Prenatal Diagnosis Proper*

In spite of conceptual, philosophical and anthropological differences on the subject, there is a surprising consensus among the ten authors examined regarding the evaluation, applications, and limits of standard PND. The moral validity of these techniques is situated within the context of "responsible" parenthood and contemporary professional medical practice. Hence, the six generally accepted indications are evaluated in themselves and in their sufficiency. With a continuous lowering of risks, and an increased perception of the fetus as patient; might other indications apply? Even so, it must be recognized that PND results are not unambivalent: hence, the key question of intentionality retains its full force --this always within a Christian framework of solidarity with the weakest.

The particular case of pre-implantation diagnosis introduces peculiar elements for consideration in view of the current theological debate, and of the present state of the art. Deontological and teleological divergences are most evident here.

6. *Shift in the Self-understanding of Medicine*

The vast majority of PND are negative; of the positive, the vast majority result in abortion: what, then, are the possibilities and limits of professional cooperation in PND? Such cooperation is situated within a broader perspective of medicine's self-understanding. Rather than an illusory radical contemporary shift, the current "rights" movement is seen within a historical continuum of medicine's first principle: not healing, but the will of the patient. That societies in past times have claudicated by uncritically subjecting to expert opinion is not questioned. What does come to the fore in the present context, is the assurance of the freedom of conscience of all parties involved, especially in the interest of dialogue within a pluralistic society which seeks to approximate consensus on issues germane to public policy. To this end, Catholic professionals and institutions, in the name of loyalty, may indeed renounce to a measure of legislative freedom available.

7. *Dialogue with the Magisterium*

Concomitantly with treating the problems, credible moral theology today demands that the proposed methods for solving them also be treated. Thus, it may well be said that whereas the six deontologist authors seek to validate magisterial teaching on the issue, the four teleologists explore some possible alternative models. Even given the Church's magisterial competence in matters of faith and morals, the deontologists cannot uncompromisingly dismiss a reasonable request for argumentation credibility and consistency. Conversely, the teleologists need to respond to the adequacy of their criticism that the official magisterium is using two distinct methodologies when interpreting social moral issues, or sexual moral issues. In reality, the ensemble of PND is more complex than that, presenting an at-times inseparable weave of sexual *and* social dilemmas. To this end, crucial as the clarification of theological and medical terminology may be, it is not sufficient in true interdisciplinary dialogue. Rather, a permanent commitment to engage in reciprocal openness and mutual re-evaluation is at the core of promoting a good life fully realized intended in the sense of a universal vocation and destiny to union with God.

PART ONE

BIO-MEDICAL CONSIDERATIONS OF PRENATAL DIAGNOSIS

CHAPTER I

PRENATAL DIAGNOSIS

A. DEFINITION

Prenatal diagnosis (PND) is: "diagnosis utilizing procedures available for the recognition of diseases and malformations in utero, and the conclusion reached."[1] Because all PND carries some degree of risk either to the mother, to the child, or to both, it is not indicated for all pregnant women.

B. INDICATIONS

More than 95% of all PND are negative.[2] However, certain couples are at a higher risk of parenting a child with some disorder, such as: advanced maternal age; prior child with a chromosomal anomaly; either parent with a translocation or other chromosomal abnormality; fragile X syndrome; either parent with a numerical chromosomal defect (aneuploidy); and other factors.

1. Maternal Age[3]

This is the most common indication for PND, at about 85% of all expectant women tested. The incidence of trisomy 21 (Down syndrome) in the general population is about 1:800. For a woman who is 35 years old it is about 1:385, and about 1:106 if she is 40.[4] The present conventional indication for amniocentesis is around 35 years of age or older.

2. Prior Abnormal Child[5]

Couples with a child born with chromosomal disorders, stillborn, or spontaneous abortion with a trisomy, are indications for PND, even if both parents exhibit a normal phenotype. Possible causes of defects may be: both parents with a heterozygous genotype for the same abnormality, parental mosaicism, structural chromosomal rearrangement during gametogenesis or at the zygote level, and a Mendelian gene with a higher rate of nondisjunction.

3. Inversions and Translocations[6]

If either parent is a carrier of a translocation or other chromosomal anomaly, PND is indicated even if heterozygous, that is, even if there is no phenotypic expression. In theory, 25% of all children with Down syndrome have one heterozygous parent for trisomy 21. Yet, the observed ratio is about 11% (10% of women and 1-2% of men[7]), since not all heterozygous trisomy 21 adults are fertile.

4. Fragile X Syndrome[8]

In some karyotypes the distal end of the long arm of the X chromosome shows a "fragile" site (staining gap). The phenotype consists of mental retardation, macro-orchidism (enlarged testes), and prognathism. The incidence in the general population is about 1:1,000, accounting for 6-10% of all retarded males. It is the second most common inherited disorder (after trisomy 21) of the mentally retarded. Thus, these couples have indications for PND.

5. Aneuploidy[9]

If either parent karyotypes a numerical chromosomal anomaly (aneuploidy), PND is indicated. In theory, 50% of all children born to parents with Down syndrome should manifest the defect.[10] Other aneuploids which are fertile and therefore indicate for prenatal diagnosis are mosaic females, such as 45,X;45,X/46,XX, and 45,X/46;XX/45,XXX. Aneuploid males (47,XYY and 47,XXY) are often sterile, but 46,XY/47,XXY mosaics may be fertile, thus indicating for PND.

6. Other[11]

Other conditions indicating for PND may be: a previous undiagnosed stillborn or spontaneously aborted fetus, parental exposure to teratogens (chemotherapy or therapeutic irradiation), parental metabolic defects, too high or too low maternal serum alpha-fetoprotein (MSAFP), delayed fertility, pregnancy from ovulation induction, and a fetus showing intrauterine growth retardation (IUGR) or decreased activity. Contemporary studies in human population genetics are constantly augmenting the families of syndromes of multiple congenital disorders which may indicate for PND.[12]

Notes

[1]Stedman's **Medical Dictionary**, 25th ed. Baltimore-Hong Kong-London-Sydney: Williams and Wilkins 1990; *diagnosis, prenatal.*

[2]See: Elias S, Annas GJ, **Reproductive Genetics and the Law.** Chicago: Year Book Medical Publishers 1987, 83.

[3]See: Elias and Annas, **Reproductive Genetics**, 84-86; Simpson JL, Elias S, "Prenatal diagnosis of genetic disorders" in: Creasy RK, Resnik R, eds, **Maternal-Fetal Medicine: Principles and Practice**, 2nd ed. Philadelphia: Saunders 1989, 78-107, 89.

[4]After the maternal age of 30, the risk of bearing a child with a trisomy rises exponentially.

[5]See: Elias and Annas, **Reproductive Genetics**, 86-87; Simpson and Elias, *Genetic disorders*, 89-90.

[6]See: De Paepe A, De Bie S, "Genetic counseling of a couple presenting respectively terminal transverse defects and congenital arthrogryposis" *GenCounsel* 2 (1991) 195-203; Elias and Annas, **Reproductive Genetics**, 87-88; Narod S, "Counselling under genetic heterogeneity: A practical approach" *ClinGen* 39 (1991) 125-131; Simpson and Elias, *Genetic disorders*, 90-91.

[7]The lower percentage in men is presumably due to sperm pre-selection. See: Elias and Annas, **Reproductive Genetics**, 88.

[8]See: Elias and Annas, **Reproductive Genetics**, 88; Simpson JL, "Transmitting genetic disorders to offspring of mentally retarded individuals: principles underlying genetic counseling" in: Evans MI, Dixler AO, Fletcher JC, Schulman JD, eds, **Fetal Diagnosis and Therapy: Science, Ethics and the Law**. Philadelphia: Lippincott 1989, 98-99.

[9]See: Elias and Annas, **Reproductive Genetics**, 88; Simpson and Elias, *Genetic disorders*, 92.

[10]The actual observed ratio is about 30%, again presumably due to natural gamete pre-selection.

[11]See: Elias and Annas, **Reproductive Genetics**, 89; Simpson and Elias, *Genetic disorders*, 92-94.

[12]See: Lurie IW, Lazjuk GI, Korotkova IA, Cherstvoy ED, "The cerebro-reno-digital syndromes: a new community" *ClinGen* 39 (1991) 104-113.

CHAPTER II

HUMAN REPRODUCTION

A. BASIC HUMAN GENETICS[1]

Chromosomes are organic macromolecules consisting of discrete subunits called genes. Each gene codes for a particular characteristic of the organism. The genetic make-up of any biological species is called the genotype, whereas the visible, physical characteristic is the phenotype. In classical Mendelian genetics, only dominant genotypes are expressed in the phenotype, whereas recessive genotypes are masked by dominant ones. A cell (or organism) which has either only dominant or only recessive genotype is homozygous, whereas one with both dominant and recessive genes together is heterozygous. Thus, the phenotype of both homozygous dominant and heterozygous genotypes are dominant type. The phenotype of a homozygous recessive is recessive. The genome is the entire genetic make-up of a species.[2]

The normal number of chromosomes in human beings is 46, with each chromosome containing several thousands of genes. These 46 chromosomes actually represent a duplicate set of 23 each. Of these 23 homologous pairs, one pair codes for sexual traits: XX for females and XY for males. XX and XY are sex chromosomes, while the other 22 pairs are somatic chromosomes or autosomes. The vast majority of somatic or body cells in the human body have a full number of chromosomes: 46. These cells are diploid. Haploid cells, by contrast, have a single set of chromosomes: 23. Haploid cells are mainly represented by reproductive cells, or gametes: eggs in females and spermatozoa in males. Genes which do not code for sexual traits, but which are nonetheless located in the sex chromosomes are sex-linked.[3]

Somatic cells regularly reproduce by mitosis, by which the number of chromosomes doubles before the parent cell divides so that each one of the two daughter cells will have a full number of chromosome pairs. This type of asexual reproduction is the normal way in which living human tissues, organs and systems grow and develop. Somatic cells are heterozygous.

Sexual cells, on the other hand, fuse instead of splitting. The single diploid cell resulting from this fusion is called a zygote. Sexual reproduction in humans involves the fusion of an egg and a sperm. Thus, it is imperative that these two gametes be haploid in order for the zygote not to end up with twice the normal number of chromosomes, or 92 (tetraploid). An egg and a sperm are produced by a process of chromosome reduction called meiosis. Overall, the production of gametes is called gametogenesis: oogenesis for the egg and spermatogenesis for sperm.

1. Human Gametogenesis[4]

Through gametogenesis each gamete receives 23 chromosomes: 22 autosomes and an X chromosome in eggs, and 22 autosomes and either an X or a Y chromosome in sperm.[5] Since none of these chromosomes are paired, all gametes are homozygous for each phenotype. This is important when analyzing human fertilization, because it means that both sperm and egg will pass whatever characteristics each carries onto the zygote 'pure and simply', that is, without a duplicate back-up. Thus, if both sperm and egg are homozygous recessive for a particular characteristic, that trait will in principle show up in the offspring. It also means that any alteration which may happen to either the genes or the chromosomes of each egg and sperm will also be 'passed on' if the altered gametes are the ones involved in fertilization. The conventional way of expressing the genome in humans is, for females: 46,XX, and for males: 46,XY. Thus, normal human eggs are 23,X, whereas human sperm may be either 23,X or 23,Y.

2. Nondisjunction and Aneuploidy[6]

During both mitosis and meiosis homologous pairs of chromosomes interchange genes by crossing-over. Once this genetic recombination has occurred, each chromosome pair separates and migrates to an opposite pole of the dividing cell, where it forms the nucleus of the new cell. Sporadically, any random number of homologous pairs of chromosomes may fail to separate during crossing-over. This is called nondisjunction, resulting in one daughter cell containing extra chromosomes, while the other cell is missing the same number. These daughter cells are aneuploid: the condition of the cell with one extra chromosome is called trisomy, whereas the condition of the cell missing one chromosome is called monosomy. Polyploidy, then, is any abnormal genome.

B. HUMAN EMBRYOLOGY[7]

For study purposes, normal embryonic development in humans may be divided into four main stages: fertilization, implantation (through the second week), embryonic development (through the eighth week), and fetal development (through the 38th week).[8]

1. Fertilization[9]

For human fertilization to occur, egg and sperm must first mature, then migrate toward one another and finally, fuse. Maturation of human egg and sperm is a long and complex development beginning at the embryonic stage and culminating only after puberty. During the embryonic stage diploid primordial sexual germ cells produce myriads of oogonia -in the developing ovaries of females-, and spermatogonia -in the developing testes of males. These undergo further differentiation into primary oocytes and spermatocytes, which through meiosis eventually produce mature eggs and sperm. But here a difference occurs between the genders: Spermatogonia remain undifferentiated into puberty, thus maintaining their capacity to produce innumerable primary spermatocytes through mitosis for the entire adult life of males. After puberty, primary spermatocytes undergo meiosis to duplicate into secondary spermatocytes, which take an average of 64 days to become mature spermatozoa. Oogonia, on the other hand, differentiate during embryonic development, so that at birth a normal female has a fixed number of primary oocytes (between one and two million). Meiosis begins in these, but is arrested until puberty. During childhood, the vast majority of oocytes regress. However, about 40,000 do make it to puberty. Of these, about 400 to 500 eventually mature, giving a woman an average of 35-40 fertile years after puberty.

Hormonal Control of Human Reproduction[10]

The female reproductive cycle is regulated mainly by the hypothalamus, pituitary, ovaries, uterus and mammary glands. During puberty the hypothalamus synthesizes a gonadotropin-releasing factor (GnRH), which signals the pituitary to release follicle-stimulating hormone (FSH) and luteinizing hormone (LH) into circulation. FSH is the first to arouse ovarian follicles into maturing, but LH is also needed to finish the process. The maturing follicle then produces estrogen, which causes the endometrium to thicken in preparation for a possible pregnancy. At about mid-cycle (14th day), the rise in estrogen triggers a surge in LH, causing a follicle growth spurt, culminating in ovulation, the expulsion of a mature egg. The remaining follicle forms the corpus luteum. If fertilization occurs, the corpus luteum secretes mainly progesterone, but also some estrogen. Progesterone maintains the endometrium during implantation and for the first 14-20 weeks of pregnancy, by which time the placenta produces enough estrogen and progesterone to sustain gestation. If no fertilization occurs, the corpus luteum degenerates and stops producing progesterone. This causes the functional layer of the endometrium to be sloughed off during menstruation.

Reproduction in males is controlled mostly by the hypothalamus, pituitary gland, testes, epididymis, seminal vesicles, prostrate gland, and bulbourethral glands. In males during puberty, LH[11] stimulates testicular Leydig cells to produce testosterone, which manages spermatogenesis. Spermatozoa then mature in the epididymis surrounding the testes. The seminal vesicles, prostrate, and bulbourethral glands are all associated with the production of seminal fluid.

Fusion of Egg and Sperm[12]

Once semen is deposited within the vagina, sperm are propelled by cervical mucous, uterine contractions, and the sperms' own flagellar motility ("capacitation") through the cervix and into both uterine tubes. An average ejaculate contains 200-600 million sperm, but only about 200 ever reach the proximity of the egg. The egg also has a journey to complete. At ovulation, an ovarian follicle releases into the infundibulum an egg "package" containing a secondary oocyte and a polar body, surrounded by an acellular layer of matrix called the zona pellucida, itself enclosed within a layer of follicular cells forming the corona radiata. This package is "swept up" by the fimbriae, where mucous, cilia and tubal contractions move the egg toward the ampulla of the oviduct. Fertilization normally occurs within the ampulla.

As sperm and egg meet, the sperm penetrates the corona radiata and the acrosomal sperm head releases enzymes, digesting the zona pellucida. This causes a chemical reaction around the entire zona which makes it impermeable to other sperm. It also signals the secondary oocyte to complete the long process of meiosis, forming a haploid female pronucleus and a second polar body. The plasma membranes of egg and sperm meet and dissolve, allowing the sperm haploid pronucleus to empty into the cytoplasm of the secondary oocyte. Finally, the two haploid male and female pronuclei fuse, forming a single diploid cell called a zygote. A normal human zygote is about 7-8 microns in diameter. In a typical 28-day human reproductive cycle (from menses to menses), ovulation occurs on day 14. The mature egg normally remains 1-3 days within the ampulla. Usually, fertilization occurs within 24 hours of intercourse, though the average sperm lifespan in the fallopian tube is about 48 hours. If two or more eggs mature simultaneously, all will most likely be fertilized, giving rise to dizygotic or fraternal twins, triplets, etc.

2. Implantation[13]

First Week[14]

Within two days the zygote cleaves mitotically, forming an even number of diploid blastomeres.[15] At about three days, a morula of 12-16 blastomeres is formed. At about four days, spaces within the morula appear, forming a blastocyst with an outer trophoblast layer, an inner embryoblast layer, and a cavity. The trophoblast will form the placenta, while the embryoblast will form the embryo. By the end of the first week, the blastocyst reaches the uterus[16], where he or she begins to implant into the endometrium, and may have grown to about 50 microns in diameter. If the zygote has not reached the uterus by this time, he or she may implant along the oviduct wall, causing an ectopic pregnancy. Occasionally, a zygote exits the uterine duct through the infundibulum and begins implanting within the mesentery, giving rise to an abdominal pregnancy. Both ectopic and abdominal pregnancies may gravely endanger the life of an expectant mother.

Second Week[17]

By the 8th day, the embryoblast begins to develop a bilaminar embryonic disc of epiblast and hypoblast, with the epiblast facing the amniotic cavity and the hypoblast facing the primary yolk sac. The trophoblast develops into the syncytiotrophoblast burying deeper into the endometrium, and the cytotrophoblast producing extraembryonic mesoderm surrounding a primary yolk sac.

By about the 10th day the embryo is fully embedded. The syncytiotrophoblast forms a primitive uteroplacental capillary circulation, while extraembryonic mesoderm surrounds the amniotic cavity and the yolk sac. Spaces develop within the extraembryonic mesoderm, becoming a coelom to enclose the embryonic structure.

By the 13th day primary chorionic villi begin extending from the cytotrophoblast into the syncytiotrophoblast and by the 14th day the embryonic hypoblast forms a circular prochordal plate, the organizer of the cranial region and where the mouth will be.

By the end of the second week the embryo is suspended by a stalk within the chorionic cavity. The surrounding chorion interacting with the endometrium is formed by trophoblasts and somatic extraembryonic mesoderm. At this stage, a normal bilaminar human embryo is less than a millimeter in length.

3. Embryogenesis

Third Week[18]

Through gastrulation the bilaminar embryo becomes a trilaminar embryonic disc from which ectoderm eventually gives rise to the epidermis and the nervous system, endoderm gives rise to the epithelial linings of the respiratory, digestive and glandular systems, and mesoderm gives rise to the muscular, skeletal, reproductive, excretory and circulatory systems.[19] The primitive streak migrates dorsally from the caudal region to form a notochordal process: cells moving inward constitute mesenchyme, while epiblast forms embryonic ectoderm and hypoblast forms embryonic endoderm. A notochord develops from the primitive knot of the streak to the oropharyngeal region. Through neurulation, a neural plate is induced[20] by the notochord and surrounding mesenchyme to form the neural tube. Neuroectoderm forms a neural crest, dividing into bisymmetrical ganglia. Mesoderm flanking the notochord forms somite pairs, which will give rise to vertebrae, ribs, ligaments and axial musculature. The intraembryonic coelom becomes a single, horseshoe cavity which gives rise to body cavities. Blood islands develop within the wall of the yolk sac and allantois. These islands derived from mesenchyme gradually fuse to form a primitive cardiovascular network, with paired endocardial heart tubes[21] and blood vessels extending into the embryo, yolk sac, umbilical cord and chorionic sac. Primary, then secondary, and then tertiary chorionic villi with mesenchymal cores branch into the endometrium, forming an arteriocapillary network. A cytotrophoblastic shell surrounds the entire structure. This complex will give rise to the placenta.[22] The human embryo is now about 2mm along the long axis and the head fold is already evident.

Fourth and Fifth Week[23]

Organogenesis begins with the three germ layers giving rise by induction to all major organ systems,[24] therefore teratogens may cause extensive congenital defects during this time. The embryo curves inwardly cranially, bilaterally, and caudally due to rapid growth of the nervous system. The head fold thickens and projects dorsally into the amniotic cavity as the rostral neuropore forms three primary brain vesicles: forebrain, midbrain and hindbrain. The heart and oropharyngeal membrane curl ventrally, forming a foregut. The tail fold projects over the cloacal membrane, including part of the yolk sac to form a hindgut. As the amniotic cavity expands and the embryo "curls" ventrally, the connecting stalk constricts to form an umbilical cord, enclosing the allantois, and with amnion as epithelium. By mid-fourth week the neural tube is formed, but is still open at the rostral and caudal neuropores. Eye and ear primordia, and the mandibular and branchial arches appear.[25] By about day 26 the neuropores close, two more pairs of branchial arches open, and the upper and lower limb buds appear. By the end of the fourth week three well-defined cavities are present: pericardial, pericardioperitoneal and peritoneal. A primitive pharynx develops internally along the foregut, matching the branchial arches. Nephrogenic cords of mesoderm form bilateral urogenital ridges. The endocardial tubes fuse into a single heart, with three paired veins: vitelline, umbilical and common cardinal veins. By the fifth week in the head and neck regions myoblasts from cervical somites migrate with their phrenic nerves into the diaphragm. The first bilateral (mandibular) branchial arches fuse distally, forming a stomodeum, or primitive mouth. The second branchial arch overgrows the third and fourth arches, forming the cervical sinus. Pharyngeal pouches, future site of head and neck glands, develop anterior to the esophagus. A thyroid gland begins developing from endoderm in the floor of the primitive pharynx. Bilateral nasal pits, eyes and external ears start forming. In the thoracic and abdominal regions bilateral lung buds arise from the caudal end of the trachea into a primitive pleural cavity. A laryngotracheal tube leads from the pharynx into the bronchial buds. Liver, stomach, pancreas, spleen, gallbladder, intestine and mesonephric kidneys all begin differentiating. The circulatory system consists of bicameral atria and ventricles, left and right atrioventricular canals, sinus venosus, aorta, venae cavae, umbilical artery and vein, and pulmonary veins. The lymphatic system forms alongside the circulatory system. From mesenchyme, chondroblasts produce cartilage and osteoblasts bone, especially in vertebral segments enclosing the neural tube, and in the digital rays and primordia of forearm bones within bilateral forearm plates. An attenuated tail is also present. By the end of the fifth week the three distinct regions of the brain are further developed: forebrain (with two lateral hemispheres), midbrain, and hindbrain (with developing medulla). Neural cellular differentiation occurs also from neuroepithelium. Optic cups and lenses, and otic vesicles are forming. The embryo is covered with epidermis, is suspended within the fluid-filled amnion,[26] and is now about 8mm CR.[27]

Sixth and Seventh Week[28]

Externally, the head contains pigmented eyes, auricular hillocks, and oral and nasal cavities. The upper lip is forming. Internally, the head contains secondary brain vesicles, the pontine flexure, and optic stalks, with cup, lens and cornea. Nasal and oral cavities connect. The palate develops. The tongue, tonsils, thymus, parathyroid and salivary glands are all forming. An epiglottis grows at the entrance of the laryngotracheal tube. Within the body trunk bilateral secondary bronchi branch into the pleural cavity. The esophagus elongates and the stomach rotates, suspended by mesenteries. A duodenal loop links midgut with hindgut, with its lumen temporarily occluded. Hemopoiesis begins within fast-growing liver lobes. Hepatic, cystic and pancreatic ducts form. The midgut loop continues herniating into the umbilical cord, with a cecal diverticulum appearing. A perineal body separates urogenital canal from anal canal. Caudally, bilateral mesonephric ducts and tubules develop into nephrogenic cords, while a ureteric bud develops. Bilateral suprarenal glands begin forming. Primordial germ cells migrate from the yolk sac into undifferentiated paired gonads developing from mesodermal epithelium within urogenital mesentery, merging into primary sex cords. The genital tubercle elongates anterior to the cloacal membrane to form a phallus in both genders. By the seventh week, the forebrain divides into two cerebral hemispheres and a thalamus, and the hindbrain develops into the pons, cerebellum and medulla. Ganglia grow along the spinal cord. The pituitary gland is forming. A peripheral nervous system forms from neural crest cells. Twelve pairs of cranial nerves result in three groups: somatic efferent cranial nerves, branchial arch nerves, and special sensory nerves. Paired sympathetic ganglia trunks form bilaterally along the vertebral column. Neurons migrating from the brain stem and sacral region of the spinal cord produce parasympathetic ganglia. Fissures within the optic stalks close, containing the hyaloid arteries and veins bathing the lens and retina. Corneas form. Semicircular ducts develop within the otic vesicles, and cartilage from the first and second branchial arches begin growing middle ear ossicles. The first and second branchial arches develop bilateral auricular hillocks. Major arteries and veins branch into the cephalic, thoracic, abdominal and sacro-iliac regions, and into the yolk sac and developing placenta. Interatrial septa and the interventricular septum fuse within a four-chambered heart. Pulmonary veins branch from the left atrium. An aorticopulmonary septum forms within the truncus arteriosus. A pericardium encloses the entire heart, and six major lymph sacs associated with venous circulation develop. A cartilaginous neurocranium molds from mesenchyme around the brain, forming a calvaria. Vertebral chondrification of the spinal cord continues, with paired costal processes appearing laterally along the thoracic region. Chondrification of the forelimbs leads to digital rays and elbows. The critical period for formation of forelimbs is from about 24 to 42 days, and for hindlimbs it extends to about 44 days. Mammary glands develop pectorally from epidermis burying into mesenchyme along the remains of bilateral mammary ridges. The embryo is now about 18mm CR.

Eighth Week[29]

The muscular system has begun differentiating into skeletal, smooth or cardiac muscles. Arms begin moving.[30] The respiratory system now includes the oral and nasal cavities, larynx, trachea, bronchi and pseudoglandular lungs. The digestive system includes the pharynx, esophagus, stomach, liver, gallbladder, pancreas, duodenum, intestine, appendix, colon and rectum. The urogenital system consists of metanephric kidneys, suprarenal glands, ureters, and bladder; urethra, developing testes or ovaries[31], phallus, and primitive genital ducts. The circulatory system contains a functioning four-chambered heart with all embryonic valves in place.[32] All major arteries and veins of the heart, head, neck, thorax, abdomen, fore and hind limbs, and umbilical arteries and veins, are present. The lymphatic system is forming in close association with the venous system, including development of the spleen. Tonsils also develop from lymph nodules along the neck region. The skeletal system contains rudiments of most major bones and joints. The skeleton is first formed by cartilaginous structures during the embryonic period, which are then ossified during the fetal period. The axial skeleton contains a vertebral column, twelve pairs of ribs, sternum and rudiments of the skull. The notochord disappears where vertebrae surround it, forming a gelatinous center of intervertebral discs. The appendicular skeleton contains rudiments of bones of the arms, hands and fingers, legs, feet and toes. The stubby tail is reabsorbed. The central nervous system consists of a brain with two distinct hemispheres[33], the thalami, pineal body, infundibulum, pontine flexure, medulla oblongata, pons and cerebellum; and the spinal cord with spinal ganglia and meninges. The peripheral nervous system consists of cranial, spinal, and visceral nerves, with corresponding ganglia. The autonomic system is dividing into sympathetic trunks and parasympathetic fibers.[34] The head now has a face with eyes oriented forward. Each eye is developing an iris, a cornea, and eyelids. Hair rudiments appear in the eyebrows. Paired nostrils, an upper lip, a mouth, a lower jaw, and bilateral ears[35] are also in place. Bent elbows and knees, unwebbed fingers and toes. Hands and feet are rotating 90 degrees downward to their normal position. An undifferentiated phallus is present in both sexes. Thus, by the end of the eighth week, a human embryo contains the rudiments of all major internal and external organs and systems which he or she will have for the rest of its life. That is why the eighth week normally marks the end of the embryonic period and the beginning of the fetal period.[36] The embryo is now about 30mm CR and may weigh about 7g.

4. Fetal Development[37]

The emphasis is now on cellular and tissue differentiation, and overall growth in size and weight: a normal ten week human fetus measures and weighs twice as much as an eight week embryo.

At 9 weeks, the head size is about half the body length, and the legs and thighs are relatively small. Both retinal membranes are fusing and the eyelids are closing. Primary ossification has begun, especially at the diaphysis of long bones and clavicles. Intestinal coils are still visible near the umbilical cord. The kidneys "ascend" to the suprarenal glands. The fetus begins producing urine, which is excreted into the amniotic fluid and some is swallowed, reabsorbed, and passed to the placenta and even onto the maternal circulation. Ovaries or testes generate from primary sex cords within the mesonephros. The urogenital groove is fusing in males to form a scrotum and glans penis, but remains open in females as labia flanking the glans clitoris.

Between 10-11 weeks, deciduous teeth develop from teeth buds.[38] Taste buds are forming on the tongue. The intestines have returned to the abdomen and peristalsis can be observed.[39] The spleen takes over erythropoiesis and the liver produces bile.

By the end of 12 weeks, the body has doubled its size, so that the head is now only about one third of the total length. Skin is developing into a complex organ system of epidermis (from ectoderm), dermis (mesoderm), and associated sweat, sebaceous, and mammary glands, hair follicles, and nails. The fetus is now about 85mm CR and weighs about 45g.

From 13 to 16 weeks, there is rapid body growth. Because ossification has begun, arms and legs lengthen[40]. The head is erect, and the pattern of scalp hair appears. All main lung structures are present, except for those involved in gas exchange.[41] The eyes, nose, mouth and ears are closer to their permanent position on the face, and motor reaction of hands and feet to cutaneous stimuli can be observed.[42] The stomach has begun peptic activity.[43] Prepuce grows around the glans penis. The fetus doubles again in length to about 140mm CR and more than quadruples its weight to about 200g.

From 17 to 20 weeks,[44] lymph sacs branch into a network of lymph nodes and sinuses. Lymphocytes originating from mesenchyme enter bone marrow to form lymphoblasts. The larynx develops.[45] Bronchioles vascularize highly and periodic breathing movement of lungs occurs.[46] The uterus forms and the vagina canalizes in females. Testes or ovaries have begun their descent through the inguinal canals.[47] The fetus accumulates brown fat, helping to maintain its body temperature by heat from oxidizing fatty acids.
The legs reach their final relative size. Eyebrows and head hair are present, and lanugo covers the entire body. Vernix caseosa, a greasy layer for protection from amniotic fluid, is secreted. The fetus is now about 190mm CR and weighs about 460g.

From 21 to 25 weeks, there is noticeable weight gain and body parts are better proportioned. Myelin sheaths form in the spinal cord and neural fiber tracts. Capillaries bulge through the thin epithelium of terminal sacs within bronchioles, and lung cells begin secreting surfactant, which decreases surface tension for terminal sacs to expand.[48] The fetus is viable, but seldom survives, since the lungs are still not capable of breathing. The fetus is now about 240mm CR and weighs about 900g.

From 26 to 29 weeks, the cerebral hemispheres are convoluting to greatly increase cortex surface. Internal, middle and external ear parts begin to function in unison.[49]. Eyelids reopen. White fat constitutes about 3.5% of body weight. At about 28 weeks, erythropoiesis passes from the spleen to bone marrow. By now, terminal sacs in the lungs are capable of gas exchange and the nervous system can regulate rhythmic breathing and control body temperature, therefore, the fetus is viable with intensive care. The fetus is now about 275mm CR and weighs about 1500g.

From 30 to 34 weeks, primitive alveoli are forming.[50] The testes continue descending. Pupillae can react to light. Sucking reflexes are observed.[51] The fetus in now about 320mm CR and weighs about 2500g. If born, he or she can usually survive.

From 35 to 38 weeks, the chest is prominent. The testes are in the scrotum or palpable along the inguinal canal. Secondary ossification begins. Hands can grasp. The head circumference is nearly that of the body; thereafter the body is slightly wider. The fetus shows a spontaneous orientation toward light. The lungs are about half filled with fluid at birth, therefore aeration is not so much the inflation of collapsed lungs as the replacement of fluid with air at birth.[52] The amount of white fat is about 16% of body weight, with 14 g of fat being added daily. It is important to distinguish between infants with low birth weight: due either to premature birth or to IUGR (which can be due to placental insufficiency). The infant is now about 360mm CR and weighs about 3400g.

Human gestation normally lasts 266 days (38 weeks) after fertilization or 280 days (40 weeks) after last menses.

C. MULTIFETAL GESTATION (MFG)[53]

Twins in the United States occur about 1:90 pregnancies, triplets about 1:8,100, and quadruplets about 1:729,000. Dizygotic (fraternal) twins develop from two zygotes.[54] Depending on their implantation site, dizygotic twins may develop separate, or fused chorionic sacs and placentas. The propensity for repeated dizygotic pregnancies tends to be hereditary. Monozygotic (identical) twins originate from a single zygote whose blastomeres have separated before implantation. They normally have almost identical genotypes[55], and develop two amniotic sacs, but share a common chorionic sac and placenta. Conjoined ("Siamese") twins derive from monozygotic twins whose blastula or gastrula fail to fully separate. Based on the severity of fusion, they may or may not be surgically separated if born alive. About 1:40 monozygotic twins are conjoined.

MFG is a high-risk condition which for the mother and child can result in: hypertension, anemia, pyelonephritis, postpartum hemorrhage, preterm labor and delivery, hydramnios, abnormal fetal presentation, cord prolapse, placenta previa or abrupta, congenital malformations, IUGR, spontaneous abortion, and perinatal mortality. Most fetal MFG morbidity and mortality happens before 30 weeks gestation, yet most complications arise later in pregnancy.[56] Factors influencing perinatal MFG morbidity and mortality are: IUGR, discordancy, anastomoses,[57] single fetal demise, congenital malformations, and chromosomal abnormalities.[58] Premature delivery is the single most important factor in perinatal MFG morbidity and mortality, with the mean for twins being 35 weeks gestation, for triplets 33, and for quadruplets 29. IUGR is the most frequent danger of premature delivery, and usually occurs in varying degrees among fetal twins (discordancy).[59] The higher weight an infant has the better the prognosis. The main factor causing discordancy is placental vascular anastomoses, where the "recipient" fetus grows larger at the expense of the "donor" fetus, whose development is further stunted by decreased amniotic fluid and space. It may be acute or chronic, and can augment during labor and delivery. Bed rest, tocolytics and serial removal of amniotic fluid (amniocentesis)[60] may help manage twin-to-twin transfusion pregnancies.

MFG siblings show higher rates of congenital malformations, such as: meromelia, single umbilical artery, and midline defects (anencephaly, heart disease). Acardia is specific to MFGs, and consists in the degeneration or absence of the heart in the "recipient" twin due to the overwhelming hemodynamic dominance of the "donor" twin.[61] If the surviving fetus has reached pulmonary maturity, a preterm delivery might be indicated.

The earlier the diagnosis of MFG, the better the prognosis. Screening may be done by physical observation of fetal size and weight-to-gestation age, palpation, and measurement of AFP (2.5 MOM or higher[62]), chorionic gonadotropin, placental lactogen, and pregnancy specific glycoproteins (amniocentesis,[63] ultrasound, Doppler[64]). Prophylactic therapies may be cerclage[65], tocolysis, and bed rest. The best delivery route (vaginal or cesarean) depends on the position of each fetus (vertex, transverse, breech). Vaginal delivery may accommodate vertex-vertex twins. For other variations, however, the Apgar scores[66] are inconclusive when compared to those of single deliveries.

Notes

[1]See: Elias and Annas, **Reproductive Genetics**, 1-16; Mange AP, Mange EJ, **Genetics: Human Aspects**, 2nd ed. Sunderland, MA: Sinauer Associates 1990, 12-78; Sutton HE, **An Introduction to Human Genetics**, 2nd ed. New York: Holt, Rinehart and Winston 1975, 17-33; Weaver RF, Hedrick PW, **Genetics**. Dubuque, IA: Brown 1989, 14-77.

[2]There is currently an international project to map the entire human genome (Human Genome Project), and software is being developed for automatizing the construction of genetic maps. See: Letovsky S, Berlyn MB, "CPROP: A rule-based program for constructing genetic maps" *Genom* 12 (1992) 435-446.

[3]An example of a sex-linked characteristic in humans in the color of the eyes.

[4]See: Elias and Annas, **Reproductive Genetics**, 16-21; Johnson KE, **Human Developmental Anatomy**. New York: Wiley 1988, 17-25; Moore KL, **The Developing Human: Clinically Oriented Embryology**, 4th ed. Philadelphia: Saunders 1988, 13-28; Sadler TW, **Langman's Medical Embryology**, 5th ed. Baltimore: Williams and Wilkins 1985, 3-18; Shostak S, **Embryology: An Introduction to Developmental Biology**. New York: HarperCollins 1991, 55-105, 133-219.

[5]Approximately half of the sperm in any single ejaculate is 23,X and the other half is 23,Y, that is why it is the sperm which determines the genetic sex of the future offspring. See: Cherry SH, **Understanding Pregnancy and Childbirth**. Indianapolis-New York: Bobbs-Merrill 1973, 4 (Note that while Cherry erroneously proposes 48 chromosomes in human cells, his description of chromosomal sex determination still holds true).

[6]See: Emery AEH, Rimoin DL, eds, **Principles and Practice of Medical Genetics**, 2nd ed. Vols. 1 and 2. New York: Churchill Livingstone 1990; Johnson, **Human Developmental Anatomy**, 26-27; Mange and Mange, **Genetics**, 107-120; Moore, **Developing Human**, 17-18.

[7]See: England MA, **Color Atlas of Life Before Birth: Normal Fetal Development**. Chicago: Year Book Medical Publishers 1990, 15-29; Johnson, **Human Developmental Anatomy**, 33-40; Mange and Mange, **Genetics**, 81-101.

[8]These dates are counted from the estimated day of fertilization. By contrast, if the point of departure is the day of last menses, then all the dates are pushed forward two weeks, making the entire human gestation period an average of 40 weeks.

[9]See: Glass RH, "Sperm and egg transport, fertilization, and implantation" in: Creasy RK, Resnik R, eds, **Maternal-Fetal Medicine: Principles and Practice**, 2nd ed. Philadelphia: Saunders 1989, 108-115; Johnson, **Human Developmental Anatomy**, 45-49; Moore, **Developing Human**, 13-31; Sadler, **Medical Embryology**, 19-28.

[10]See: Johnson, **Human Developmental Anatomy**, 25-26: Moore, **Developing Human**, 19-26; Shostak, **Embryology**, 166-171.

[11]LH is also called interstitial-cell-stimulating hormone (ICSH) when it occurs in males. Johnson, **Human Developmental Anatomy**, 25.

[12]See: Glass, *Sperm and egg*, 108-115; Moore, **Developing Human**, 28-31; Shostak, **Embryology**, 229-259.

[13]See: England, **Life before Birth**, 35-36; Gasser RF, **Atlas of Human Embryos**. Hagerstown, MD: Harper and Row 1975, 1-14; Johnson, **Human Developmental Anatomy**, 49-55; Moore, **Developing Human**, 31-49; Sadler, **Medical Embryology**, 30-36; Shostak, **Embryology**, 653-678.

[14]Embryonic development is a dynamic process which is influenced by a complex of internal and

external factors. Thus, these time frames are only approximations; the more gestational time passes, the greater will be the variation in the appearance of specific tissues, organs, and events. See: England, **Life before Birth**, 35; Gasser, **Human Embryos**, 1-5; Johnson, **Human Developmental Anatomy**, 49-50; Moore, **Developing Human**, 31-37; Sadler, **Medical Embryology**, 29-31; Shostak, **Embryology**, 307-352.

[15]Since blastomeres are pluripotential, if they separate they may give rise to monozygotic or identical siblings.

[16]The zygote spends about three days travelling through the uterine tube before reaching the uterus. See: Glass, *Sperm and egg*, 110.

[17]See: England, **Life before Birth**, 35-36; Gasser, **Human Embryos**, 7-14; Johnson, **Human Developmental Anatomy**, 51-54; Moore, **Developing Human**, 38-49; Sadler, **Medical Embryology**, 39-46; Shostak, **Embryology**, 577-602.

[18]This is the time of the first missed menstrual period. This section is based on: Gasser, **Human Embryos**, 15-24; Johnson, **Human Developmental Anatomy**, 54-55; Moore, **Developing Human**, 50-64; Sadler, **Medical Embryology**, 48-56; Shostak, **Embryology**, 631-651.

[19]"The specificity of the germ layers is not rigidly fixed. The cells of each germ layer divide, migrate, aggregate, and differentiate in rather precise patterns as they form the various organ systems (*organogenesis*)." Moore, **Developing Human**, 69. See also: England, **Life before Birth**, 38-39; Johnson,

[20]Induction is the process by which adjoining cells, tissues and organs influence one anothers' development. See: Moore, **Developing Human**, 69-72.

[21]Contractions of the heart begin at about day 22. See: Moore, **Developing Human**, 3 (timetable).

[22]Mesoderm of chorionic villi and body stalk derive only from the primitive streak, which can be detected as early as the 12th day. See: England, **Life before Birth**, 36, 40-50; Johnson, **Human Developmental Anatomy**, 93-102; Moore, **Developing Human**, 104-122.

[23]See: Gasser, **Human Embryos**, 25-101; Johnson, **Human Developmental Anatomy**, 79-87; Moore, **Developing Human**, 65-73; Sadler, **Medical Embryology**, 58-77.

[24]Ectoderm normally gives rise to the central and peripheral nervous systems, the sensory epithelia of the eye, inner ear and nose, the epidermis, hair and nails, mammary glands, pituitary gland, subcutaneous glands, and teeth enamel. Mesoderm gives rise to cartilage, bone, dermis and connective tissue, striated and smooth muscles, the heart, blood and lymph vessels, kidneys, testes, ovaries and genital ducts, the serous membranes lining body cavities, the spleen, and the cortex of the suprarenal gland. Endoderm gives rise to the epithelial lining of the gastrointestinal and respiratory tracts, the parenchyma of the tonsils, thyroid and parathyroid glands, thymus, liver and pancreas, the epithelial lining of the urinary bladder, most of the urethra, and the epithelial lining of the tympanic cavity, tympanic antrum, and auditory tube. See: England, **Life before Birth**, 39; Moore, **Developing Human**, 70; Shostak, **Embryology**, 580.

[25]The branchial apparatus, which is present in humans only during embryonic development, consists of branchial arches, pharyngeal pouches and branchial grooves, and is the site of most congenial malformations of the head and neck during embryonic development. See: Moore, **Developing Human**, 170-206.

[26]Amniotic fluid eventually consists of embryonic epithelial cells, lanugo, vernix caseosa, proteins, fats, carbohydrates, hormones, enzymes, pigments, fetal urine and about 99% water. See: England, **Life before Birth**, 42.

[27]CR= crown to rump measure. Ultrasound today permits further refinements of CR measure,

which is used for determining gestation age. See: Goldstein SR, "Embryonic ultrasonographic measurements: crown-rump length revisited" *AJObGyn* 165 (1991) 497-501.

[28]See: Gasser, **Human Embryos**, 103-239; Johnson, **Human Developmental Anatomy**, 115-120; Moore, **Developing Human**, 72-82.

[29]See: England, **Life before Birth**, 18; Gasser, **Human Embryos**, 241-297; Moore, **Developing Human**, 78-86; Shostak, **Embryology**, 687-774.

[30]See: England, **Life before Birth**, 171.

[31]While chromosomal sexual differentiation occurs at fertilization, gonadal sexual differentiation occurs at about the seventh week of embryonic development, mainly due to the presence of the testis-organizing factor regulated by the Y chromosome. Thus, in the absence of Y chromosomes the previously-undifferentiated gonads of the human embryo will now develop into ovaries. See: Moore, **Developing Human**, 262-265.

[32]Before birth, higher pressure blood from the right atrium shunts into the left atrium through the foramen ovale. After birth, higher pressure blood returning from the now functioning lungs into the left atrium forces the septum primum to fuse with the septum secundum, thus sealing the foramen ovale. See: Moore, **Developing Human**, 294-300.

[33]"Electrical activity [of cerebrum] is shown when studied in abortuses." Shiota K, "Central nervous system" in: Nishimura H, ed, **Atlas of Human Prenatal Histology**, 1st ed. Tokyo-New York: Igaku-Shoin 1983, 22.

[34]Spontaneous fetal movement is observed. See: Shiota, *Nervous system*, 40.

[35]The human ear is a composite of three sets of organs with a relative independent origin and early development one from the other. Internal ear: semicircular ducts, saccule and cochlea; middle ear ossicles and tympanic membrane; external ear auricle and acoustic meatus. The three gradually migrate from the first branchial arch toward a common region of the head, and connect to one another. See: England, **Life before Birth**, 90-93; Johnson, **Human Developmental Anatomy**, 351-357; Moore, **Developing Human**, 412-418.

[36]"The transition from an embryo to a fetus is not abrupt, but the name change is meaningful because it signifies that the embryo has developed into a recognizable human being." Moore, **Developing Human**, 87.

[37]See: England, **Life Before Birth**, 51-211; Gasser, **Human Embryos**; Johnson, **Human Developmental Anatomy**, 125-357; Moore, **Developing Human**; 159-436; Nishimura H, ed, **Atlas of Human Prenatal Histology**, 1st ed. Tokyo-New York: Igaku-Shoin 1983; Sadler, **Medical Embryology**, 79-86; Shostak, **Embryology**, 687-774.

[38]See: Semba R, Tanaka O, Tanimura T, "Digestive system" in: Nishimura H, ed, **Atlas of Human Prenatal Histology**, 1st ed. Tokyo-New York: Igaku-Shoin 1983, 176.

[39]See: Semba *et al*, *Digestive system*, 205.

[40]Intramembranous ossification occurs from mesenchyme which condenses and differentiates into osteoblasts, which in turn produce osteoid tissue within a matrix (where Calcium phosphate deposits). Endochondral (intracartilaginous) ossification occurs in pre-existing cartilaginous structures from primary and secondary ossification centers. The primary center is located at the diaphysis (body) of the matrix, where cartilage cells hypertrophy, become calcified, and die. The periosteum surrounds the diaphysis, invading it with hemopoietic (bone marrow) and osteoblastic cells. This process elongates the bone until the secondary center has done the same within the epiphyses (ends of the bone). By about 20 years of age the diaphysis has fused with the epiphyses, ending bone formation. See: Moore, **Developing Human**, 334-337.

[41]Due to nonfunctional lungs, fetal circulation is somewhat different from that of a newborn in order to facilitate gas exchange: Well-oxygenated blood returns from the placenta to the fetus by an

umbilical vein, where some of it goes through the hepatic sinusoids and the rest bypasses the liver through the ductus venosus into the inferior vena cava, mixing with some deoxygenated blood returning from the lower body. This still well-oxygenated blood passes into the right atrium, where most of it shunts through the foramen ovale into the left atrium, and is then pumped by the left ventricle into the aorta. The remaining blood mixes with deoxygenated blood returning from the superior vena cava into the right atrium, and is then pumped by the right ventricle into the pulmonary trunk, where it returns through the ductus arteriosus to the descending aorta. Some well-oxygenated blood goes from the aorta into the head, neck and fore limbs, whereas the remaining blood on the descending aorta mixes with deoxygenated blood coming from the ductus arteriosus. About half of this partly-oxygenated blood returns to the placenta through the umbilical arteries, whereas the other half goes to the abdomen and lower limbs. Fetal lungs only receive some partly-deoxygenated blood, which is sufficient, since they are still non-functioning. At birth, the three fetal shunts -the foramen ovale, the ductus venosus and the ductus arteriosus- are occluded, so that oxygenated and deoxygenated blood remain separated. See: Moore, **Developing Human**, 326-327.

[42]See: Shiota, *Nervous system*, 40.

[43]See: Semba *et al*, *Digestive system*, 200.

[44]Fetal movement ("quickening") is commonly felt by the mother during this time.

[45]"A series of cries occurs, if fetus is born." Tanimura T, "Respiratory system" in: Nishimura H, ed, **Atlas of Human Prenatal Histology**, 1st ed. Tokyo-New York: Igaku-Shoin 1983, 242.

[46]See: Tanimura, *Respiratory system*, 250.

[47]Testes continue descending for several weeks into scrotum, but ovaries only reach the pelvic brim.

[48]It is rather a sufficient quantity of surfactant and adequate pulmonary vasculature more than presence of terminal sacs or primitive alveoli which is responsible for the survival of premature fetuses. See: Moore, **Developing Human**, 213.

[49]"Fetus can respond to acoustic stimuli." Tanaka O, "Sense organs" in: Nishimura H, ed, **Atlas of Human Prenatal Histology**, 1st ed. Tokyo-New York: Igaku-Shoin 1983, 64.

[50]But 95% of alveoli actually develop after birth. See: Moore, **Developing Human**, 214.

[51]See: Shiota, *Nervous system*, 24.

[52]This fluid leaves the lungs by three routes due to pressure on it's thorax during delivery: through the newborn's mouth and nose; into it's pulmonary capillaries, and; into it's lymphatic system, and pulmonary arteries and veins. Moore, **Developing Human**, 214.

[53]This section on multifetal gestation is based on: Adam C, Allen AC, Baskett TF, "Twin delivery: Influence of the presentation and method of delivery on the second twin" **AJObGyn** 165 (1991) 23-27; Donnenfeld AE, Van de Woestijne J, Craparo F, Smith CS, Ludomirsky A, Weiner S, "The normal fetus of an acardiac twin pregnancy: perinatal management based on echocardiographic and sonographic evaluation" *PrenatDiag* 11 (1991) 235-244; Evans MI, Bronsteen RA, "Multiple gestation" in: Evans MI, Dixler AO, Fletcher JC, Schulman JD, eds, **Fetal Diagnosis and Therapy: Science, Ethics and the Law**. Philadelphia: Lippincott 1989, 242-266; Fowler MG, Kleinman JC, Kiely JL, Kessel SS, "Double jeopardy: twin infant mortality in the United States, 1983 and 1984" *AJObGyn* 165 (1991) 15-22; Johnson, **Human Developmental Anatomy**, 107-109; Moore, **Developing Human**, 122-129; Nora JJ, Fraser FC, **Medical Genetics: Principles and Practice**, 3rd ed. Philadelphia: Lea and Febiger 1989, 261-267; Pridjian G, Nugent CE, Barr M, "Twin gestation: influence of placentation on fetal growth" *AJObGyn* 165 (1991) 1394-1401; Romero R, Pilu G, Jeanty P, Ghidini A, Hobbins JC, **Prenatal Diagnosis of Congenital Anomalies**. Norwalk, CT: Appleton and Lange 1988, 403-411; Shostak, **Embryology**, 678-679.

[54]Fertilization of two eggs which mature simultaneously.

[55]Some genetic variation may be found in monozygotic twins. See: Watson WJ, Katz VL, Albright SG, Rao KW, Aylsworth AS, "Monozygotic twins discordant for partial trisomy 1" *ObGyn* 76 (1990) 949-951.

[56]28 weeks after fertilization.

[57]Anastomoses happens when blood vessels of twins sharing a common or fused placenta intermingle, allowing for the transfusion of blood from one fetus to another.

[58]Chromosomal abnormalities may appear independently in each fetus of MFG just as in singletons, even in monozygotic siblings due to postzygotic nondisjunction.

[59]Discordancy is any birth weight difference between siblings of the same gestation, and may vary from 15-25% difference. See: Evans and Bronsteen, *Multiple gestation*, 244.

[60]See: Elias S, Gerbie AB, Simpson JL, Nadler HL, Sabbagha RE, Shkolnik A, "Genetic amniocentesis in twin gestations" *AJObGyn* 138,2 (1980) 169-174.

[61]The phenotype of an acardiac twin can range from a mass of undifferentiated tissue to a fairly formed fetus.

[62]Since 2.5 MOM AFP is also the high value for normal singleton pregnancies, it only detects 50% of twins. See: Evans and Bronsteen, *Multiple gestation*, 243.

[63]See: Elias *et al*, *Twin gestations*, 169-174.

[64]The use of frequency-shifted ultrasound maternal and fetal blood flow wave form analysis. Stedman's **Medical Dictionary**: *ultrasonography, doppler.*

[65]See: Treadwell MC, Bronsteen RA, Bottoms SF, "Prognostic factors and complication rates for cervical cerclage: a review of 482 cases" *AJObGyn* 165 (1991) 555-558.

[66]"Evaluation of a newborn infant's physical status by assigning numerical values (0 to 2) to each of 5 criteria: 1) heart rate, 2) respiratory effort, 3) muscle tone, 4) response stimulation, and 5) skin color; a score of 10 indicates the best possible condition." Stedman's **Medical Dictionary**: *score, Apgar.*

CHAPTER III

HUMAN EMBRYONIC DISORDERS[1]

Twenty five to 50% of all spontaneous abortions and stillbirths contain some kind of genetic anomaly in their karyotype,[2] since many of these defects are incompatible with life. However, some disorders do survive through the entire gestational period onto birth. Five to 7% of all live births involve some kind of congenital defect, ranging from gross (anatomical) to molecular (physiological). Gross malformations tend to develop during the embryonic stages,[3] whereas molecular ones during the fetal stages.

A. ETIOLOGY

The cause of birth defects may be genetic, environmental, or more often, multifactorial (a combination of the two).

B. GENETIC FACTORS[4]

About 1:150 living persons carries a chromosomal disorder,[5] which may vary from a single gene to entire chromosomes. Chromosomal anomalies may be numerical or structural.

1. Abnormal Number of Chromosomes[6]

Aneuploidy

Meiotic nondisjunction gives rise to an uneven distribution of chromosomes within gametes. Monosomy is when a single chromosome is missing, whereas trisomy occurs when there is an extra chromosome in the karyotype[7]. Monosomy X0[8] is the most common cytogenetic abnormality in spontaneously aborted fetuses, and the incidence in live births is about 1:2,500 newborn females. These Turner syndrome females exhibit webbed necks, lymphedema of hands and feet, short stature, absence of sexual maturation, and broad, shield-like chests with widely spaced nipples. Yet, because their autosomes are unaffected, they have quite normal mental development. The three most common autosomal trisomies are Down syndrome (trisomy 21), Edwards syndrome (trisomy 18), and Patau syndrome (trisomy 13).[9] Trisomy 21 occurs in about 1:700 births, usually with mental deficiency, brachycephaly, flat nasal bridge, upward slant to palpebral fissure, protruding tongue, simian crease, clinodactyly of the 5th finger, and congenital heart defects. About 60% are spontaneously aborted, and at least 20% are stillborn.[10] Trisomy 18 arises in about 1:3,000 births, exhibiting mental deficiency, growth retardation, prominent occiput, short sternum, ventricular septal defect, micrognathia, low-set malformed ears, flexed fingers, hypoplastic nails, and rocker-bottom feet. Trisomy 13 occurs in about 1:5,000 births, displaying mental deficiency, severe CNS malformations, sloping forehead, malformed ears, scalp defects, microphthalmia, bilateral cleft lip and/or palate, polydactyly, and posterior prominence of the heels. Due to the severe abnormalities of neonates with trisomy 18 or 13, they rarely survive beyond a few months after birth.[11] Trisomy of sex chromosomes is a fairly common condition, occurring about 1:1,000, but is usually not detected until after puberty. Kleinfelter syndrome males (47,XXY) have typically small testes, hyalinization of seminiferous tubules, aspermatogenesis, are often tall with disproportionately long lower limbs, and their intelligence is less than in normal siblings.[12] Other sex chromosome trisomies are: 47,XXX females, who are normal in appearance, usually fertile, and 15-25% are mildly mentally retarded; 47,XYY males, who are also normal in appearance, often tall, and frequently show aggressive behavior.

Mosaicism

If nondisjunction occurs during early cleavage of the zygote, some blastomeres may end up with a greater number of chromosomes, whereas others contain the normal number. This gives rise to cell layers with different genotypes within the same embryo, which in turn leads to a patch-like pattern of less severe anomalies, depending on the organ system(s) affected.

Polyploidy

Polyploidy arises from cells containing multiples of the haploid number of chromosomes. The prevalent type in humans is triploidy (69 chromosomes).[13] Polyploid embryos usually abort spontaneously, but a few triploid fetuses have been known to be born, only to die soon thereafter due to severe abnormalities.

2. Structural Chromosomal Abnormalities

These may result from translocations, deletions, duplications or inversions. Translocations occur when a piece of a chromosome is added to a nonhomologous chromosome. Reciprocal translocations do not lead to abnormal development, but unilateral ones do.[14] Deletions may happen when a chromosome loses a piece, as in Cri du chat syndrome. These show a deletion in the short arm of chromosome 5, and develop a weak cat-like cry, microcephaly, severe mental retardation, and congenital heart disease.[15] Duplications of chromosome segments may involve part of a gene, a whole gene, or a series of genes. Since there is no loss of genome, they tend to be less harmful. Inversions reverse the genetic sequence of given chromosomes, at times causing structural or functional defects. Damaged chromosomes may be transmitted in an autosomal recessive fashion, and may give rise to growth retardation, somatic anomalies, and a propensity for neoplasia. Examples are: Bloom's syndrome, ataxia telangiectasia, and Fancomi's anemia.

Fragile X Syndrome[16]

This syndrome usually causes a higher spontaneous abortion rate, mental retardation, macroorchidism, and prognathism. It is related to a "fragile site" (staining gap) on the long arm of the X chromosome (Xq27), and can be detected with cytogenetic analysis. However, it doesn't follow strict Mendelian laws, since not all affected males display corresponding phenotype, while some heterozygous females do.

3. Mutant Genes[17]

Mutation may be of a single gene, or of several genes. Also, it may occur in autosomes, or it may be sex-linked. In autosomal dominant inheritance one parent is heterozygous for a particular mutation, whereas the other parent does not carry such mutation: In theory, 50% of progeny will be carriers of the particular mutation. Examples are: Acrocephalosyndactyly, aortic supravalvular stenosis, brachydactyly, cleft lip and palate, craniosynostoses, deafness, ectodermal dysplasias, epidermolysis bullosa, Huntington disease, arachnodactyly, muscular dystrophy, Noonan syndrome, and polycystic kidney.[18] In autosomal recessive inheritance, both parents are heterozygous carriers of the mutation, therefore: 25% of progeny will be affected by the mutation, 50% will be heterozygous carriers, and 25% will be unaffected. Since these mutations are not sex-linked, in principle they occur at equal rates in male and female progeny. Examples are: adrenocortical disorders, albinism, amino acid errors (maple syrup, PKU), tyrosinemia, sickle cell anemia, thalassemia, ataxia, cystic fibrosis, deafness, dwarfism, galactosemia, hypothyroidism, Tay-Sachs disease, mucolipidoses, muscular atrophy and dystrophy, Cockayne syndrome (premature senility), and retinitis pigmentosa.[19] Sex-linked mutations also have dominant-recessive patterns, but they tend to be more complicated. For instance, they tend to occur mostly on the X chromosome, since the Y chromosome seems to contain no functional genes.[20] In theory this means that whereas females may be either homozygous or heterozygous for a mutation, males can only be homozygous (having only one X chromosome). Examples are: ichthyosis, Duchenne muscular dystrophy, incontinentia pigmentosa, Menkes syndrome, Lesch-Nyhan syndrome, Hunter syndrome, mental retardation, and hemophilia A.[21] In practice, the picture is not as precise, since at times genes do not give rise to a full phenotypic expression,[22] or a single genetic trait may behave as if it was polygenic or multifactorial in origin.[23] Examples of multifactorial inheritance disorders are: anencephaly, cardiovascular diseases, cleft and lip palate, spina bifida, mental retardation, diabetes mellitus, epilepsies, pyloric stenosis, and peptic ulcers.[24]

4. Inborn Errors of Metabolism[25]

Many fetal metabolic disorders result in spontaneous abortions or stillbirths, but a few survive until birth and later. Most are autosomal recessive, but some are X-linked or autosomal dominant. They may involve lipid metabolism (Gangliosidosis), carbohydrate or glycoprotein metabolism (Fucosidosis, Galactosemia), mucopolysaccharide metabolism (Hunter syndrome, Hurler syndrome, Sly syndrome), amino acid and organic acid metabolism (Arginase deficiency, Cystinosis, Maple syrup urine disease), and other deficiencies (Adenosine deaminase deficiency, Congenital adrenal hyperplasia, Lesch-Nyhan syndrome, Hypophosphatasia, Cystic fibrosis, Xeroderma pigmentosum).[26]

C. COMMON HUMAN MENDELIAN DISORDERS[27]

Tay-Sachs Disease (Gangliosidosis Type 1)

The fetus fails to produce an enzyme that metabolizes sphingolipids, which accumulate and eventually interfere with normal neurological development, resulting in death by 3 to 4 years after birth. This autosomal recessive disorder is rarely found in the gentile population, but frequently among Jews, especially Ashkenazy (about one heterozygous in every 27).

Cystic Fibrosis (CF)[28]

CF is a chronic dysfunction of exocrine and mucus-producing glands (pancreas, bile ducts, intestine, and bronchi), causing malnourishment, bronchitis and pneumonia, ending in death from respiratory failure between 20 and 30 years of age. It is the most frequent Mendelian disorder among Caucasians, occurring about 1:1,500 births. It follows recessive transmission and is found in autosome 7q, therefore RFLPs could help detection, but CVS is most reliable. When both parents are heterozygotes, low levels of fetal alkaline phosphatases in amniotic fluid have been detected.

Duchenne Muscular Dystrophy (DMD)

DMD is a gradual muscle deterioration in males, appearing in children as a weakness at the waist and pseudohypertrophy of the calves, leading to difficulty in climbing stairs and a waddling gait. Contractures gradually spread to the trunk and appendages, confining the adolescent to a wheelchair. Affected adults may eventually develop cardiomyopathy and pulmonary infections due to dystrophy of respiratory muscles, usually leading to an early death. DMD children also show some degree of mental retardation. It is the most frequent childhood dystrophy, occurring in about 1:3,300 males. Since it is X-linked recessive (with about 33% new spontaneous mutation rate), RFLP probes on the short arm of the X chromosome (Xp21) can detect heterozygotes.

Hemophilia A (Classical Hemophilia)

It occurs when there is deficient production of coagulation factor VIII, resulting in a predisposition for traumatic or spontaneous bleeding, which can cause crippling hemarthroses. Internal hemorrhages can result in death. It is an X-linked recessive disorder affecting males almost exclusively, at a rate of about 1:7,000 to 1:10,000. The gene for procoagulant factor VIII (VIII:C) has now been cloned, making DNA probes available for detecting heterozygotes.

Congenital Adrenal Hyperplasia (CAH)

CAH causes female virilization during embryogenesis. Because the adrenal glands begin functioning during the third trimester, female CAH fetuses undergo virilization of external genitalia: enlarged clitoris, partial fusion of the labio-scrotal folds, and a phallic urethra. Internal female reproductive organs remain unaffected, however. CAH is the most frequent adrenal biosynthesis disorder, occurring in about 1:5,000 to 1:15,000 (1:700 in Alaskan Yupik Eskimos). In about 67% of cases it also reduces renal salt resorption ("salt wasting"), which untreated can lead to death. It is autosomal recessive, and the mutation is located at a single locus on the short arm of chromosome 6, which allows for the use of RFLP probes and heterozygote detection. Treatment of CAH is now possible by treating heterozygous expectant mothers with dexamethasone to about 8-10 weeks gestation.

Beta-Thalassemias

These are anemias with diminished synthesis of beta-globin. The deficiency may range from very mild to fatal. It is most common in Mediterranean countries, the Middle East and Southeast Asia, but not restricted to these areas. Though all Beta-thalassemias are due to mutations in the beta-globin locus of chromosome 16, the great variety of mutations makes PND difficult. Thus, for some kinds it is possible to use direct DNA analysis (Beta-39,Sardinia), whereas for others RFLPs of heterozygous parents may be used. If the parents are homozygous normal, the only technique may be PUBS.

Alpha-Thalassemias

These include a group of four anemias, this time due to insufficient synthesis of alpha-globin. It also ranges from mild to fatal, and is observed world-wide, but especially in Africa, the Philippines, and Southeast Asia. They are due to mutations on any one of four alpha-globin loci on chromosome 11. The severity of the condition depends on the mutation site. Since all four loci have been identified, prenatal diagnosis can be achieved by direct DNA analysis.

Sickle Cell Anemia

It results from a single amino acid substitution in Beta-globin, which produces characteristic sickle-shaped erythrocytes and accelerated hemolysis. Affected homozygotes manifest severe anemia and pain due to microvascular occlusions, together with bone necrosis and an increased susceptibility to infections. Since the specific nucleotide sequence point mutation is known, this allows for PND by direct DNA analysis.

Phenylketonuria (PKU)[29]

PKU women fail to metabolize phenylalanine into tyrosine, leading to an accumulation of the former and a deficit of the latter. In pregnancy, these imbalances may cause in the fetus mental retardation, IUGR, microcephaly, and malformations of the heart and central nervous system. It is autosomal recessive.

D. ENVIRONMENTAL FACTORS

1. Teratogens[30]

These are agents capable of causing congenital defects, such as chemical substances, radiation, or infectious diseases. They are most harmful during the time of most rapid cell growth and differentiation, that is, during organogenesis (15-60 days).[31]

Chemical Teratogens[32]

These cause less than 2% of all birth defects.[33] However, when they are present, they can cause extensive damage.

a. Social Drugs

Alcohol may cause IUGR, mental retardation, microcephaly, ocular and joint anomalies, short palpebral fissures, and congenital heart disease (Fetal alcohol syndrome, FAS). Alcohol abuse affects 1-2% of women of childbearing age,[34] and is thought to be the most common agent of mental retardation. The average minimal incidence of FAS is about 1-3:1,000 births.[35] Nicotine is not known to cause birth defects, but it does affect fetal growth (low birth weight and miscarriage) by constricting uterine blood vessels.[36] Caffeine does not appear to be teratogenic, though there is presently no substantial evidence that it may not be.[37] There is some evidence that Lysergic Acid Diethylamide (LSD) and Phencyclidine (PCP, "Angel Dust") may be teratogenic.[38] Marijuana does not seem to be teratogenic, but may be instrumental in causing IUGR and mental retardation.[39] Cocaine and heroin are not known not to be teratogenic.[40]

b. Prescription Drugs[41]

Androgenic hormones, such as testosterone, may cause virilization of females and ambiguous genitalia, whereas progesterones and estrogens, such as in oral contraceptives, may develop vertebral, anal, cardiac, tracheo-esophageal, renal and limb malformations (VACTERAL syndrome). Antibiotics, such as tetracyclines, may cause tooth defects and diminished growth of long bones.[42] Streptomycin may cause deafness. Chloramphenicol does not seem to be toxic to the fetus, but to newborns (Gray syndrome: abdominal distention, cyanosis, vascular collapse). Penicillin seems not to be teratogenic.[43] Anticoagulants, except for heparin, may cause hemorrhage in the fetus because they all cross the placental membrane. Warfarin causes hypoplasia of the nasal cartilage and defects of the CNS, mental retardation, optic atrophy, and microcephaly.[44] Anticonvulsants, such as trimethadione (Tridione) and paramethadione (Paradione) may be teratogenic. Phenytoin (Dilantin) causes IUGR, microcephaly, mental retardation, ridged metopic suture, inner epicanthal folds, eyelid ptosis, broad depressed nasal bridge, and phalangeal hypoplasia (Fetal hydantoin syndrome). Phenobarbital may not be teratogenic.[45] Antineoplastic agents (tumor-inhibiting drugs) are considered to be highly teratogenic, such as: Aminopterin, producing a wide range of skeletal defects, IUGR, malformations of the CNS (meroanencephaly); Busulfan, producing stunted growth, skeletal abnormalities, corneal opacities, cleft palate, and hypoplasia of various organs; Methotrexate, causing multiple skeletal defects (face, skull, limbs and vertebral column).[46] Vitamin A in large doses may cause thymic aplasia, cleft palate, craniofacial dysmorphism, and neural tube defects.[47] Aspirin in large doses may be teratogenic. Thyroid drugs, may cause thyroid enlargement and cretinism. Tranquilizers may be teratogenic. Thalidomide affects the limbs, ranging from amelia to micromelia, the ears, forehead, heart, and urinary and digestive systems.[48] Lithium carbonate may affect the heart and great vessels.

c. Environmental Chemicals[49]

A number of environmental chemical substances may be teratogenic in large amounts, such as: heavy metals (lead, mercury, cadmium)[50], solvents (hexanes, ketones, ethers, acetone, toluene, ethanols and butanol), and hydrocarbons (pyrenes, dioxins and biphenyls; TCDD, PCBs, PBBs)[51].

Radiation[52]

Large amounts of ionizing radiation may cause microcephaly, spina bifida cystica, cleft palate, skeletal and visceral abnormalities, and mental retardation. Any exposure above 10,000-25,000 millirads may be considered dangerous. However, exposure to diagnostic levels does not seem to cause malformations.[53]

Maternal Diseases

Maternal diabetes mellitus is known to cause fetal cardiovascular, genitourinary, and musculoskeletal defects.[54]

Infections[55]

Some viruses and microorganisms cross the placental membrane into the embryonic environment, where they may act as teratogens, depending on the time of infection (organogenesis; 15-60 days). Rubella Virus (German Measles) can cause cataracts, cardiac malformations, and deafness, and occasionally, chorioretinitis, glaucoma, microcephaly, microphthalmia, and tooth defects.[56]

Cytomegalovirus, probably the most common infection of the human fetus, usually ends in abortion during early development. In later development it may cause IUGR, microcephaly, blindness, microphthalmia, cerebral palsy, and hepatosplenomegaly.[57] Herpes Simplex virus may cause microcephaly, microphthalmia, retinal dysplasia, and mental retardation. If the fetus is not infected during gestation, it can be at delivery by contact with the birth canal. Therefore, a cesarean delivery may be indicated. Varicella virus (Chickenpox and shingles) may cause skin scarring, muscle atrophy and mental retardation.[58] Toxoplasma gondii, a parasite, damages the brain and eyes, causing microcephaly, microphthalmia, and hydrocephaly.[59] Treponema pallidum (Syphilis) may cause deafness, abnormal teeth and bones, hydrocephalus, mental retardation, lesions of the palate and nasal septum, and abnormal facies (frontal bossing, saddlenose, and a poorly developed maxilla).[60]

2. Mechanical Forces

Overall, the fetus is protected from mechanical forces by the amniotic fluid, but external pressures can cause damage, for instance, when early rupture of embryonic membranes may result in bands, fibers or scar tissue which affect normal growth.[61].

E. CONGENITAL MALFORMATION OF HUMAN ORGAN SYSTEMS[62]

These can occur by too little growth, little resorption, too much resorption, resorption in the wrong place, normal growth in the wrong place or local overgrowth of tissues or structures.[63]

Primitive Mesenteries and Diaphragm[64]

Congenital Diaphragmatic Hernia is when the pleuroperitoneal membranes fail to fuse during the 6th week[65], allowing viscerae into the thorax during the 10th week, encroaching on development of heart and lungs. At birth, it prevents the lungs from aerating fully. If lung hypoplasia is severe, some alveoli may rupture while breathing, causing pneumothorax. It occurs about 1:2,000 births, and may be a life-threatening breathing ailment. Other hernias may be: epigastric, hiatal, retrosternal and pericardial.

Branchial Apparatus, Head and Neck[66]

a. Branchial Malformations[67]

First Arch syndrome results in malformations of the eyes, ears, mandibles (micrognathia), and cleft palate. Thymic aplasia and absence of parathyroid glands may cause hypoparathyroidism, a higher rate of infections, defects of the mouth, nasal clefts, thyroid hypoplasia, and cardiac anomalies.

b. Cleft Lip and Palate[68]

Cleft lip is the most common facial defect, occurring about 1:1,000 births, more often in males. It may be mild or severe, unilateral or bilateral, and isolated or involving the palate. Cleft palate occurs about 1:2,500 births, more often in females. It may include the lip and may also be mild or severe, bilateral or unilateral. Cleft lip/palate may be due to abnormal autosomes (trisomy 13), sex-linked, teratogenic or multifactorial.

Lower Respiratory System[69]

Tracheoesophageal fistula is the most common defect of the lower respiratory system, affecting about 1:2,500 births. It is associated with esophageal atresia in about 90% of cases. If so, food in the blind esophagus is regurgitated, the stomach and intestines fill with air upon breathing, and gastric juices may reflux into the lungs, causing pneumonia or pneumonitis. Respiratory distress syndrome in premature infants is due to an insufficient surfactant, where alveoli of underinflated lungs are full of a glassy fluid, causing hyaline membrane disease. Lung hypoplasia occurs when abdominal viscerae herniate into the thorax through a diaphragmatic hernia. Lung agenesis (rare) may result from underdevelopment of bronchial buds. Unilateral agenesis is compatible with life (existing lung hyperexpands).

Digestive System[70]

Esophageal atresia impedes the fetus from swallowing amniotic fluid and eliminating it through the placenta, causing polyhydramnios. This condition may be caused by teratogens. Esophageal stenosis generally occurs in the distal third of the esophagus. Also, a short esophagus may pull the stomach through a diaphragmatic hiatus, causing a hiatal hernia. Congenital hypertrophic pyloric stenosis occurs about 1:150 male or 1:750 female infants, and may be of genetic origin. Duodenal stenosis and atresia also cause polyhydramnios and vomiting. An annular pancreas can cause duodenal obstruction. Extrahepatic biliary atresia is potentially life-threatening if not corrected surgically. It appears about 1:20,000 infants and manifests in jaundice soon after birth. Omphalocele happens when the intestines fail to return to the abdomen during the tenth week, but may be triggered by incomplete closure of the lateral folds as early as the fourth week. It occurs about 1:6,000 births, and one third to one half of these infants show other congenital malformations, such as malrotation, Meckel's diverticulum, or cardiovascular defects. Umbilical hernias form when part of the intestines return into an imperfectly closed umbilicus, and is thus less severe than omphalocele. They become manifest when crying, straining or coughing. Nonrotation of the midgut can cause volvulus of intestines and subsequent obstruction of the superior mesenteric artery. Meckel's diverticulum is a remnant of the yolk sac which is still attached to the intestinal wall, containing all layers of the ileum and pieces of gastric and pancreatic tissue, which can secrete acid. This acid inflames the affected area, which may seem as appendicitis. If the diverticulum opens to the umbilicus through a fistula, it can cause ulceration and bleeding. Congenial aganglionic megacolon (Hirschsprung's Disease) causes dilation in a portion of the colon due to the absence of autonomic ganglion cells. The dilated colon is incapable of peristalsis, impeding intestinal contents to move through. Imperforate anus happens about 1:5,000 births, and is more frequent in males; mostly due to incomplete separation of the cloaca into urogenital and anorectal canals. Other low anorectal defects are: anal agenesis, stenosis and membranous atresia. High anorectal defects are: anorectal agenesis, with or without fistula to the bladder, urethra, or vagina, and rectal atresia, with the rectum and anal canal widely separated.

Urogenital System[71]

Kidney and ureter defects are common (3-4% of all births). Renal agenesis may be unilateral or bilateral. Unilateral agenesis happens about 1:1,000 births, and is compatible with life; bilateral agenesis occurs about 1:3,000 and is not compatible with life due to rapid accretion of urine after birth. Bilateral polycystic kidneys usually result in death, but some newborns are saved with hemodialysis and kidney transplants. Duplication of ureters and, rarely the kidneys, may occur. Ectopic ureters may empty into the urethra, seminal vesicles, or the vagina, causing incontinence. Urachal sinuses or cysts may occur along the urachus. Exstrophy of the bladder may cause epispadias. This severe defect is rare, occurring about 1:10,000 to 50,000 births. Congenital adrenal hyperplasia leads to an overproduction of androgens. This causes virilization in females and may lead to precocious sexual development in males.

Genital System[72]

Genetic sex is determined by the Y chromosome at fertilization, whereas anatomical sex is controlled by androgens during the fetal period. Hermaphroditism is when there is an inconsistency between the genetic sex and external genitalia. Female pseudohermaphroditism (46,XX) is due to virilizing adrenal hyperplasia, causing hypertrophy of the clitoris, partial closure of the labia majora, and a persistent urogenital sinus (adrenogenital syndrome). These females develop normal ovaries. Male pseudohermaphroditism (46,XY) is due to insufficient testosterone, and causes underdeveloped testes and phallus. True hermaphroditism presents both testicles and ovaries (or an ovotestis), but are usually nonfunctional. External genitalia are ambiguous, so individuals may appear as males or females. It is extremely rare, and 80% are genetic females (46,XX). Testicular feminization occurs when the labioscrotal and urogenital cells are resistant to testosterone, preventing virilization. These individuals develop a female phenotype, albeit their 46,XY genotype. Though the external genitalia are female, the vagina is usually truncated from the uterus, which may be rudimentary or absent. It is rare (about 1:50,000 births), and seems to be transmitted as a sex-linked recessive gene which controls the cellular androgen receptor mechanism. Hypospadias may be caused by insufficient androgens. It occurs about 1:300 male births, and is associated with chordee. Absence of vagina and uterus from lack of development of the sinovaginal bulbs occurs in about 1:4,000 female births. Cryptorchidism usually results in sterility. It occurs about 1:30 premature male births, and about 1:300 full term male births, and may be unilateral or bilateral. Inguinal hernias are found more often in males, especially with cryptorchidism. Hydrocele can occur from a persistent processus vaginalis.

Cardiovascular System[73]

Defects of the heart are most common, accounting for about 25% of all congenital malformations. There exists a wide range, from most mild (dextrocardia) to most severe (ectopia cordis).

a. Atrial Septal Defects (ASD)

Probe patent foramen ovale is the most common atrial defect, (about 25% of the population), and is compatible with life, but may lead to a functional pathology when present with other heart defects. Other types of ASD are: secundum type, endocardial cushion, sinus venosus, and common atrium.

b. Ventricular Septal Defects (VSD)

These are the most common of heart malformations, accounting for about 25% of all congenital heart disease. Membranous VSD is an interventricular septum foramen. Rarely, the entire septum may be missing (cor triloculare biatriatum). Persistent truncus arteriosus leaves the aorta and pulmonary trunk partially communicated. Pulmonary atresia is when the trunk is occluded at the valve due to severe anomaly of the truncus arteriosus, whereas stenosis occurs with fused valve cusps or a malformed infundibulum, resulting in hypertrophy of the right ventricle. Aortic stenosis or atresia is from a fused aortic valve. Patent ductus arteriosus (PDA) allows venous and arterial blood to mix. It is more common in females, and from rubella-infected mothers. Most premature infants have a PDA for a day. Transposition of great arteries usually occurs with ASD or VSD, resulting in death in a few months after birth if untreated. Tetralogy of Fallot includes: pulmonary stenosis, VSD, overriding aorta, and hypertrophy of the right ventricle.

Skeletal System[74]

Klippel-Feil Syndrome (Brevicollis) may be due to absent or fused vertebrae, causing a short neck with limited movement, while hemivertebrae force scoliosis of the vertebral column. Acrania results from no calvaria. Usually other sections of the vertebral column and CNS are also absent (meroanencephaly). It occurs about 1:1,000 births, and is incompatible with life.

Craniosynostosis is caused by premature closure of skull sutures and results in a deformed calvaria. Microcephaly involves a normal-sized or slightly small calvaria at birth, but the fontanelles and sutures close early. Rachischisis is when the neural folds fail to fuse, exposing the CNS. Other defects of the craniovertebral junction are fairly common, appearing about 1:100 births. They may include: basilar invagination around the foramen magnum, assimilation of the atlas with the occipital bone, atlantoaxial dislocation, Arnold-Chiari malformation, and separate dens or odontoid process. Achondroplasia (dwarfism) is caused by abnormal endochondral ossification of long bones (limbs) and is an autosomal dominant trait. It occurs about 1:10,000 births. Hyperpituitarism may result in gigantism or acromegaly, while hypothyroidism causes cretinism. It is very rare and related to insufficient iodine.[75] There are a great variety of congenital limb malformations,[76] such as cleft hands and feet ("Lobster-Claw"), brachydactyly (short fingers), syndactyly (webbing), polydactyly, talipes (clubfoot), absence of the radius, and dislocation of the hip (occurring mostly at delivery). Though crippling to different degrees, all are generally compatible with life.[77]

Muscular System

Absence of formation of one or more muscles is fairly common, and usually without much clinical consequence, since surrounding muscles tend to substitute. Absence of other muscles is more serious, as in the case of the abdomen, which can cause pneumonia, and of the anterior abdominal wall, which can result in defects of the digestive, urinary and reproductive systems. Absence of certain muscles may lead to muscular dystrophy.

Nervous System[78]

Neural tube defects derive mostly from impartial closure of either neuropore during the 4th week. If it involves the caudal neuropore, it will affect the spinal cord, resulting in various types of spina bifida. If it involves the rostral neuropore, it will affect the brain.

a. Spinal Cord

Spina bifida oculta is the failure of a vertebral arch to completely fuse medially, usually in the lumbo-sacral region. It occurs about 1:10 births and is of no clinical consequence. Spina bifida cystica occurs about 1:1,000 births, and its degree of severity depends on the extent of the defect, and the amount and type of tissue extruding. If it contains meninges it is a meningocele (less severe), if it includes the spinal cord or nerve roots it is a meningomyelocele (more severe), and if the spinal cord is open it is a myeloschisis (most severe). Spina bifida cystica usually causes dermal anesthesia and muscle paralysis. If the defect occurs in the sacro-lumbar region, it may cause saddle anesthesia. It is sometimes associated with craniolacunia, resulting in meroanencephaly.

b. Brain

Defects may be histological or morphological. Histological malformations may lead to mental retardation, especially by exposure to viruses or radiation from the 8th to the 16th week. Cranium bifidum is when the calvaria fails to form properly. It usually occurs at the posterior fontanelle or at the base of the foramen magnum. If it is small, only the meninges herniate, forming a meningocele. If large, part of the brain also herniates causing a meningoencephalocele. If it includes a ventricle, it is a meningohydroencephalocele. It occurs in about 1:2,000 births. Exencephaly and anencephaly[79] are severe brain defects which result from the absence of the calvaria. In meroanencephaly (anencephaly) the exencephalic brain degenerates into a spongy, vascular tissue, which usually results in death within a few hours after birth. Since a meroanencephalic fetus is incapable of swallowing and eliminating amniotic fluid, polyhydramnios and a high level of AFP may indicate the defect. It occurs about 1:1,000 births, and is four times more frequent in females. It may be caused by genetic or environmental (teratogenic) factors.

Microcephaly usually results from an underdeveloped brain, causing the calvaria to remain very small in relation to a normal-sized face. These infants are severely mentally retarded. It may rarely also result from premature synostosis of cranial sutures, and can be caused by genetic or environmental agents. Hydrocephalus results from an enlargement of cerebral ventricles due to an excess of cerebrospinal fluid (CSF). It may be caused by aqueductal stenosis, and may be inherited, but is more often due to fetal viral infections. It is related to atrophy of the cortex and white matter, and spina bifida cystica. Arnold-Chiari malformation is a projection of the medulla and cerebellum into the foramen magnum, preventing normal absorption of CSF, and also causing distention of the ventricular system. It often occurs together with meningomyelocele, myeloschisis, and hydrocephaly. It occurs about 1:1,000 births. Corpus callosum agenesis may be complete or partial. It causes seizures and mental deficiency, but may also be asymptomatic.[80]

c. Eye

Most anomalies result from a defective closure of the optic fissure during the 6th week, such as coloboma of the eyelid, iris, and retina. Ptosis causes the eyelid to droop over the eye. Congenital glaucoma is usually the result of a recessive genetic mutation, but also from a maternal rubella infection. Congenital cataract typically causes blindness. It is inherited as a dominant trait, but also from rubella infections. Other congenital conditions are: a detached retina, aphakia, aniridia, cryptophthalmos, microphthalmos, anophthalmos, or cyclopia.

d. Ear

Congenital deafness may be due to a malformation of sound-conducting structures of the external and middle ears, or by a defect in neurosensory organs of the internal ear. The critical time of major morphological deformities is 4-9 weeks, and of functional anomalies or minor morphological defects 9-16 weeks. Even though the main cause of congenital deafness is genetic, maternal rubella infection may also produce it. Auricular anomalies are usually minor (appendages), but may indicate more serious internal congenital defects. Atresia of the external acoustic meatus may also affect the middle and internal ear (first arch syndrome). It is genetically transmitted as an autosomal dominant trait.

Integumentary System

a. Skin

Ichthyosis results in dryness and scaling. Lamellar ichthyosis impedes development of sweat glands, which causes extreme discomfort in hot weather. It is autosomal recessive. Congenital ectodermal dysplasia is rare, and may also lead to absence of hair and dental malformations. Albinism is transmitted as an autosomal recessive trait.

b. Hair and Nails

Congenital alopecia is due mainly to poor follicle growth, whereas hypertrichosis to an overabundance of follicles. Anonychia results from a malformation of proximal nail folds. It is extremely rare and may occur in any digit.

c. Mammary glands

Athelia and amastia may happen due to lack of mammary ridges or when a mammary bud fails to form. These are rare defects. Polythelia and polymastia may also develop anywhere along the mammary ridges, unilaterally or bilaterally. These are fairly common, occurring as often as 1:100 female births. Gynecomastia is mostly due to excess estrogen. It may be caused by an extra X chromosome (Klinefelter syndrome, 47,XXY).

d. Teeth

Enamel hypoplasia may be due to injury of ameloblasts in oral ectoderm, and leads to pits and fissures in the enamel. This can be caused by teratogens, such as tetracycline, and by infections or malnutrition during pregnancy. Amelogenesis imperfecta is due to a calcium deficiency (hypocalcification), rendering the enamel soft and the teeth yellow or brown. It occurs about 1:20,000 births. Dentinogenesis imperfecta is when the enamel wears down, exposing the dentin. The teeth appear brown to gray-blue. Both are autosomal dominant.

F. VERY LOW BIRTH WEIGHT (VLBW)[81]

A fetus weighing 500-1,500 g being born between 25-32 weeks gestation[82] is considered VLBW and at high risk, particularly to perinatal hypoxia, acidosis, and birth trauma. Long term problems may be: mental and neurological handicaps, somatic growth retardation, and major organ system disorders. Survival rate of VLBW fetuses is mostly related to birth weight and gestational age. Major direct causes of VLBW can be: fetal hormonal or enzymatic imbalance, restricted intrauterine blood flow (abruptio placentae or true knot of umbilical cord), dysfunctional adrenal receptors, abnormal fetal skeletal and muscular development, and insufficient oxygen and nutrients in fetal blood. Causes of premature labor may be: IUGR (intra-uterine growth retardation), hypertension or preeclampsia, multifetal pregnancy, maternal smoking, sickle cell anemia, diabetes, infectious diseases, chronic alcohol and drug abuse, maternal age (less than 17 or over 34), race (black), low weight for height, incompetent cervix, low maternal birth weight, isoimmunization, oligohydramnios, and premature rupture of membranes (PROM: in about 1/3 of all VLBW preterm deliveries). There are two types of IUGR: a decreased growth potential in the fetus, usually due to some related congenital anomaly (type I); or a restriction of fetal growth due to decreased oxygen and nutrient supply (uteroplacental insufficiency) to an otherwise normally-developing fetus with no other anomaly (type II).

The major concern in VLBW is immaturity of organ systems, especially respiratory, circulatory, renal, gastrointestinal and nervous systems. Two main causes of VLBW neonatal mortality are intraventricular hemorrhage (IVH) and respiratory distress syndrome (RDS). RDS is the single most frequent VLBW neonatal morbidity, especially due to perinatal asphyxia and related complications. It is triggered mainly by a chronic reduction in uterine blood flow, which causes fetal hypoxia, itself leading to fetal myocardial depression and metabolic acidosis.

The single most critical VLBW mortality factor is insufficient surfactant in the lungs of the neonate. IVH in the neonate ranges from mild to severe. IVH prognosis can be enhanced by minimizing perinatal asphyxia and managing other perinatal and postnatal conditions. Therefore, the earlier IVH is diagnosed, the better the prognosis. IVH can be detected in utero by ultrasound.

The longer preterm labor can be delayed, the better the prognosis of VLBW infants. Delivery delay may be attempted by: tocolysis, cerclage, beta-sympathomimetic agents, prostaglandin synthetase inhibitors, calcium channel blockers, and bed rest. Some of these methods do pose serious side effects for both fetus and mother, thus risk-benefits must be estimated for each case.

Positive prognosis of VLBW neonates depends on accurate diagnosis of fetal weight by gestational age, which can be done with invasive and non-invasive PND techniques. Such diagnosis also helps determine the best route of delivery (vaginal or cesarean), and the eventual need of specific expertise, protocol and equipment at time of delivery (transfusion, resuscitation).

Notes

[1] General references for this chapter on human embryonic disorders are: Miller JR, Lowry RB, "Birth defects registries and surveillance" in: Wilson JG, Fraser FC, eds, **Handbook of Teratology: Comparative, Maternal, and Epidemiologic Aspects**. New York: Plenum 1977, 227-242; Wilson JG, **Environment and Birth Defects**. New York: Academic 1973, 97-109.

[2] See: Johnson, **Human Developmental Anatomy**, 373.

[3] Particularly during organogenesis (15 to 60 days of gestation). See: Moore, **Developing Human**, 142-144.

[4] This section on genetic factors is based on: Elias and Annas, **Reproductive Genetics**, 25-30 (Mendelian inheritance); Nora and Fraser, **Medical Genetics**, 20-94; Sadler, **Medical Embryology**, 118-122; Simpson, *Transmitting genetic disorders*, 94-101.

[5] See: Simpson, *Transmitting genetic disorders*, 94.

[6] See: Elias and Annas, **Reproductive Genetics**, 16-25; Nora and Fraser, **Medical Genetics**, 29-71.

[7] "The chromosome characteristics of an individual or of a cell line, usually presented as a systematized array of metaphase chromosomes from a photomicrograph of a single cell nucleus arranged in pairs in descending order of size and according to the position of the centromere." Stedman's **Medical Dictionary**: *karyotype*.

[8] This happens when the fertilizing sperm is missing the sex chromosome, which means that only the X chromosome of the egg will be present. See: Elias and Annas, **Reproductive Genetics**, 21-22.

[9] See: Elias and Annas, **Reproductive Genetics**, 16-21; Nora and Fraser, **Medical Genetics**, 28-54.

[10] See: Moore, **Developing Human**, 136.

[11] There are reports, however, of chromosome 18 duplication with apparent normal phenotypes. Wolff DJ, Raffel LJ, Ferré MM, Schwartz S, "Prenatal ascertainment of an inherited dup(18p) associated with an apparently normal phenotype" *AJMedGen* 41 (1991) 319-321.

[12] See: Elias and Annas, **Reproductive Genetics**, 23-25; Nora and Fraser, **Medical Genetics**, 54-71.

[13] This may occur either from the simultaneous fertilization of an egg by two sperms, or by the

second polar body failing to separate from the oocyte during the second meiotic division. Connor and Ferguson-Smith estimate that 66% of triploid embryos result from double fertilization. See: Moore, **Developing Human**, 138.

[14]For instance, 3-4% of persons with Down syndrome exhibit the extra 21 chromosome attached to another, that is, they have a translocated 21 trisomy.

[15]See: Elias and Annas, **Reproductive Genetics**, 21.

[16]See: Elias and Annas, **Reproductive Genetics**, 88; Romain DR, Chapman CJ, "Fragile site Xq27.3 in a family without mental retardation" *ClinGen* 41 (1992) 33-35; Toncheva D, "Fragile sites and spontaneous abortions" *GenCounsel* 2 (1991) 205-210.

[17]See: Elias and Annas, **Reproductive Genetics**, 25-30; Nora and Fraser, **Medical Genetics**, 76-87.

[18]See: Nora and Fraser, **Medical Genetics**, 130-158.

[19]See: Elias and Annas, **Reproductive Genetics**, 57-60; Nora and Fraser, **Medical Genetics**, 159-190.

[20]See: Goodfellow PN, Goodfellow PJ, Pym B, Banting G, Pritchard C, Darling SM, "Genes on the human Y chromosome" in: Haseltine FP, McClure ME, Goldberg EH, eds, **Genetic Markers of Sex Differentiation**. New York: Plenum 1987, 99-111.

[21]See: Nora and Fraser, **Medical Genetics**, 190-200.

[22]This is called penetrance or expressivity. See: Wolff *et al*, *Prenatal ascertainment*, 319-321.

[23]See: Elias and Annas, **Reproductive Genetics**, 106-109.

[24]See: Nora and Fraser, **Medical Genetics**, 230-247.

[25]This section on inborn errors of metabolism is based on: Elias and Annas, **Reproductive Genetics**, 89-90; Nora and Fraser, **Medical Genetics**, 95-118.

[26]See: Johnson, **Human Developmental Anatomy**, 380.

[27]References for this section on common human mendelian disorders are from: Elias and Annas, **Reproductive Genetics**, 62-66; Evans *et al, First trimester*, 17-36; Simpson and Elias, *Prenatal diagnosis*, 94-103; Simpson, *Transmitting genetic disorders*, 94-101.

[28]See: Verlinsky Y, Rechitsky S, Evsikov S, White M, Cieslak J, Lifchez A, Valle J, Moise J, Strom CM, "Preconception and preimplantation diagnosis for cystic fibrosis" *PrenatDiag* 12 (1992) 103-110.

[29]See: Biddle FG, Fraser FC, "Maternal and cytoplasmic effects in experimental teratology" in: Wilson JG, Fraser FC, eds, **Handbook of Teratology: Comparative, Maternal, and Epidemiologic Aspects**. New York: Plenum 1977, 18-19; Elias and Annas, **Reproductive Genetics**, 54-57.

[30]See: Anderson RL, Golbus MS, "Chemical teratogens" in: Evans MI, Dixler AO, Fletcher JC, Schulman JD, eds, **Fetal Diagnosis and Therapy: Science, Ethics and the Law**. Philadelphia: Lippincott 1989, 114-139; Beck F, Lloyd JB, "Comparative placental transfer" in: Wilson JG, Fraser FC, eds, **Handbook of Teratology: Comparative, Maternal, and Epidemiologic Aspects**. New York: Plenum 1977, 155-186; Dencker L, Danielsson BRG, "Transfer of drugs to the embryo and fetus after placentation" in: Nau H, Scott Jr WJ, eds, **Pharmacokinetics in Teratogenesis: Interspecies Comparison and Maternal/Embryonic-Fetal Drug Transfer**. Boca Raton, FL: CRC 1987, 55-69; Krauer B, "Physiological changes and drug disposition during pregnancy" in: Nau and Scott, **Pharmacokinetics in Teratogenesis**, 3-12; Sever JL, Brent RL, eds, **Teratogen Update: Environmentally Induced Birth Defect Risks**. New York: Liss 1986, 1-201; Spielmann H, Vogel R, "Transfer of drugs into the embryo before and during implantation" in: Nau and Scott, **Pharmacokinetics in Teratogenesis**, 45-53.

---

[31]Teratogens are known to critically affect the normal development of the central nervous system from the third to the
16th week of gestation, the ears from the fourth to the ninth, the eyes from the forth to the eighth, the heart from the third to the sixth, the upper and lower limbs from the fourth to the sixth, the teeth and palate from the sixth to the eight, and the external genitalia from the seventh to the ninth week. See: Moore, **Developing Human**, 143.

[32]See: Dencker and Danielsson, *Transfer of drugs*, 55-69; Elias and Annas, **Reproductive Genetics**, 200-214; Krauer, *Drug disposition*, 3-12; Sadler, **Medical Embryology**, 113-114; Spielmann and Vogel, *Transfer of drugs*, 45-53.

[33]See: Brent in Moore, **Developing Human**, 145.

[34]See: Golbus in Moore, **Developing Human**, 146.

[35]See: Abel EL, Sokol RJ, "Alcohol" in: Evans MI, Dixler AO, Fletcher JC, Schulman JD, eds, **Fetal Diagnosis and Therapy: Science, Ethics and the Law**. Philadelphia: Lippincott 1989, 140-149; Elias and Annas, **Reproductive Genetics**, 208-210; Mulvihill JJ, "Fetal alcohol syndrome" in: Sever JL, Brent RL, eds, **Teratogen Update: Environmentally Induced Birth Defect Risks**. New York: Liss 1986, 13-18.

[36]See: Elias and Annas, **Reproductive Genetics**, 210-212; Werler MM, Pober BR, Holmes LB, "Smoking and pregnancy" in: Sever JL, Brent RL, eds, **Teratogen Update: Environmentally Induced Birth Defect Risks**. New York: Liss 1986, 131-139.

[37]See: Sullivan FM, Smith SE, McElhatton PR, "Interpretation of animal experiments as illustrated by studies on caffeine" in: Nau H, Scott Jr WJ, eds, **Pharmacokinetics in Teratogenesis: Interspecies Comparison and Maternal/Embryonic-Fetal Drug Transfer**. Boca Raton, FL: CRC 1987, 123-127.

[38]See: Moore, **Developing Human**, 149.

[39]See: Moore, **Developing Human**, 149.

[40]See: Johnson, **Human Developmental Anatomy**, 380; Tabor BL, Soffici AR, Smith-Wallace T, Yonekura ML, "The effect of maternal cocaine use on the fetus: change in antepartum fetal heart rate tracings" *AJObGyn* 165 (1991) 1278-1281.

[41]See: Elias and Annas, **Reproductive Genetics**, 204; Sadler, **Medical Embryology**, 115-117.

[42]See: Cohlan SQ, "Tetracycline staining of teeth" in: Sever JL, Brent RL, eds, **Teratogen Update: Environmentally Induced Birth Defect Risks**. New York: Liss 1986, 51-52.

[43]In reports of possible teratogenicity, benefits outweigh risks. See: Rosa FW, "Penicillamine" in: Sever JL, Brent RL, eds, **Teratogen Update: Environmentally Induced Birth Defect Risks**. New York: Liss 1986, 71-75.

[44]See: Warkany J, "Warfarin embryopathy" in: Sever JL, Brent RL, eds, **Teratogen Update: Environmentally Induced Birth Defect Risks**. New York: Liss 1986, 23-27.

[45]See: Goldman AS, Zackai EH, Yaffe SJ, "Fetal trimethadione syndrome" in: Sever JL, Brent RL, eds, **Teratogen Update: Environmentally Induced Birth Defect Risks**. New York: Liss 1986, 35-38; Hanson JW, "Fetal hydantoin effects" in: Sever JL, Brent RL, eds, **Teratogen Update: Environmentally Induced Birth**

[46]See: Warkany J, "Aminopterin and methotrexate: Folic acid deficiency" in: Sever JL, Brent RL, eds, **Teratogen Update: Environmentally Induced Birth Defect Risks**. New York: Liss 1986, 39-43.

[47]See: Rosa FW, Wilk AL, Kelsey FO, "Vitamin A congeners" in: Sever JL, Brent RL, eds, **Teratogen Update: Environmentally Induced Birth Defect Risks**. New York: Liss 1986, 61-70.

[48]See: Newman CGH, "Clinical aspects of thalidomide embryopathy: a continuing preoccupation" in: Sever JL, Brent RL, eds, **Teratogen Update: Environmentally Induced Birth Defect Risks**. New York: Liss 1986, 1-12.

[49]See: Elias and Annas, **Reproductive Genetics**, 213-214; Silbergeld EK, Mattison DR, Bertin JE, "Occupational exposures and female reproduction" in: Evans MI, Dixler AO, Fletcher JC, Schulman JD, eds, **Fetal Diagnosis and Therapy: Science, Ethics and the Law**. Philadelphia: Lippincott 1989, 149-171.

[50]See: Weiss B, Doherty RA, "Methylmercury poisoning" in: Sever JL, Brent RL, eds, **Teratogen Update: Environmentally Induced Birth Defect Risks**. New York: Liss 1986, 119-121.

[51]See: Rogan WJ, "PCBs and cola colored babies: Japan, 1968, and Taiwan, 1979" in: Sever JL, Brent RL, eds, **Teratogen Update: Environmentally Induced Birth Defect Risks**. New York: Liss 1986, 127-130.

[52]See: Elias and Annas, **Reproductive Genetics**, 214-216; Sadler, **Medical Embryology**, 112-113.

[53]"The recommended limit of maternal exposure of the whole body to radiation from all sources is 500 millirads for the entire gestational period." Moore, **Developing Human**, 153. See also: Brent RL, "Radiation teratogenesis" in: Sever JL, Brent RL, eds, **Teratogen Update: Environmentally Induced Birth Defect Risks**. New York: Liss 1986, 145-163.

[54]See: Mills JL, "Malformations in infants of diabetic mothers" in: Sever JL, Brent RL, eds, **Teratogen Update: Environmentally Induced Birth Defect Risks**. New York: Liss 1986, 165-176; Briddle and Fraser, *Experimental teratology*, 19-21;

[55]See: Sadler, **Medical Embryology**, 110-112.

[56]See: Korones SB, "Congenital rubella: An encapsulated review" in: Sever JL, Brent RL, eds, **Teratogen Update: Environmentally Induced Birth Defect Risks**. New York: Liss 1986, 77-80; South MA, Sever JL, "The congenital rubella syndrome" in: Sever JL, Brent RL, eds, **Teratogen Update: Environmentally Induced Birth Defect Risks**. New York: Liss 1986, 81-91.

[57]See: Lynch L, Daffos F, Emanuel D, Giovangrandi Y, Meisel R, Forestier F, Cathomas G, Berkowitz RL, "Prenatal diagnosis of fetal cytomegalovirus infection" *AJObGyn* 165 (1991) 714-718; Reynolds DW, Stagno S, Alford CA, "Congenital cytomegalovirus infection" in: Sever JL, Brent RL, eds, **Teratogen Update: Environmentally Induced Birth Defect Risks**. New York: Liss 1986, 93-95.

[58]Balducci J, Rodis JF, Rosengren S, Vintzileos AM, Spivey G, Vosseller C, "Pregnancy outcome following first-trimester varicella infection" *ObGyn* 79 (1992) 5-6; Fuccillo DA, "Congenital varicella" in: Sever JL, Brent RL, eds, **Teratogen Update: Environmentally Induced Birth Defect Risks**. New York: Liss 1986, 101-105.

[59]See: Foulon W, Naessens A, Mahler T, De Waele M, De Catte L, De Meuter F, "Prenatal diagnosis of congenital toxoplasmosis" *ObGyn* 76 (1990) 769-772; Larsen Jr JW, "Congenital toxoplasmosis" in: Sever JL, Brent RL, eds, **Teratogen Update: Environmentally Induced Birth Defect Risks**. New York: Liss 1986, 97-100.

[60]See: Grossman III JH, "Congenital syphilis" in: Sever JL, Brent RL, eds, **Teratogen Update: Environmentally Induced Birth Defect Risks**. New York: Liss 1986, 113-117.

[61]See: Moore, **Developing Human**, 153; Romero *et al*, **Congenital Anomalies**, 411-414.

[62]See: Johnson, **Human Developmental Anatomy**, 79-357; Moore, **Developing Human**, by chapters; Romero *et al*, **Congenital Anomalies**, 1-431; Sadler, **Medical Embryology**, 133-366.

[63]See: Moore, **Developing Human**, 142.
[64]See: Romero *et al*, **Congenital Anomalies**, 209-232.
[65]All week estimates given in this section of congenital malformation of human organ systems are from fertilization. To estimate weeks of gestation, add 2 weeks.
[66]See: Romero *et al*, **Congenital Anomalies**, 81-123.
[67]See: Romero *et al*, **Congenital Anomalies**, 113-123.
[68]See: Romero *et al*, **Congenital Anomalies**, 81-112.
[69] See: Romero *et al*, **Congenital Anomalies**, 195-207.
[70]See: Romero *et al*, **Congenital Anomalies**, 233-254.
[71]See: Romero *et al*, **Congenital Anomalies**, 255-299.
[72]See: Romero *et al*, **Congenital Anomalies**, 301-309.
[73]See: Romero *et al*, **Congenital Anomalies**, 125-194.
[74]See: Romero *et al*, **Congenital Anomalies**, 311-384.
[75]See: Warkany J, "Iodine deficiency" in: Sever JL, Brent RL, eds, **Teratogen Update: Environmentally Induced Birth Defect Risks**. New York: Liss 1986, 177-179.
[76]See: Romero *et al*, **Congenital Anomalies**, 411-414.
[77]"Many severe limb malformations occurred from 1957 to 1962 as a result of maternal ingestion of thalidomide. This drug, widely used as a sedative and antinauseant, was withdrawn from the market in December 1961. Since that time, similar limb malformations have rarely been observed." Moore, **Developing Human**, 358.
[78]See: Romero *et al*, **Congenital Anomalies**, 1-79.
[79]Meroanencephaly describes this condition better than anencephaly, since a rudimentary brain stem is present. See: Moore, **Developing Human**, 392.
[80]"In two sisters with agenesis of the corpus callosum, the only symptoms were seizures, recurrent in one but only occasional and minor in the other. Their I.Q.'s were average." Moore, **Developing Human**, 393.
[81]See: Dekker GA, Sibai BM, "Early detection of preeclampsia" *AJObGyn* 165 (1991) 160-172; Lin C-C, "Medical considerations in obstetric management" in:
[82]23-30 weeks after fertilization.

CHAPTER IV

PRENATAL INTERVENTIONS

A. MENDELIAN DISORDERS[1]

Parental and fetal cells may be analyzed to detect genetic disorders transmitted in classical Mendelian ratios. The analysis can be cytogenetic or molecular. The disorders may be autosomal or sex-linked, and may be metabolic, anatomic, or both.

Cytogenetic Analysis (FTS, PUBS)[2]

Some disorders may be detected by sampling specific fetal tissues, such as blood, liver or skin. Hemoglobinopathies include sickle cell anemia, alpha and beta-thalassemia, and hemophilia. Hepatopathies include urea cycle defects, such as ornithine transcarbamulase (OTC) deficiency. Dermatopathies may include epidermolysis bullosa and congenital harlequin ichthyosis.

Molecular Analysis[3]

Fetal DNA anomalies range from absence of DNA to a change in a single nucleotide (point mutation). Two basic methods are used, depending on whether the molecular basis is known or not.

a. Known Molecular Sequence

If the defect involves the absence of DNA and fetal DNA fails to hybridize for the normal sequence, one can conclude that the fetus is affected by a deficiency. This technique detects all alpha-thalassemia, some DMD, and a few beta-thalassemia. If the defect involves a point mutation, codon-specific restriction enzymes or oligonucleotide hybridization is used to pinpoint the site of the disorder, such as in sickle cell anemia.

b. Unknown Molecular Sequence

Restriction fragment length polymorphisms (RFLPs) are innumerable, ostensibly innocuous DNA sequence differences found in all individuals of the same species. These RFLP markers are inherited as co-dominant alleles. If a fetus codes for the same RFLP marker as its heterozygous parents, he or she may well have inherited the defect. Limitations arise when the distance from mutant gene to marker is not known. Due to a higher chance of recombination, this distance is inversely proportional to its reliability. Also, if all members of a family show the same RFLP pattern, normal and affected members are not distinguishable. This type of linkage analysis can detect beta-thalassemia, DMD, hemophilia A and B, Huntington's chorea, PKU-related cystic fibrosis, and polycystic kidney disease, and is becoming more useful as the human genome is mapped further.

B. PRENATAL DIAGNOSIS (PND)[4]

Various PND techniques are currently used in obtaining samples for cytogenetic and molecular analysis and other information. These may be invasive or noninvasive to the fetus and its environ. Invasive are: amniocentesis, chorionic villi sampling, fetal skin sampling, percutaneous umbilical blood sampling, and pre-implantation diagnosis. Noninvasive are: maternal and paternal DNA analysis, maternal serum alpha-fetoprotein assays, analysis of fetal cells in maternal blood, ultrasound, and magnetic resonance imaging.

1. Invasive Techniques[5]

Amniocentesis

Amniocentesis is a technique by which amniotic fluid is obtained. The fluid and living fetal cells floating within are analyzed for fetal chromosomal and DNA status, and enzyme levels.

About 20-30 cc of amniotic fluid is aspirated through a 20 to 22 gauge spinal needle inserted transabdominally. Ultrasound is concurrently used to indicate fetal location, biparietal diameter, placental position, amniotic fluid location, fetal cardiac movement, and number of fetuses present. Some authors also recommend injecting about 300 microg of Rh-immune globulin into the amniotic sac to prevent possible Rh sensitization.[6] Since it requires about 200 ml of fluid within the amniotic sac, it is typically done between 13-15 weeks after conception.[7] As noted above, by 15 weeks (second trimester) the fetus already contains all the major organs and systems he or she will have for the rest of its life, the mother may be visibly pregnant, and she may have also already felt fetal movements ("quickening"). Associated risk of spontaneous abortion following amniocentesis is about 0.5%, which is compatible with that of high risk mothers (age 35 and older). Minor fluid leakage is reported in 1-2% of cases, usually self-limited and clinically inconsequential.

Chorionic Villi Sampling (CVS)[8]

In CVS 10-25 mg of fetal chorionic villi are aspirated transcervically or transabdominally for biopsy. In transcervical CVS a fetoscope or flexible biopsy forceps is used, guided by ultrasound. Associated risk of spontaneous abortion is somewhat higher than that in amniocentesis, depending on the time of gestation when it is done. Cervical pathologies (herpes, gonorrhea) and Rh sensitization contraindicate. Transabdominal CVS may be done with an 18 gauge spinal needle guided with ultrasound. It is safe with cervical pathologies, and the risk of abortion is slightly less than that of amniocentesis. An advantage of CVS is that it can be done between 7-9 weeks after conception[9] (first trimester), allowing an earlier diagnosis and possible treatment of the fetus. Amniocentesis, in addition to providing living fetal cells, also provides amniotic fluid and fetal metabolic byproducts, such as alpha-fetoprotein, which is associated with neural tube defects. An advantage of both is that fetal cells are obtained for rapid karyotype (within 24-28 hrs), due to the presence of trophoblasts in various stages of mitosis.

However, neither amniocentesis nor CVS are 100% infallible. Some problems associated with both techniques may be:

-no fetal cell growth in vitro due to an insufficient amount of cells extracted, or damaged cells

-contamination with maternal cells, which have a different karyotype and can thus give false information

-defects in chorionic villi cells, which not always means an abnormal fetus, since the fetus comes from a different cell layer

-chromosomal abnormalities which may arise in vitro due to spontaneous mutations or other unforeseen factors

-it has also been observed that some phenotypes do not arise in spite of apparent defective genotype

Also, an abnormal chromosome number does not necessarily mean a fatal condition, such as in the case of extra sex chromosomes. Indeed 47,XXY and 47,XYY males, and 47,XXX females may show some physiological and anatomical variants, but none are usually either grossly malformed or severely mentally retarded.

Fetal Tissue Sampling (FTS)

FTS involves the removal of a small sample of fetal skin, usually from the dorsal surface, using biopsy forceps through a 14 gauge sleeve guided by ultrasound. It is used for detecting specific fetal dermatologic pathologies. A liver biopsy can also be done to check for albumin synthesis from 14 weeks gestation. A 2-3% associated risk of spontaneous abortion has been reported.

Percutaneous Umbilical Blood Sampling (PUBS)

In PUBS a 25 to 23 gauge spinal needle is inserted into the umbilical cord vein guided by ultrasound. Originally used for treating acute erythroblastosis *in utero*, it can now be used also for obtaining fetal serum and cells. These cells can provide karyotype in 48-72 hours (short-term lymphocyte cultures).

Alpha-Fetoprotein (AFP)

AFP is the most abundant protein in fetal plasma during early embryogenesis, reaching its peak between 12-14 weeks gestation, before it is replaced by albumin. As the fetal liver begins producing albumin, AFP diffuses into fetal urine and is excreted into the amniotic fluid. Some AFP traverses the amnion into the maternal bloodstream. A high level of AFP is related to neural tube defects (NTD), such as spina bifida and meroanencephaly. But it is also associated with other congenital diseases[10], complicating its use for NTD diagnosis. Yet, since acetylcholinesterase (ACHE) has also been found in amniotic fluid of fetuses with NTDs, assaying for ACHE together with AFP allows accurate diagnosis.

Pre-Implantation Diagnosis[11]

Preimplantation diagnosis is any technique by which cells are biopsied either from an early conceptus (first stages of cleavage) or from a blastocyst (which may contain about 100 cells). If the cells are carefully removed, the remaining blastocyst continues to develop normally. These cells are then analyzed for defects by looking either at enzymes in the cytoplasm, or at the genes. One possible way to obtain a viable conceptus is by pre-implantation uterine lavage. Alternatively, pre-implantation cells may also be procured through *in vitro* fertilization, or from the first polar body (attached to the oocyte, within the zona pellucida). Genetic defects may be checked by DNA amplification through polymerase chain reaction. The goal is to obtain genotyping for single gene, or anatomic and metabolic disorders.

2. Noninvasive Techniques[12]

Maternal Serum Alpha-Fetoprotein Assay (MSAFP-A)

AFP diffusing into maternal circulation constitutes maternal serum alpha-fetoprotein (MSAFP), which increases gradually during pregnancy, beginning at about week 13, peaking at week 30, and then declining. High MSAFP has been associated with NTDs. Conversely, low MSAFP is associated with aneuploidy (trisomy 21).[13] Factors affecting the level of MSAFP are: time of gestation, maternal weight, race,[14] diabetes, and multiple pregnancies. Therefore, corrections are made for all these in order to arrive at an accurate multiple of median (MOM) measure. The standard cut-off point for further testing is 2.5 MOM.[15] Optimal time for MSAFP assay is 15-18 weeks gestation.

When the genetic history of a couple indicates the possibility of a NTD or trisomy, the level of AFP may be determined by amniocentesis. However, since the vast majority of NTDs occur without any previous history,[16] MSAFP assay provides a non-invasive method of screening for NTDs.

Analysis of Fetal Cells in Maternal Blood[17]

Fetal lymphocytes and other cells may be found occasionally in the bloodstream of pregnant women. The DNA, RNA and enzymes of these cells could be analyzed for detecting genetic defects and other anatomic and metabolic abnormalities.

Ultrasound[18]

a. Transabdominal[19]

Ultrasound is a method of visualizing the placenta, embryonic membranes, and the embryo or fetus. It may be used in: determining fetal and cranial size for estimating gestational age; determining the position of the placenta; guiding needles and forceps used in invasive methods (amniocentesis, CVS, PUBS); detecting congenital abnormalities; observing heart and fetal movement; identifying multiple pregnancies, conjoined twins and fetal death. It is also used as a preliminary visualization which may lead to further testing and analysis. Ultrasound for diagnosis of congenital malformations may be used in detecting: the absence of normally present structures (renal agenesis, oligohydramnios, allobar holoprosencephaly, cleft lip and palate, anencephaly): the presence of additional structures distorting normal contour (teratomas, cystic hygromas, hydrops fetalis); dilatation behind an obstruction (unilateral and bilateral ureteral dilatation, hydrocephalus, duodenal atresia); herniations through structural defects (diaphragmatic hernia, meningomyelocele, cephalocele, meningocele, omphalocele); abnormal fetal biometry (microcephaly, skeletal dysplasias, orbital hypotelorism and hypertelorism, polycystic kidneys); and absent or abnormal fetal motion (clubfoot, cardiac anomalies).

b. Transvaginal[20]

Transvaginal ultrasound offers specific diagnostic advantages due to the proximity of the transducer to the observed organs. It permits high resolution visualization of the female pelvis, and can confirm successful implantation, thus helping to estimate gestational age and ruling out an ectopic pregnancy. During the second week from fertilization, it can detect the gestational sac; during the third week, the yolk sac and fetal pole; during the fourth week, a pulsating heart; during the fifth week, precise CR length; during the sixth week, embryonic membranes and embryonic movement; during the seventh week, distinct embryonic parts (head, trunk, and limbs) and the placenta (CVS); from 9-11 weeks, different brain, face and lip parts and sizes; from week 10, bone development in appendages, thoracic measurements, fetal eye lens, movements and size, and unilateral or bilateral defects; from week 11, umbilical veins, abdomen, stomach, intestines, kidneys, bladder and gender. Comparing normal and abnormal developmental nomograms can help in early diagnosis of defects.

On the average, ultrasound diagnosis can be done 1-3 weeks earlier by transvaginal method as contrasted to transabdominal. However, transvaginal diagnosis is less accurate during the second and third trimesters due to the increasing distance between transducer and "target" organ as the fetus grows. The transvaginal transducer can also be fitted with a needle guide to aid in follicle retrieval, amniocentesis, and CVS without penetrating the abdomen or bladder, and without anesthesia.

Magnetic Resonance Imaging (MRI)[21]

Fast-scan magnetic resonance imaging is now being used to visualize the fetus. This techniques allows for a higher resolution and less distortion than ultrasound.

C. FETAL THERAPY[22]

One of the uses of prenatal diagnosis is its growing potential for pregnancy management and fetal therapy. Fetal therapy may be attempted either through medication or through surgery.

Medical Therapy[23]

Human embryos and fetuses can now be treated for some anomaly by administering medication to the mother. These include: glucocorticoids to arrest preterm labor, propylthiouracil to prevent IUGR, and medication to prevent fetal tachycardia. Also, some metabolic diseases have been treated, such as: methylmalonic acidemia (vitamin B deficiency) and thrombocytopenia treated with vitamin B supplements; multiple carboxylase deficiency treated with biotin; congenital adrenal hyperplasia treated with dexamethasone, which suppresses fetal adrenal activity.

Fetal Surgery[24]

Fetal surgery is first decided by detecting some congenital abnormality *in utero* (level I ultrasonography), leading to a careful evaluation of prognosis (level II ultrasonography). Examples of fetal surgery are: PUBS transfusion to avert erythroblastosis fetalis; affixing a ventriculoamniotic shunt to relieve hydrocephaly (aqueductal stenosis); clearing fetal urinary tract obstructions to relieve oligohydramnios and hydronephrotic kidneys. Fetal surgery might also help prevent diaphragmatic hernias, spina bifida, and gastroschisis.

Gene Therapy[25]

Gene therapy consists in treating a genetic disease by seeking to replace or correct defective mutant gene(s). If the therapy involves somatic cells, the correction (or potential damage) remains within the treated individual organism. However, if the therapy is done on germ cells, the correction (or potential damage) will likely be passed to future generations.

Somatic cell gene therapy is presently being attempted in bone marrow to correct immune deficiencies and other metabolic disorders (bone marrow stem cell transplantation). Possible modes of transfer may be: viral vectors; chemical intake of DNA; fusion of DNA-loaded membrane vesicles (red blood cell ghosts); physical microinjection or electroporation.

Notes

[1]See: Elias and Annas, **Reproductive Genetics**, 89-90; Simpson, *Transmitting genetic*

disorders, 94-101; Simpson and Elias, **Prenatal Diagnosis**, 94-98.

[2]See: Rebello TM, Gray CTH, Rooney DR, Smith JH, Hackett GA, Loeffler FE, Horwell DH, Beard RW, Coleman DV, "Cytogenetic studies of amniotic fluid taken before the 15th week of pregnancy for earlier prenatal diagnosis: a report of 114 consecutive cases" *PrenatDiag* 11 (1991) 35-40.

[3]See: Elias and Annas, **Reproductive Genetics**, 90-106; Petit P, Moerman P, Fryns JP, "The fetal phenotype of partial trisomy of the long arm of chromosome 4 (4q22-4qter)" *GenCounsel* 2 (1991) 163-165.

[4]See: Nora and Fraser, **Medical Genetics**, 251-260; Simpson and Elias, **Prenatal Diagnosis**, 78-107; Seeds JW, Cefalo RC, "Prenatal diagnosis: clinical considerations" in: Malherbe J-F, ed, **Human Life: Its Beginnings and Development**. Paris: L'Harmattan 1988, 117-124; Serra A *et al*, "La diagnosi prenatale di malattie genetiche. Esperienze, prospettive, problemi" *ProgrMed* 37 (1981) 1-18; Serra A, "La diagnosi prenatale di malattie genetiche" *MedMor* 4 (1984) 433-448.

[5]See: Evans MI, Belsky RL, Greb A, Clementino N, Syner FN, "Alpha-fetoprotein: maternal serum and amniotic fluid analysis" in: Evans MI, Dixler AO, Fletcher JC, Schulman JD, eds, **Fetal Diagnosis and Therapy: Science, Ethics and the Law**. Philadelphia: Lippincott 1989, 46-54; Evans MI, Quigg MH, Koppitch III FC, Schulman JD, "First trimester prenatal diagnosis" in: Evans MI, Dixler AO, Fletcher JC, Schulman JD, eds, **Fetal Diagnosis and Therapy: Science, Ethics and the Law**. Philadelphia: Lippincott 1989, 17-36; Larsen Jr JW, MacMillin MD, "Second and third trimester prenatal diagnosis" in: Evans MI, Dixler AO, Fletcher JC, Schulman JD, eds, **Fetal Diagnosis and Therapy: Science, Ethics and the Law**. Philadelphia: Lippincott 1989, 36-43; Smidt-Jensen S, Philip J, "Comparison of transabdominal and transcervical CVS and amniocentesis: sampling success and risk" *PrenatDiag* 11 (1991) 529-537.

[6]Maternal Rh immunization is not universally accepted. See: Beeson JH, "Controversies surrounding antepartum Rh immune globulin prophylaxis" in: Evans MI, Dixler AO, Fletcher JC, Schulman JD, eds, **Fetal Diagnosis and Therapy: Science, Ethics and the Law**. Philadelphia: Lippincott 1989, 172-180.

[7]15 to 17 menstrual weeks.

[8]See: Baumann P, Jovanovic V, Gellert G, Rauskolb R, "Risk of miscarriage after transcervical and transabdominal CVS in relation to bacterial colonization of the cervix" *PrenatDiag* 11 (1991) 551-557; Doran TA, "Chorionic villus sampling as the primary diagnostic tool in prenatal diagnosis: should it replace genetic amniocentesis?" *JReprMed* 35,10 (1990) 935-940.

[9]9 to 11 weeks after menstruation.

[10]Congenital skin defects, conjoined twins, duodenal atresia, exstrophy of cloaca, tetralogy of Fallot, fetal teratoma, gastroschisis, hemangioma of umbilical cord, hydrocephalus, Meckel syndrome, nuchal bleb, esophageal atresia, osteogenesis imperfecta, pilonidal sinus, Rh-isoimmunization, and Turner syndrome. See: Evans *et al, Alpha-fetoprotein*, 47.

[11]See: Handyside AH, "Preimplantation diagnosis by DNA amplification" in: Chapman M, Grudzinskas G, Chard T, eds, **The Embryo. Normal and Abnormal Development and Growth**. London: Springer-Verlag 1991, 81-90; Handyside AH, Lesko JG, Tarín JJ, Winston RML, Hughes MR, "Birth of a normal girl after *in vitro* fertilization and preimplantation diagnostic testing for cystic fibrosis"

[12]See: Crandall BF, Robinson L, Grau P, "Risks associated with an elevated maternal serum alpha-fetoprotein level" *AJObGyn* 165 (1991) 581-586; Evans *et al, Alpha-fetoprotein*, 46-54; D'Amelio R, Giorlandino C, Masala L, Garofalo M, Martinelli M, Anelli G, Zichella L, "Fetal echocardiography using transvaginal and transabdominal probes during the first period of

pregnancy: a comparative study" *PrenatDiag* 11 (1991) 69-75; Evans *et al, First trimester*, 17-36; Haddow JE, Holman MS, Palomaki GE, "Can gestational dates routinely derived from very early ultrasound be used to interpret maternal serum alpha-fetoprotein measurements?" *PrenatDiag* 12 (1992) 65-68.

[13]See: Evans *et al, Alpha-fetoprotein*, 50.

[14]Blacks in the United States tend to show as much as 20% higher MSAFP values than whites, justifying the need for correction of values according to race. See: Evans *et al, Prenatal Diagnosis*, 49-50.

[15]See: Evans *et al, Alpha-fetoprotein*, 48.

[16] "...about 97% of all affected fetuses [with neural tube defects] come from pregnancies not previously suspected to be at risk." Evans *et al, Alpha-fetoprotein*, 47.

[17]See: Yeoh SC, Sargent IL, Redman CWG, Wordsworth BP, Thein SL, "Detection of fetal cells in maternal blood" *PrenatDiag* 11 (1991) 117-123.

[18]See: Benacerraf BR, Gelman R, Frigoletto, Jr. FD, "Sonographic identification of second-trimester fetuses with Down's syndrome" *NEJM* 317,22 (1987) 1371-1376.

[19]See: Chervenak FA, Isaacson G, "Ultrasound detection of fetal anomalies" in: Evans MI, Dixler AO, Fletcher JC, Schulman JD, eds, **Fetal Diagnosis and Therapy: Science, Ethics and the Law**. Philadelphia: Lippincott 1989, 60-71; Johnson, **Human Developmental Anatomy**, 361-362; Simpson and Elias, **Prenatal Diagnosis**, 78-107.

[20]See: Bronshtein M, Mashiah N, Blumenfeld I, Blumenfeld Z, "Pseudoprognathism: An auxiliary ultrasonographic sign for transvaginal ultrasonographic diagnosis of cleft lip and palate in the early second trimester" *AJObGyn* 165 (1991) 1314-1316; Dolkart LA, Reimers FT, "Transvaginal fetal echocardiography in early pregnancy: normative data" *AJObGyn* 165 (1991) 688-691; Drugan A, Timor-Tritsch IE, "Transvaginal ultrasonography" in: Evans MI, Dixler AO, Fletcher JC, Schulman JD, eds, **Fetal Diagnosis and Therapy: Science, Ethics and the Law**. Philadelphia: Lippincott 1989, 71-83; Timor-Tritsch IE, Monteagudo A, Warren WB, "Transvaginal ultrasonographic definition of the central nervous system in the first and early second trimesters" *AJObGyn* 164 (1991) 497-503.

[21]See: Fedele L, Dorta M, Brioschi D, Giudici MN, Candiani GB, "Magnetic resonance imaging in Mayer-Rokitansky-Küster-Hauser syndrome" *ObGyn* 76 (1990) 593-596; Garden AS, Griffiths RD, Weindling AM, Martin PA, "Fast-scan magnetic resonance imaging in fetal visualization" *AJObGyn* 164 (1991) 1190-1196; Herzog TJ, Angel OH, Darram MM, Evertson LR, "Use of magnetic resonance imaging in the diagnosis of cortical blindness in pregnancy" *ObGyn* 76 (1990) 980-982.

[22]See: Copel JA, Kleinman CS, "Diagnosis and management of fetal heart disease" in: Evans MI, Dixler AO, Fletcher JC, Schulman JD, eds, **Fetal Diagnosis and Therapy: Science, Ethics and the Law**. Philadelphia: Lippincott 1989, 412-421; Elias and Annas, **Reproductive Genetics**, 243-271; Evans and Schulman, *Fetal therapy*, 403-412; Hogge WA, Golbus MS, "Surgical management of fetal malformations" in: Evans MI, Dixler AO, Fletcher JC, Schulman JD, eds, **Fetal Diagnosis and Therapy: Science, Ethics and the Law**. Philadelphia: Lippincott 1989, 395-403.

[23]See: Copel and Kleinman, *Fetal heart disease*, 412-421; Elias and Annas, **Reproductive Genetics**, 262-267; Evans and Schulman, *Fetal therapy*, 403-412; Kaaja R, Julkunen H, Ämmälä P, Teppo A-M, Kurki P, "Congenital heart block: successful prophylactic treatment with intravenous gamma globulin and corticosteroid therapy" *AJObGyn* 165 (1991) 1333-1334; Kofinas AD, Simon NV, Sagel H, Lyttle E, Smith N, King K, "Treatment of fetal supraventricular tachycardia with flecainide acetate after digoxin failure" *AJObGyn* 165 (1991) 630-631; Watson WJ, Katz VL, "Steroid therapy for hydrops associated with antibody-mediated congenital heart

block" *AJObGyn* 165 (1991) 553-554.

[24]See: Elias and Annas, **Reproductive Genetics**, 243-250; Hogge and Golbus, *Surgical management*, 395-403.

[25]See: Anderson WF, "Gene therapy" in: Evans MI, Dixler AO, Fletcher JC, Schulman JD, eds, **Fetal Diagnosis and Therapy: Science, Ethics and the Law**. Philadelphia: Lippincott 1989, 421-430; Elias and Annas, **Reproductive Genetics**, 267-269.

PART TWO

TEN NORTH AMERICAN CATHOLIC MORAL THEOLOGIANS

CHAPTER V

BENEDICT M. ASHLEY, OP, and KEVIN D. O'ROURKE, OP

A. A THEOLOGICAL VERSUS A HUMANISTIC VALUE SYSTEM

Ashley's basic value system is set forth most clearly in his book,[1] where he seeks to explicate his unified Christian theory of the human body, as contrasted with a dualistic Humanistic theory (influenced by Platonic idealism).

He begins by acknowledging existence as a human body living in a world of living and non-living bodies. Seeking to ethically evaluate this bodily existence, he recognizes the dilemma of interpretation, a dilemma which may be considered to be only philosophical--by those who believe that we create ourselves--, but which he considers to be theological--since we are creative creatures.[2] He explores the Christian notion of an expanding horizon where we seek to creatively "enter into" one another's worlds. As an example of this Christian convergence of horizons, he cites the ecumenical movement: a convergence between the Holy Spirit and the human body. Yet, due to the vastness of the ecumenical dialogue, he limits himself to the dialogue between two contrasting theological horizons: Humanist and Christian.[3]

He holds that our bodily existence is susceptible to either a Humanist or a Christian interpretation. The former he considers dualistic and based upon the Cartesian distinction of mind/body, which reduces contemporary humanist philosophy to language analysis and leads to subjectivism.[4] But he also believes that the Christian theology of the body was originally influenced by Platonic idealistic dualism,[5] with its pernicious dualistic theology continuing to influence Christianity today.[6] By contrast, a complimentary, holistic theology of the body-soul developed, beginning with biblical times, continuing through the Eastern and Western Christian Fathers, and into the European Middle Ages.[7] Aristotelianism provided an alternative reading of reality to Platonism, a reading that influenced Medieval, Renaissance and Reformation Christian theologies.[8] Thus, he argues that today "... a Christian anthropology must retain the Platonic defense of human spirituality and interior life, but it ought also to support Aristotle's criticism of Platonic dualism and accept the Aristotelian concept of the soul as the vital principle of the body and the body as the necessary instrument of the soul in thinking and willing."[9]

He, then, seeks to ground his anthropology in Scripture, which speaks of the creation of the human person in the image of God, culminating in the manifestation of that image in the person of Jesus Christ, as witnessed by the Christian community.[10] Thus, his anthropology is one of basic human needs, which are fulfilled in Christ, since He is the fulfillment of humanity.[11] He deduces six universal needs as basic to all human life: food, security, sexual expression, information, society and creativity.[12] Following an analysis of these six needs, within a radical process theology of the body, he proposes that human ethics is the ethics of co-creative stewardship.[13] Morality, then, is what makes it possible for us to meet our basic human needs.[14]

He applies this basic value system to issues of family life in an article that touches upon prenatal life and conflict situations.[15] In it he states that the new reproductive technologies call us to question whether we wish to follow a Christian or a Humanist value system. He contends that while the common belief is that the United States is fundamentally a Christian society, it is really Humanist. While there is considerable overlap between both systems, a Humanist system tends to put us in absolute control of nature. This control is done through technology, which would portend that in regard to the family, society has the power to define what it is or should be.[16]

In contrast, a Christian value system holds that the entire dynamism of family life is guided according to the plan of God. Hence, Ashley sustains that nature follows God's design, and that human action on nature should be according to the intrinsic values of that plan: "The Christian is guided by norms consistent with reproduction's natural processes and the family's natural biological and psychological bonds."[17] He implies that the new reproduction technologies are a distortion of the natural way in which human persons beget children, that they view children as a commodity which can be obtained at a certain (technological) price, and that they fail to respect the natural family bonds and values established by God, the creator of nature.[18]

Similarly, O'Rourke's basic value system speaks of the notion of "sanctity of life," which he expounds in an article on prenatal life and conflict situations.[19] He begins by stating that Christians may convey strong emotions against abortion, but these must nonetheless be backed-up by solid theological reasons. He does so by succinctly stating that whereas direct abortion is in violation of natural law and divine positive law, indirect abortion may be allowed to protect a good such as another human life.[20] He also notes the two medical cases which presently qualify as indirect abortion.[21]

Then, he briefly recounts how the Church, from its beginnings, has consistently upheld the intrinsic value of innocent human life, a value which cannot be compromised to lesser values. The reason behind this teaching is the Church's belief that human life has been uniquely created by God in an act of love, an act which establishes a personal relationship between God and each human being, which is called "sanctity of life." Hence, this sanctity of human life does not depend on any merit or worth won, or bestowed on by others and is not dependent on the "quality of life."[22] He does not deny that there are other compelling reasons for opposing abortion, but restates that the basic Catholic reason is the unique relationship between God and each individual.[23]

O'Rourke further delineates his basic value system when he grounds this opposition to abortion on a common natural law which is reasonably accessible to all peoples. He points at the grave obligation to provide realistic alternatives to abortion, *i.e.* financial, social, and spiritual help, and to uphold the sanctity of human life in other instances, such as war, capital punishment, imprisonment, and social reform.[24]

O'Rourke's basic Christian value system of moral absolutes is also elucidated is his article on experimentation on prenatal life.[25] While seeking to avoid the ethical issues involved in research on the earliest stages of development, he states that the term "pre-embryo" is inadequate because from fertilization onward one is already dealing with human, not pre-human, life.[26] He also asserts that, ethically speaking, the difference between therapeutic and nontherapeutic embryo research is a most important distinction.[27]

Noting the different evaluations of human embryo research by government commissions of various nations with capacity for such research, he affirms that these are not due to discrepancies over the nature of the human embryo, but rather over whether damage to the embryo may be permitted for the sake of advancing human knowledge (balance of rights).[28] He opposes such a utilitarian method, since the value of human life is not granted by society.[29] In the final analysis, a utilitarian method dehumanizes because it sacrifices certain inalienable rights of the individual for social or State benefit.[30]

These basic values have led Ashley and O'Rourke to develop a position of prudential personalism,[31] which they contrast with proportionalism.[32] It is appropriate, then, at this point to examine their philosophical and anthropological presuppositions in regard to this personalistic vision.

B. THE ACTUALIZATION OF FUNCTIONAL POTENTIALITIES

Ashley and O'Rourke's anthropological and philosophical views on human life are discernible in their works on health-care ethics.[33] Here they define the human person as one who has the "need and capacity for intelligent freedom."[34] Personhood encompasses all of human life, from conception, and not just those moments when we are consciously self-aware.[35]

This leads to a developmental theory of the human person, who is in constant actualization,[36] occurring within a given community.[37] They acknowledge that some distinguish between human being and human person, but they reject such distinction as morally irrelevant when it comes to treating a human patient, who is by definition a person.[38] This includes the unborn, since he or she has the potential to actualize its humanity by functional potentialities, especially of self-development. This presupposes the presence of minimal structures, which modern embryology acknowledges in the zygote if human development is understood in an epigenetic, and not in a preformist, way.[39] By contrast, human personhood cannot be attributed to either the unfertilized egg or the sperm (both haploid), for neither possesses the genetic information necessary for self-development into a human being (diploid).[40]

Ashley continues to expose his anthropological presuppositions in his book on his theology of the human body, where he maintains that while we belong to a single biological species, we are culturally diverse. We are communicators, and we are self-aware.[41] He seeks a holistic view of the human person,[42] acknowledging that our bodies serve our brains, and that our bodily selves belong and interact with the rest of the bodily universe which is composed of matter and energy in kinetic interaction.[43] He, then, defines human persons as "creative, communicating, socially intelligent animals, motivated by unconscious and conscious emotions and purposes, capable of achieving scientific knowledge through which we can control our own behavior, our environment and our own evolution."[44]

In his world-picture, influenced by Teilhard, he delineates a radical process interpretation of science and of humanity.[45] Yet he seeks to avoid two reductionisms of process philosophies: "all is matter" and "all is energy,"[46] while admitting a certain duality in physical reality.[47] He states that: "The natural unit [of such a world-picture] most empirically evident to a scientist is himself or herself, not as a mind, but as a thinking body presupposed to every act of observation or experimentation."[48] He understands the primary matter of this primary natural unit to be pure potentiality (consistent with the principle "nothing causes itself"), hence, radically open to process by being acted upon. The best example, he says, is the embryo, whose development is caused by induction and by energy from without.[49] Thus, because natural processes are directional, they are teleological.[50]

He argues that, contrary to critics, this interpretation of radical process is consistent with Aristotelian philosophy, which views the human person as becoming,[51] and which interprets "matter as the capacity to undergo process and of energy as the dynamic actualization of primary units of matter interacting with each other to produce new units out of the old..."[52] As bodily beings, we are subject to natural process, which makes us historical beings, "...exercising our creative freedom within history and helping to shape it."[53] Regarding the relationship between the human body and nature, he states that: "The human person is an animal, but transcends the animal by intelligence and freedom. Consequently 'life according to reason' is not determined by nature or natural instincts, but by our intelligent understanding of our own nature, including our own bodies, which permits us to control our own actions freely and creatively."[54] He sees natural law in terms of basic human needs,[55] which are transcultural. Thus, he answers yes to his original question "can we create ourselves?", but not merely by the use of science and technology, as Humanists and Marxists believe, rather by participating in God's own creative activity.[56]

The fact that we are created in the image of God does not detract from the fact that we are the product of natural selection, an evolution which has brought us to the possibility of harmonious coexistence with our present surrounding environment.[57] This capacity to coexist with the environment and indeed, to control it to a certain extent, is largely due to our capacity to process information in a thoughtful way, a way unique to humans. Because information begins to be processed at fertilization, he believes that a human being is such from the moment of conception.[58]

Further insights into Ashley's anthropological and philosophical presuppositions can be gained where he touches on other topics related to the human body, such as defending the natural, biological basis of the human family as species-specific,[59] and reconstructing the human person.[60] Regarding artificial reproduction, he concurs with *Donum vitae* in condemning these techniques, not because they are artificial, but because they give rise to abnormal children on several counts: by depriving the child of a personal identity and human relationships that develop in normal human families, and by severing normal flesh and blood linkage vital for the child's sense of security, which in turn is needed for his or her psychological and religious development. Nonetheless, such abnormality does not detract from the child's full humanity as image of God.[61]

O'Rourke's anthropological and philosophical presuppositions are also observed in a co-authored work on medical ethics.[62] In it he distinguishes between informed consent and proxy consent, noting two conditions needed for the latter: "(1) the patient or research subject cannot offer informed consent; and (2) the person offering the consent must determine what the incompetent person would have decided were he or she able to make the ethical decision."[63] Applied to neonatal life, he states:

> Hence, parents of a neonate with serious birth anomalies may not say, 'Let the baby die; he will be a burden to us.' Rather, they must make a decision in accord with the good of the child, weighing especially the fact that in most cases we judge life to be a gift worth preserving, even if living may involve working with handicaps or infirmities.[64]

He also points out that the distinction between "ordinary" and "extraordinary" means something different to the medical doctor than to the ethicist. For the physician, ordinary applies to standard procedures, whereas extraordinary applies to experimental ones.[65] For the ethicist, the patient's condition must also be known to distinguish between the two, since a person has a general obligation to prolong human life, given certain limits[66]: "Ethically speaking, then, ordinary means of preserving life are the medicines, treatments, and operations that offer a reasonable hope of benefit for the patient or that can be obtained or used without excessive expense, pain, or burden."[67]

Addressing the "quality of life"/"sanctity of life" controversy, he now holds that these are opposites only in oversimplified arguments, for a patient's quality of life is indeed relevant to his sanctity, but what is more important is that medical decisions be based on reason and justice.[68]

Regarding human genetic reconstruction, he disapproves "radical transformations," but approves more normal ones, as long as they improve basic human function. He maintains that: "Transformation would be forbidden, however, (a) if human intelligence and creativity are endangered and (b) if the fundamental functions that constitute human integrity are suppressed."[69]

Finally, he acknowledges the beginning of human life presently to be a philosophical question: "The following query sums up this aspect of the issue [in vitro fertilization]: Is the zygote human life with potential or potential human life?"[70]

Ashley and O'Rourke, also, address the issue of anencephalics, admitting a dilemma: if the brain is so damaged that one can legitimately doubt the existence of the primary organ necessary for such brain development, then one may logically doubt whether a human person is present any longer.[71] However, they caution prudence here, since the exact loci of intellectual activity and potentiality have not yet been clearly identified. In other words, anencephalics may be considered nonpersons if they lack the potentiality for free, intelligent activity from the beginning of their development, but since this is at present impossible to determine, they should receive the benefit of the doubt in favor of personhood.[72]

C. EPIGENETIC VERSUS PREFORMIST HOMINIZATION

Ashley and O'Rourke's theory of immediate hominization comes forth in several of their medical ethics works.[73] They argue that if contemporary embryological evidence is applied to Aquinas' classical theory of delayed hominization, this theory is now obsolete.[74] They note that Aquinas, who based his hylomorphic system on Aristotle's epigenetic theory, could only posit a human soul on matter which is capable of being informed by such a soul, which can only occur when the "primary organ" is present.[75] Hence, they distinguish between epigenetic and preformist development.[76]

Ashley maintains that both Aristotle and Aquinas opted for delayed hominization because of insufficient biological knowledge.[77] It is now known that the mother normally contributes, not just uninformed matter, but fully half of the genetic information (oocyte haploid nucleus, its primary organ) of the new entity (zygote). Semen too, is not just passive matter to be mixed with the mother's passive matter and externally activated by spirit, but active material normally containing the other half of genetic information (sperm haploid nucleus). The efficient cause, then, of the new entity (zygote) may well be the sperm. The "primary organ" of the new (diploid) zygote is its own nucleus.[78]

Regarding the objection of no individuality before implantation because there is as yet no differentiation, he counters that from fertilization there already exists in the zygote a metabolic polarity and bilaterality (fundamental to the development of the embryo and subsequent stages) such that at the first cell division some cytoplasmic differentiation occurs within the resulting daughter cells. At the morula stage, though the cells may be individually totipotential if separated, as a whole they relate collectively so as to constitute heterogeneous parts, with regulatory cells probably at the superior pole. Epigenetic polar and bilateral continuity is maintained at the blastocyst stage (when implantation occurs) as the cluster of cells at the morula's superior pole form the posterior lip of the blastopore, the new "primary organizer."[79] Thus, by updating Thomistic epigenetic philosophy according to contemporary embryology, it is plausible to trace a primary organ epigenetically from completed fertilization to implantation.[80]

Against those who complain about high pregnancy wastage, they counter that, first, not all these spontaneous abortions are in fact completed or normal fertilizations, and thus possibly not ensouled. Second, infant mortality has at times also been as high as 50%, yet no one would question that those children were indeed human beings.[81]

Hence, Ashley's economic epigenetic hominization theory would hold the zygote to be a new human being, with its nucleus the primary organ and with differentiation occurring from first cleavage, blastomeres retaining certain totipotentiality before implantation such that, if separated, "they become a new substance with its own form, by a process analogous to asexual reproduction, budding or cloning."[82] God may now ensoul the new twin, just as with the first twin at completed fertilization. Both twins are children of the same male parent, since he provided the instrumental cause (sperm) to initiate their development (the one directly; the other mediately). Conversely, if individual identity happens only after twinning is impossible, then: 1) if the morula or blastula is undifferentiated, what causes it to differentiate according to well-established plans? 2) if twin embryos receive individuality only after twinning, whence this individuality? It fails to account for the twinning process itself, a process of (further) individuation.[83]

Regarding recombination, he maintains a similar interpretation: "The individuality of the embryo depends on its primary organ. If cells are separated form the morula and then rejoined to it, they become a part of the living substance when they fall under the directive influence of the primary organ, as does a transplant into an adult body."[84]

Thus, the proposed sequence of "governing parts" ("primary organs" elsewhere) is: nucleus for the zygote; active pole for the blastula; neural streak for the embryo; brain for the fetus, all in continuity.[85] But this center of organization of information (nucleus, primitive streak, brain) does not work in isolation, rather in interaction with the environment, at every stage of development. Accordingly, the human fetus has minimal necessary interaction with its mother.[86]

D. THE INTENTIONALITY OF THE MORAL ACT

For Ashley and O'Rourke, the intentionality of the act is basically what determines its morality.[87] An example may be seen in their discussion of abortion.[88] They first distinguish between spontaneous and procured, and then within procured, between direct[89] and indirect.[90] One may never intend the direct killing of an innocent person.

If the humanity of the embryo is doubtful *vis-à-vis* the certain humanity of the mother, can one use probabilism to justify abortion? They sustain not because once it is certain that the woman is pregnant, there is no longer any doubt about the existence of the fetus, with an equal right to life as the mother.[91] In sum, after weighing arguments for and against abortion, they conclude that the principle of proportion grounds the intrinsic and absolute right to life of the unborn as well as of the born.[92]

A similar example is seen in their refusal to allow for abortion after rape by considering the embryo an unjust aggressor, since 1) it is not attacking its mother but following normal development, and 2) even if the embryo was seen as an aggressor, one may not directly intend his or her death.[93]

In another article, O'Rourke reviews several contemporary ethical systems.[94] After rejecting emotivism,[95] legalism,[96] cultural relativism,[97] and fideism,[98] he espouses reasoned analysis.[99] He believes that this latter is the most effective way of achieving consensus in a pluralistic society regarding abortion and other controversial medical issues, "a process of patient and comprehensive examination of the ethical issues through reasoned analysis."[100]

E. PRENATAL DIAGNOSIS AND PROPORTIONAL BENEFITS

Ashley and O'Rourke recognize the definite importance of genetic prenatal diagnosis, such as amniocentesis and chorionic villi sampling, and note four possible applications: 1) for scientific research, 2) to help parents who are carriers make responsible reproductive decisions, 3) to allow for *in utero* or early birth therapy, and 4) to provide parents information resulting in abortion of defective fetuses.[101] The fourth is not morally acceptable, but the first three are, provided that there is benefit to the embryo proportionate to the risks of each technique, that the results are not misunderstood or exaggerated, that informed consent is properly obtained, that screening is not compulsory, that carrier or affected populations (born or unborn) are not stigmatized, and that responsible parenthood is promoted.[102]

They disapprove of compulsory negative eugenics, since: heterozygotes can also transmit defects; most heterozygotes are presently not detectable; even if detectable, they also carry many good traits; and spontaneous mutations are constantly being added to the gene pool.[103] Hence, carriers should be provided with genetic information necessary for responsible reproductive decisions, but not forcibly screened or prevented from procreation.[104] Accordingly, they offer nine recommendations for genetic counseling,[105] based on the guidelines of the Institute of Society, Ethics and the Life Sciences.[106] They add that it is also important to consider the cost of such eugenic programs.[107]

Referring specifically to amniocentesis, they find it presently justifiable only if some proportionate benefit to the fetus results, but not to decide on aborting, and observe a deeper shift involved:

> Thus, since amniocentesis involves risk of spontaneous abortion (although the risk has been reduced with the help of sonography to less than 1 percent), it cannot be used unless there are also proportionate benefits for the fetus. At present, therapeutic help for a genetically deficient fetus is limited, but more progress in this field is noted each year (Hendren and Lillehi, 1988; NIH, 1987). Some ethicists maintain that amniocentesis benefits the fetus because it helps the parents prepare more adequately for the birth (Dube, 1983). In sum, amniocentesis is indicated only when a pregnancy is thought to be at increased risk for a particular disorder (Kahn, 1987). Recently, Roy (1984) has pointed out a more profound ethical issue that may result from prenatal screening: 'Prenatal diagnosis delivers the knowledge required to exercise the kind of quality control over the unborn that amounts to a control over birth...The earlier long-standing belief of a theocratic reproductive culture in the equality of all human beings based on the identity of their origin and destiny has given way to an emphasis on the empirical inequalities of human beings (p.16).'[108]

However, they do uphold the responsibility of Catholic hospitals to provide for that genetic counseling which is oriented toward saving prenatal life, since otherwise couples are only left with the option of consulting those who might advocate abortion.[109]

F. PARENTAL AND MEDICAL RESPONSIBILITIES

Noting a definite shift in American society from traditional Christian values where all human life was considered sacred in and of itself, toward a secular humanism where human life can be subject to pragmatic manipulation, Ashley and O'Rourke's understanding of medicine regarding prenatal diagnosis seeks to focus on the duties of parents and the medical profession in protecting prenatal life.

Hence, regarding those who maintain that a defective child can be aborted because every child has a right to be born free of defects, they point to a contradiction in such argument: "It certainly is a right for a child to be free of every defect which medicine has the power to prevent or correct. It is paradoxical, however, to believe that this right is protected by destroying the child who has not been saved from defect."[110] Therefore, they reject the Humanist dictum; "it is better never to be than to be a defective," and state that if parents have begotten a child with defects, they have the responsibility to care for him or her, but not to destroy the child, and counselors have the duty to help prospective parents make responsible procreative decisions, which might include not to procreate.[111] Yet, they also note that every conception carries unknown risks. Thus, to pretend for parents to beget only perfect children is as reprehensible as to encourage them to reproduce fatalistically.[112] They state:

> Some argue that if serious reasons exist to believe a fetus is gravely defective, the parents should be persuaded to agree to abort the child if this suspicion is confirmed by amniocentesis. Otherwise, they argue, it is difficult to justify the risks of the amniocentesis procedure. If abortion is ethically unacceptable, the counselor should not recommend prenatal screening that is potentially dangerous to the infant unless this is justified by the possibility of intrauterine therapy proportionate to the risks or of some benefit to the infant because the parents will be better prepared to care for the child. A recent survey of fetal surgery expresses that the main value of antenatal diagnosis lies in prompt postnatal treatment of major malformations before complications develop (Hendren and Lillehi, 1988).[113] The desire to satisfy the parents' curiosity concerning the sex of the child does not seem to be a sufficient reason for subjecting the infant to even minimal risk of harm.[114]

They go on to indicate that the main role of genetic counselors is to help parents interpret genetic information and to support them in their ethical decisions. And, while recognizing the right of every individual not to submit to genetic diagnosis, they also encourage adults who suspect a birth defect in their own lives to undergo evaluation so as to plan their lives accordingly.[115] Recognizing that persons with birth defects do have a right to procreate,[116] they also mention society's obligation to educate regarding genetic hazards in order to promote voluntary negative eugenics.[117]

In addition, O'Rourke also touches on four relevant issues associated with genetic screening[118]: confidentiality, autonomy, beneficence and justice.[119] Confidentiality enhances the physician-patient relationship by protecting information exchanged therein, but sometimes it may be necessary to break it to protect others.[120] Regarding autonomy, he maintains that since the norm for genetic screening is voluntary, an individual's informed choice whether to undergo testing should be respected, "except in those programs where beneficial treatment is available."[121] Beneficence is the principle which seeks to provide benefit rather than harm to a patient. As such, if little or nothing can be done for an individual at risk, testing should not be obligatory, since some persons may want to know about their condition, while others may not. Voluntary programs would provide for both.[122] By justice, he means an equitable distribution of risks and benefits in a screening program.[123] This includes developing care protocols and support systems beyond testing, making sure the people understand the information received, and assuring access to applicable services. He also states: "Genetic information that is given with an assumption of moral failure or blame, especially for couples who decide to have children, is unacceptable."[124]

In a brief article, O'Rourke also touches on the moral responsibilities of parents regarding medical treatment of their children.[125] The case involves a couple who withheld their seven year-old ill daughter from ordinary, beneficial medical treatment because of religious beliefs. He says that the family unit must be protected because it is the basis of society, and that parents are primarily responsible for the care of their children.[126] However, if parents abuse their children, society has a right to intervene, which illustrates another ethical assumption, "namely, that parents do not 'own' their children. Rather, parents are stewards, caretakers, of their children, enablers who help their children grow in knowledge and virtue. Above all, life and death decisions concerning children are not to be made for the benefit of the parents."[127]

Granted that the discussion at hand is with born children, he also raises the future possibility of society seeking to ensure that pregnant women respect their unborn children, especially as more is learned about the effects of alcohol, tobacco and drugs on fetal development.[128] He likewise asks the question, but does not answer, of more "invasive" intervention upon a negligent mother.[129] He concludes by upholding the right and duty of parents to be the primary caretakers of their children, stating that: "Only when the family patently neglects its responsibilities should society intervene."[130]

G. TWO DISTINCT TELEOLOGIES

From the aforesaid it can be deduced that Ashley and O'Rourke seek to validate magisterial teaching in their analysis of contemporary medicine when applied to moral dilemmas in prenatal diagnosis.

This can be further observed in Ashley's article on exceptionless norms.[131] He attributes today's polarization of Catholic medical ethics to two divergent views of human nature: objectivist and subjectivist. While each one has something to contribute, he prefers objectivism because subjectivism tends to be dualistic due to an exaggerated emphasis on historical change and process.[132] Yet one must incorporate three valid subjective insights: 1) facts are relative to the observer; 2) the observer is always situated within a particular place, time and culture; 3) the observer must also be sensitive to historical development, including the Biblical tradition.[133]

For him, one's understanding of the human person remains central when assessing medical technology. Subjective ethics emphasizes the person's historicity, relativizing human values according to cultural and personal influences.[134] This leads to a proportionalistic dualism wherein "the moral meaning of an act arises not from the act's objective structure but from the subject's creative purposes within the cultural and historical world. With the subjective view, we can never distinguish the intrinsic, objective morality of an act from the meaning a particular value system gives it; this is cultural relativism."[135] He concludes by stating his belief that the Church's moral teaching, while incorporating the present subjective insights of the importance of the person, culture and history, will continue to be fundamentally objective.[136]

Likewise, O'Rourke follows magisterial lines in his analysis of medical research on human subjects.[137] He contrasts two ethical systems: one following the Church's teaching, whereas the other following a secular, autonomous, utilitarian approach. While these two systems share some common principles,[138] they disagree regarding the philosophical and anthropological foundations for these principles, which leads to different applications when in comes to prenatal life.[139] He points to some specific differences, as in the evaluation of potential risk and benefit of a particular procedure, noting that the Church's evaluation is based on the principle of double effect (whereby intentions need moral justification), while the other system follows a utilitarian approach (whereby actions are justified simply if they result in more overall good than harm). Underlying these differences are two distinct teleologies: "When both the Church and the [utilitarian] study groups[140] require informed consent to protect the 'dignity of the person,' for example, the Church bases its view of human dignity on the belief that man and woman are made in the image and likeness of God, whereas the study groups' documents usually base their view on the principle of autonomy."[141] While autonomy is not contrary to Church teaching, it does not stress the patient's natural need of community, nor his or her ultimate goal of eternal life.[142]

He submits that the application of these principles to prenatal life leads the Church to oppose nontherapeutic research on human embryos. The study groups, on the other hand, are divided on the issue. Again, the basis for these differences are found in distinct philosophical and anthropological interpretations of human actions. For the Church, actions are not necessarily good simply because they result in good effects, rather certain actions are intrinsically good or evil in themselves, according to objective evidence.[143] As an example of exceptionless ethical norm he cites: "Do not kill innocent human beings."[144] By contrast, the study groups follow a utilitarian approach where they merely seek to balance overall risks and benefits.[145] He concludes by pointing out the growing disparity of these two ethical systems, and wonders whether, in view of certain past events involving research on human beings, a utilitarian approach sufficiently protects the human person as subject of medical research.[146]

Always along these lines, Ashley wrote an article where he criticizes McCormick's most recent book,[147] especially McCormick's criticism of *Dv*, in the second part of the book: *Practical and Pastoral Questions*. The main criticism is again based on maintaining the natural bond between children and their parents, which Ashley claims is weakened by using *in vitro* fertilization.[148] Once more, he states his belief in the purposefulness of human nature, and technology's subservience to it,[149] and criticizes McCormick's theory of delayed hominization as contrary to current biological evidence.[150] He then asks why McCormick seems to question the position of *Dv* (and other magisterial documents), which McCormick himself admits to being based on a long tradition, while his own position seems to be so tenuous? Ashley speculates that this is because, deep down, McCormick, like many of the "revisionists," has been unable to make the proper transition from an older legalist system (whose purpose was to soften the rigors of the law) to a presently more pastoral one.[151] Lastly, he criticizes the first section of the book, on *Fundamental Moral Theology*, concluding that McCormick, while admitting to limits on dissent from magisterial teaching, fails to establish any real, tangible demarkation of such limits.[152] The ultimate consequence of such a position is a further weakening of the family.[153]

Notes

[1]Ashley BM, **Theologies of the Body: Humanist and Christian**. Braintree, MA: Pope John XXIII Medical-Moral Research and Education Center 1985.

[2]Ashley, **Theologies**, 3-11.

[3]Whereas the voice **Humanistic** would better describe what Ashley seeks to convey, this text uses **Humanist** in fidelity to Ashley's terminology. See: Ashley, **Theologies**, 11-15.

[4]Ashley, **Theologies**, 51-89.

[5]"Plato and his followers expressed their deep conviction that the true human self is the spiritual soul and that the soul's earthly existence in the body is a kind of death or exile or imprisonment." Ashley, **Theologies**, 103.

[6]Ashley, **Theologies**, 104.

[7]"...recognizing that the human body is not simply the prison of the soul." Ashley, **Theologies**, 135.

[8]Ashley, **Theologies**, 148-187.

[9]Ashley, **Theologies**, 238. Two other contributions of Humanism to Christian anthropology are: a positive evaluation of the material world to which we belong, and a positive evaluation of that technological control of nature which advances the Reign of God. Ashley, **Theologies**, 238-239.

[10]In another article, Ashley contends that, contrary to popular belief, the Bible can provide moral guidance to contemporary dilemmas regarding the human body, especially those raised by the new reproductive technologies and genetic engineering. A proper Scriptural anthropology leads us to a vision of the human person as the image of God, co-creator with God, and entrusted with stewardship over the rest of creation. This covenant relationship between God and humanity is confirmed in the person of Jesus Christ. Ashley BM, "Constructing and reconstructing the human body" *Thom* 51,3 (1987) 501-520.

[11]"The goal of human life which is the first principle of any teleological ethics must include the satisfaction in an integral manner of these basic needs as the primary condition of a good human life and indeed of any Christian life, since 'grace perfects nature.' If Jesus is the existential embodiment of his own ethics and therefore its goal and first principle, these basic needs and their right fulfillment must be manifest in Him." Ashley, **Theologies**, 374-397; here 396.

[12]Ashley, **Theologies**, 396.

[13]Ashley, **Theologies**, 415-467.

[14]Ashley, **Theologies**, 458.

[15]Ashley BM, "A child's rights to his own parents: a look at two value systems" *HospProgr* 61,8 (1980) 47-49.

[16]"For humanists the child is a product of human power which can be modified to meet changing consumer demands. The child's rights are not inherent in the child's nature; society confers these rights in terms of its own evolving priorities." Ashley, *A child's rights*, 47-48; here 48.

[17]Ashley, *A child's rights*, 49.

[18]Ashley, *A child's rights*, 48-49.

[19]O'Rourke KD, "'Because the Lord loved you': theological reasons for the sanctity of life" *HospProgr* 54,8 (1973) 73-77.

[20]He follows Grisez' distinctions, whereby a direct abortion "is any procedure by which the normal course of the development of the child before birth is purposely interfered with; the procedure has the intention of preventing the continuation of normal development and subsequent normal birth." (Grisez G, **Abortion: The Myths, The Realities and The Arguments** New York: Corpus 1970, 7.) By contrast, an indirect abortion "is an act nonabortive in its purpose and which only incidentally causes the death of the fetus." (Grisez, **Abortion**, 183.) O'Rourke, *Because*, 73-74.

[21]Ectopic pregnancy and cancerous (pregnant) uterus. O'Rourke, *Because*, 74.

[22]Applying this reasoning to people who are carriers of birth defects, he notes that since human life is a mystery, no one is in a position to judge which life is "useless" and which is not, and that whereas human suffering is not a good in itself, it is part of God's providence and therefore has a grace-potential. O'Rourke, *Because*, 74-75.

[23]O'Rourke, *Because*, 76.

[24]O'Rourke, *Because*, 76.

[25]O'Rourke KD, "Developments in biotechnology: ethical perspectives" *LinacreQ* 56,4 (1989) 11-17.

[26]O'Rourke, *Biotechnology*, 12-13.

[27]"Therapeutic research is designed to provide a curative or diagnostic benefit for the subject of research. Non-therapeutic research does not provide a benefit to the subject, but rather is designed to provide new knowledge which may benefit some other subject in the future." O'Rourke, *Biotechnology*, 13.

[28]O'Rourke, *Biotechnology*, 12-15.

[29]"Opposed to this method of ethical evaluation is an outlook which considers the human being worthy of respect, and protection, even if acquiring new knowledge must be delayed or sacrificed. In this system of ethical evaluation, some goods or rights are considered so significant that they cannot be balanced with other rights nor be sacrificed for other goods. These rights are not granted by the human community but are considered to be from nature and prior to consideration by the human community." O'Rourke, *Biotechnology*, 15.

[30]O'Rourke, *Biotechnology*, 16.

[31]Personalism defines the human person as "embodied intelligent freedom," thus seeking to maintain the essential body-mind unity of the classical teleology of incarnate beings. Ashley BM, O'Rourke KD, **Health Care Ethics: A Theological Analysis**. St. Louis, MO: The Catholic Hospital Association 1978, 5.

[32]They hold that proportionalists rigidly distinguish between the premoral (or ontic) and the moral act, accusing classical moral theology of "physicalism" or "biologism." Proportionalism, however, is dualistic in that the physical act is dismissed as having only ontic value, and herein its central problem; how is one to evaluate ontic value? Ashley and O'Rourke, **Health Care Ethics** (1982), 171.

[33]Ashley BM, O'Rourke KD, **Health Care Ethics: A Theological Analysis**. St. Louis, MO: The Catholic Hospital Association 1978; 1982; 1989. See also; Ashley BM, O'Rourke KD, **Ethics of Health Care**. St. Louis, MO: Catholic Health Association 1986, 18.

[34]Ashley and O'Rourke, **Healthcare Ethics** (1989), 4.

[35]"Does this mean that a human person exists only when that person is actually functioning in self-awareness and freedom? This conception would be altogether too static. The human person is

not a pure intelligence, but a bodily being, sharing with the natural world, emerging through evolution out of that world, yet never being separated from it. Consequently, our human self-awareness and freedom emerge only at high points of a very complex process, much of which is subconscious and part of the determination of nature. When a unique human organism comes into existence at conception, his or her uniqueness is already genetically determined by a novel combination and fusion of different traits never previously combined. At this moment a unique human body comes into being and is continuously identifiable." Ashley and O'Rourke, **Health Care Ethics** (1978), 11.

[36]"...human personhood is never completely actualized in this earthly life, but is always in the process of growth..." Ashley and O'Rourke, **Health Care Ethics** (1978), 15.

[37]"Community, in its turn, exists to assist each of its member-persons in this process of growth. Thus, as soon as a person comes into bodily existence as a unique human organism, it enters into this actualizing process and has a right to help from the human community to complete this process. In other words, to *be* a person is to be in the process of actualizing personhood (Eller, 1975). The community, therefore, does not confer on or impute personhood to the sleeping, unself-conscious infant or fetus but responds to its silent demand to live and grow." Ashley and O'Rourke, **Health Care Ethics** (1978), 15.

[38]"Such a view [distinguishing between human being and human person] is very difficult to reconcile with any scientific account of the unity of human nature and does violence to ordinary language. According to such usage, to be a human person is not to be here and now functioning as an intelligent, free, moral agent but to have that innate power to develop such capacities and to exercise them more or less effectively under favorable and appropriate conditions. We are actually persons, in the sense of having human rights, even when we are not actually, but only potentially, moral agents." Ashley and O'Rourke, **Health Care Ethics** (1982), 5.

[39]Ashley and O'Rourke, **Health Care Ethics** (1978), 221-226. For an explanation of their epigenetic theory, see the next section on: Epigenetic versus Preformist Hominization.

[40]Ashley and O'Rourke, **Health Care Ethics** (1978), 226.

[41]Ashley, **Theologies**, 20-22.

[42]"Thus, we humans as individuals achieve maturity and sociability only by developing the total self, conscious ego and wider unconscious self, in a suitable family and societal environment where we can achieve harmony between personal autonomy and inter-personal communications." Ashley, **Theologies**, 22.

[43]Ashley, **Theologies**, 20-40.

[44]Ashley, **Theologies**, 40.

[45]"To summarize: the world-picture revealed by modern science is most plausibly interpreted as that of a somewhat loosely organized universe whose history from the Big-Bang to its entropic death we can broadly trace. In the midst of this vast but finite time and space our little earth occupies a remarkable negentropic counter-eddy in which we can track the evolution of life as an intelligible but not predictable history. This history exhibits the operation at every point of a few fundamental natural forces working with a beautiful, but not invariable, regularity, which have finally produced the enormously complex little organism we call a human being through a remarkable sequence of historical events, each of which might have taken a very different course in any other, even slightly, different environment subject to any other interferences than those which have actually occurred through various chance encounters within the solar system and from beyond." Ashley, **Theologies**, 259.

[46]Ashley, **Theologies**, 260-264.

[47]"It must be admitted that physical reality always exhibits a certain duality; not the dualism of Descartes' mind and matter, but the polarity of matter and energy." Ashley, **Theologies**, 263.

---

[48]Ashley, **Theologies**, 277.

[49]Ashley, **Theologies**, 285.

[50]"To summarize: natural changes or processes can be adequately understood only if we attempt to determine empirically in each case (1) the subject in which this process takes place (primary matter if the change is a radical production of new primary units, some existing unit if the change is superficial); (2) the agent which produces the change, which sometimes proximately is internal to the unit, one part acting on the other, but which ultimately is always some other unit than the unit undergoing the process; (3) the new organization which the process tends to produce in the subject, in the case of radical change the new unity which constitutes the new unit, in the case of superficial change any modification of the existing subject unit; (4) if the change is a process, in the strict sense, the teleology of the process, *i.e.*, the final product whether this be a new unit, or some *constructive* modification of the existing unit." Ashley, **Theologies**, 287.

[51]"Often Aristotle is accused of proposing a philosophy of 'substance' as against a philosophy of 'process', or a philosophy of 'being' as against one of 'becoming,' or a 'static' as against a 'dynamic' philosophy. This is an anachronistic retrojection of the cartesian notion of substance on Aristotle whose notion was essentially different." Ashley, **Theologies**, 289.

[52]Ashley, **Theologies**, 333-334.

[53]Ashley, **Theologies**, 345.

[54]Ashley, **Theologies**, 370.

[55]"Once again this is an appeal to 'natural law', *i.e.*, to basic human needs." Ashley, **Theologies**, 372.

[56]Ashley, **Theologies**, 693.

[57]Ashley, *Constructing*, 505-511.

[58]"This information first guides the single cell to begin a process of division and subdivision. At no time is this clump of cells simply a collection, because it is always a self-constructing organism whose homeostasis and development is guided by the information present first in a dominant cell, and then in a dominant set of cells. Already within the tiny mass called the blastula a metabolic gradient exists differentiating a more passive from a more active pole, the governing part which will finally become the human head." Ashley, *Constructing*, 507. See also next section on hominization.

[59]Ashley, *Constructing*, 510-511.

[60]Ashley has no basic moral argument with accepted procedures (organ transplants and prostheses), provided the necessary principles of totally, benevolence and non-maleficence are observed. Ashley, *Constructing*, 511-512. He does have moral reservations, however, when the reconstruction becomes so radical that the human person actually ceases to be human, such as with some types of genetic or technological reconstructions. Ashley, *Constructing*, 513-516.

[61]Ashley, *Constructing*, 517-519.

[62]O'Rourke KD, Brodeur D, **Medical Ethics: Common Ground for Understanding**. St. Louis, MO: Catholic Health Association of the United States 1986.

[63]Also, it should only be given for the good of the individual patient, not for a class good or for the good of society at large. O'Rourke and Brodeur, **Medical Ethics**, 54.

[64]O'Rourke and Brodeur, **Medical Ethics**, 55.

[65]O'Rourke and Brodeur, **Medical Ethics**, 70.

[66]As limits they list that one is not obliged to do something useless, or "when the means to prolong life would involve a grave burden to the person insofar as striving for the more important values of life are concerned." O'Rourke and Brodeur, **Medical Ethics**, 70, both quotes.

[67]O'Rourke and Brodeur, **Medical Ethics**, 71.

[68]O'Rourke and Brodeur, **Medical Ethics**, 75-76.
[69]O'Rourke and Brodeur, **Medical Ethics**, 105.
[70]O'Rourke and Brodeur, **Medical Ethics**, 139.
[71]"Hence, it would be overscrupulous to attribute personhood and human rights to a defective fetus if we could establish with a high degree of scientific probability that it is so radically defective genetically or in the course of development has suffered so severe a trauma that it lacks the active potentiality to develop the brain structures necessary for at least some minimal activity of human thought and freedom." Ashley and O'Rourke, **Health Care Ethics** (1978), 230.
[72]Ashley and O'Rourke, **Health Care Ethics** (1978), 229-231. This commentary is absent in the third edition. Instead, a small section is added under the new heading of "Other Issues," (within the section on organ transplants), where they maintain that anencephalics are human beings whose therapeutic care may be withheld due to the inability to overcome their pathology, but that their vital organs should not be harvested until total brain death has occurred. Ashley and O'Rourke, **Healthcare Ethics** (1989), 310.
[73]Ashley BM, "A critique of the theory of delayed hominization", in: McCarthy DG, Moraczewski AS, **An Ethical Evaluation of Fetal Experimentation: An Interdisciplinary Study. Appendix** I. St. Louis, MO: Pope John XXIII Medical-Moral Research and Education Center 1976, 113-133. See also: O'Rourke, *Biotechnology*, 11-17; O'Rourke and Brodeur, **Medical Ethics**, 229-230.
[74]Ashley, *A critique*, 113-114.
[75]Regarding this "primary organ," he states that: "(a) the other parts need not be differentiated; (b) the primary organ need be present only in primordial form; (c) it need only be functioning to bring about the embryological development of itself and the whole, while its ultimate highest and specifying functions may still be in abeyance, awaiting the various auxiliary organs necessary for such functioning." Ashley, *A critique*, 114-117; here 117.
[76]"The organism develops *epigenetically* because of this original lack of differentiation. (In the theory of *preformism* the parts would exist in differentiation from the start, but in miniature.)" Ashley, *A critique*, 116.
[77]Both believed that the female's only contribution to the new human was a chemical medium (menstrual blood), which had to be informed by mingling with male semen, a process which took time. Ashley, *A critique*, 117-121.
[78]"It seems plausible enough, therefore, that we retain the Thomistic view that the semen (*i.e.*, the sperm) is the *efficient cause* of the production of the new entity we call the zygote, and that it does this by virtue of an instrumental power received from the male parent. The empirical sign of its character as efficient cause is that the ovum remains in a resting state until the entry of the sperm initiates the fertilization process. That its power is instrumental seems consistent with the fact that the sperm is produced by the male parent as a functional instrument of self-reproduction, that it is an imperfect organism, haploid, and living only briefly, unable to nourish or reproduce itself. It also is evident that the sperm is able to perform its function in virtue of its own primary organ (its nucleus), which can thus be regarded as the seat of the instrumental power." Ashley, *A critique*, 121-123; here 122.
[79]Ashley, *A critique*, 123-124.
[80]Ashley, *A critique*, 124-125.
[81]Ashley, *A critique*, 126. See also; Ashley and O'Rourke, **Healthcare Ethics** (1989), 211-213.
[82]Ashley, *A critique*, 127.
[83]He criticizes the theory of delayed hominization because it fails to explain the presence of

embryologically confirmed primary organs prior to the development of the brain. Thus, what makes a human such is not the presence of the structure necessary for the potential of free and intelligent activity (the brain), but the actual potentiality to develop such structure; the nucleus of the zygote has such active potentiality. Ashley, *A critique*, 126-127. See also: Ashley and O'Rourke, **Health Care Ethics** (1978), 228-229. The third edition also contains a reference to the Australian Research Commission which, though not explicitly granting the fertilized egg personal status, does seem to acknowledge that a fertilized egg is a human subject: "No Marker event advance carried such weight that different principles should apply to distinguish the fertilized ovum from that which all would agree is a human subject." Australian Research Commission, *Human Embryo Experimentation in Australia*, Senate Select Committee on Human Experimentation Bill, Australian Government Printing Office, 1985, 25.

[84]Ashley, *A critique*, 128.

[85]Ashley, *Constructing*, 507-508.

[86]Ashley, *Constructing*, 507-508.

[87]Granted that they hold certain human actions to be intrinsically evil, these actions are such precisely because they believe that it is humanly impossible to execute them without intending to do evil.

[88]"Abortion is the termination of a pregnancy with resulting death of the human fetus." Ashley and O'Rourke, **Healthcare Ethics** (1989), 214.

[89]"A *direct abortion* is one in which the direct, immediate intention of the procedure is to destroy the human fetus at any stage after conception or to expel it when it is not viable." Ashley and O'Rourke, **Healthcare Ethics** (1989), 214.

[90]"An *indirect abortion* is one in which the direct, immediate purpose of the procedure is to treat the mother to ratify threatening pathology, but in which the death of the fetus is an inevitable result that would have been avoided had it been possible." Ashley and O'Rourke, **Healthcare Ethics** (1989), 214-215.

[91]"Furthermore, these rights require particular advocacy precisely because the child is helpless in its own defense." Ashley and O'Rourke, **Health Care Ethics** (1978), 237.

[92]Ashley and O'Rourke, **Healthcare Ethics** (1989), 214-225.

[93]Though they use this example in the case of rape, the same logic would apply to fetuses with defects; they are victims, not aggressors. Ashley and O'Rourke, **Health Care Ethics** (1982), 238.

[94]O'Rourke KD, "Various ethical systems" *Par* 11,2 (1986) 12-13.

[95]"An ethical theory that relies mainly on subjective, emotional response. According to this theory, something is right or wrong because 'I feel it is right or wrong.'" O'Rourke, *Ethical systems*, 12.

[96]"An ethical system which maintains that the law determines what is ethical. In health care, this method is often used with a view toward avoiding malpractice litigation." O'Rourke, *Ethical systems*, 12.

[97]"An ethical method which decrees that actions are ethical if they correspond to the customs of a society or a segment of society." O'Rourke, *Ethical systems*, 12.

[98]"A method of ethical decision making based upon the religious faith of an individual or a church." O'Rourke, *Ethical systems*, 13.

[99]"A method of judging ethical issues by reasoning about the effect of the action itself upon the important values of life, and the consequences of the action upon persons involved. This system seeks to discern whether or not the action and its consequences contribute to human fulfillment and happiness." O'Rourke, *Ethical systems*, 13.

[100]O'Rourke, *Ethical systems*, 13.

[101]Ashley and O'Rourke, **Healthcare Ethics** (1989), 320.

[102]Ashley and O'Rourke, **Healthcare Ethics** (1989), 320-325. They also note that the right of married couples to engender children is conditioned by their ability to care for them. See also: Ashley and O'Rourke, **Healthcare Ethics** (1989), 320-327.

[103]Ashley and O'Rourke, **Healthcare Ethics** (1989), 321-322.

[104]Ashley and O'Rourke, **Healthcare Ethics** (1989), 322-325.

[105](1) The program should be tested beforehand by a pilot program, and then constantly evaluated; (2) there should be community participation in planning and executing such program; (3) clearly stated policies should regulate the information obtained, and privacy should be safeguarded; (4) programs should be on a voluntary basis; (5) information about the screening program should be accessible to all, especially to those groups most susceptible; (6) programs should only be instituted if the tests can provide relatively unambiguous information; (7) principles regarding experimentation with human subjects should be observed; (8) those who undergo screening should be informed beforehand, regarding the nature, cost, risks, and availability of therapy; and (9) concomitant counseling should be provided. Ashley and O'Rourke, **Healthcare Ethics** (1989), 322-323.

[106]Research Group on Ethical, Social, and Legal Issues in Genetic Counseling and Genetic Engineering, "Ethical and social issues in screening for genetic diseases" *NEJM* 286 (1972) 1129-1132.

[107]Ashley and O'Rourke, **Healthcare Ethics** (1989), 323.

[108]Ashley and O'Rourke, **Healthcare Ethics** (1989), 321; Roy D, "Created equal: the moral challenge of prenatal diagnosis," *CanCathHCRev* (Summer 1984), 13-18; here 16.

[109]They also note that counselors are now bound by law to advise parents about prenatal diagnosis if they suspect the child to carry some defect. Ashley and O'Rourke, **Healthcare Ethics** (1982), 316-321.

[110]Ashley and O'Rourke, **Healthcare Ethics** (1989), 325.

[111]"Prospective parents, therefore, have to consider these factors: (1) their own need to have children as the completion of their mutual love, (2) their own capacity to care for these children, and (3) the risk that each particular child may suffer from grave handicaps requiring special care, including the possibility that this child will be faced in turn with the question as to whether he or she should pass on defective genes to the next generation." Ashley and O'Rourke, **Healthcare Ethics** (1989), 325-326.

[112]Ashley and O'Rourke, **Healthcare Ethics** (1989), 325-327.

[113]These authors cite a number of possible fetal surgeries today (shunts), but conclude that: "Despite the growing interest in the treatment of the fetus *in utero*, we believe that the main value of antenatal diagnosis lies in prompt postnatal treatment of major malformations [esophageal atresia, diaphragmatic hernia, extracorporeal membrane oxygenation, pectus excavatum, gastroesophageal reflux, Hirschsprung's disease, ulcerative colitis and familial polyposis, imperforate anus, biliary atresia, choledochal cyst, parenteral alimentation, childhood cancer (neuroblastoma, Wilms' tumor, rhabdomyosarcoma, lymphoma), trauma] before complications develop." Hendren H, Lillehi C, "Pediatric surgery" *NEJM* 319,2 (1988) 89-96, here 94.

[114]Ashley and O'Rourke, **Healthcare Ethics** (1989), 324.

[115]Ashley and O'Rourke, **Healthcare Ethics** (1989), 323-326.

[116]Since: "(1) The balance of factors cannot be reduced to objective certitude, especially because weighing of personal needs and capacities is involved. (2) The value of personal responsibility in the use of sex and living of family life greatly outweigh the damage done society by the increased

genetic load, which cannot be significantly lightened in the short run and about which insufficient information exists to lighten significantly in the long run. (3) If the parents prove mistaken in their decision, society can and should assume the responsibility for adequate care of the children, a burden that is not great compared to many other health problems." Ashley and O'Rourke, **Healthcare Ethics** (1989), 327. However, they also hold that the parents' right to reproduce is not an absolute right. Ashley and O'Rourke, **Health Care Ethics** (1982), 322.

[117]Ashley and O'Rourke, **Healthcare Ethics** (1989), 327.

[118]O'Rourke KD, Brodeur D, **Medical Ethics: Common Ground for Understanding**, Volume II. St. Louis, MO: Catholic Health Association of the United States 1989.

[119]O'Rourke and Brodeur, **Medical Ethics II**, 79-86.

[120]O'Rourke and Brodeur, **Medical Ethics II**, 80-82.

[121]O'Rourke and Brodeur, **Medical Ethics II**, 83.

[122]O'Rourke and Brodeur, **Medical Ethics II**, 83-84.

[123]O'Rourke and Brodeur, **Medical Ethics II**, 84.

[124]O'Rourke and Brodeur, **Medical Ethics II**, 84-85.

[125]O'Rourke KD, "Parents and children: medical decision-making" *Par* 14,1 (1989) 14-15.

[126]O'Rourke, *Parents and children*, 14.

[127]O'Rourke, *Parents and children*, 14.

[128]O'Rourke, *Parents and children*, 15.

[129]"Whether or not society has the right to protect a fetus through surgery not desired by a pregnant woman, (surgery being considered usually as an 'invasive' action) will be the subject of an acrid discussion in a few years if present trends continue." O'Rourke, *Parents and children*, 15.

[130]O'Rourke, *Parents and children*, 15. See also: O'Rourke KD, "An ethical evaluation of federal norms for fetal experimentation" *LinacreQ* 43 (1976) 17-24.

[131]Ashley BM, "Ethical decisions: why 'exceptionless norms'?" *HealthProgr* 66,3 (1985) 50-53, 66.

[132]Ashley, *Ethical decisions*, 50-53.

[133]Ashley, *Ethical decisions*, 53.

[134]He also holds that in subjectivist ethics such human values are known intuitively, not empirically. Ashley, *Ethical decisions*, 53.

[135]Ashley, *Ethical decisions*, 66.

[136]"Nevertheless, Catholic medical ethics will retain firmly its grounding in absolute, concrete, exceptionless moral norms that are transcultural and transhistorical." Ashley, *Ethical decisions*, 66.

[137]O'Rourke KD, "Two ethical approaches to research on human beings" *HealthProgr* 69,8 (1988) 48-51,58.

[138]"- Research on human subjects is a vital part of scientific medicine.
"- Ethical research requires the informed consent of the subject or proxy.
"- Research on human subjects is therapeutic or nontherapeutic.
"- The risk of harm involved in research must be considered in regard to the potential benefit.
"- Research on human beings should be allowed only after appropriate research on animals.
"- Researchers should practice equity in selecting subjects and scientific problems to be studied.
"- The human subject or proxy should be free to withdraw from the research program at any time." O'Rourke, *Two ethical approaches*, 48.

[139]O'Rourke, *Two ethical approaches*, 48-50.

[140]The Australian Study Group; the International Bioethics Summit Conference; the U.S. President's Commission for the Study of Ethical Problems in Medicine and Biomedical and

Behavioral Research; and the Warnok Committee.
[141]O'Rourke, *Two ethical approaches*, 49.
[142]O'Rourke, *Two ethical approaches*, 49-50.
[143]"This objective evidence is derived form studying the human person's nature and purpose, which requires considering the needs, functions, and bodily integrity of the human person." (Principle of Totality) O'Rourke, *Two ethical approaches*, 50.
[144]O'Rourke, *Two ethical approaches*, 50.
[145]"According to this ethical approach, which is common in our society, no actions are good or evil in themselves, no exceptionless norms exist, and an action is good as long as the person performing the action believes 'it results in more good than harm.'" O'Rourke, *Two ethical approaches*, 50-51; here 51.
[146]O'Rourke, *Two ethical approaches*, 51.
[147]Ashley BM, "The chill factor in moral theology: an in-depth review of *The Critical Calling: Reflections on Moral Dilemmas Since Vatican II* by Richard A. McCormick, S.J., (Washington, DC: Georgetown University Press 1989)" *LinacreQ* 57,4 (1990) 67-77.
[148]"McCormick passes over this question in silence." Ashley, *Chill factor*, 71.
[149]"...hence technology can only morally further the divine purposes written in the human person in its bodily nature, not over-ride them." Ashley, *Chill factor*, 72-73.
[150]Ashley, *Chill factor*, 73-74.
[151]Ashley, *Chill factor*, 74.
[152]Ashley, *Chill factor*, 74-76.
[153]"If McCormick's criticisms took adequately into account the real problems which face the magisterium today in maintaining the Church's moral tradition in the face of the serious moral decadence of our society and the influence it is having on sexual morality and family life, they would be convincing. Instead, he seems to have an unbounded confidence that this tradition will be strengthened by severely restricting the Church's disciplinary restraints and trusting peer-pressure within the academy to maintain theological sobriety.

Now, I am sure that Father McCormick, like most of us in the field of bioethics, would hesitate to put full confidence in the medical profession to police itself. Why, then, such confidence in the theological profession? He certainly does not seem to have it in the theologians of the Roman Curia. No doubt the doctrine of checks and balances has application here, and the Magisterium needs some outside criticism. Certainly, it gets a good deal these days, as witness this book. At the same time, when theology grows feverish, a little cool breeze from the Tiber may not only chill but refresh and invigorate." Ashley, *Chill factor*, 77.

CHAPTER VI

CHARLES E. CURRAN

A. DEFENDING THE WEAKEST

One of Curran's recurring basic values is seeking a holistic view of the human person.[1] Accordingly, he holds that mere physical or biological data is not sufficient to define human life,[2] or to analyze the morality of a human act.[3] Rather, he believes that at times there are other basic values commensurate with life which are also worth defending or upholding.

Another of his basic values is considering the dignity of human life to derive, not from any human accomplishment, but from God's gift:

> The prohibitions of murder and direct abortion flow from this basic understanding of the respect for life. In the case of abortion, note that the concept of dignity, sanctity or respect for life based primarily on creation and not on what one does, makes or accomplishes has played a very significant role. Even in the womb the fetus is considered a human being with all the dignity and respect of human life, for such dignity depends primarily on God's gracious gift. The question of abortion seems to illustrate quite well the differences that can emerge when there are differing views of the basis for the dignity of human life. Just because the fetus is not seen, or because it produces nothing or contributes nothing to society does not mean that it has less dignity or value than other human beings.[4]

Along these lines, he holds that Christians are called to defend the weakest in society, such as the human fetus, and are likewise called to accept "less than perfect" persons as fellow members of humanity.[5]

Yet Curran also develops a theory of compromise, given certain conflict situations: "The theory of compromise recognizes the existence of human sinfulness in our world because of which we occasionally might be in a position in which it seems necessary to do certain things which in normal circumstance we would not do."[6]

Further basic values may be detected in another work,[7] where he gives an evaluation of contemporary biomedical technology. Analyzing recent biomedical advances, he contends that a classicist view of natural law sees the individual and the community conforming to rigid laws of nature fixed by God, whereas a historical view envisions humankind in constant change and development.[8] Biomedical technology confirms this dynamic creativity of the human person. These advances in effect give us a new power and control over human and family life. Yet, he is critical of a technology that tends to fascinate and dominate the human person.[9] Thus, contemporary biomedical advances have led some theologians to an anthropological revision of traditional moral theology, which too readily identified the human act's physical and moral aspects. But by this he does not intend to deny our obvious physical reality, for our very existence is a bodily existence. What he seeks is the proper balance in light of our faith.[10] Hence, technology is but one aspect of the human dimension, which means that biomedical technology should always remain at the service of a greater humanization.[11]

Addressing the issue of genetic interventions more directly, he warns against sinful abuse, especially regarding positive eugenics, for, who is to say what makes a better human being? Also, are we simply to destroy the mishaps?[12] Referring even more specifically to the issue of children born with defects, he holds that a Christian attitude of hope must leave us open and vulnerable to accepting "less-than-perfect" persons. Such Christian anthropology translates into a loving compassion for those weakest in our midst. Identifying the human fetus precisely as the weakest among us, he seeks to uphold its dignity, and states: "A utilitarian methodology which is willing to sacrifice one or another individual for the greatest good is opposed to such a Christian understanding."[13]

B. A RELATIONAL MODEL

Curran's philosophical and anthropological presuppositions are already evident in his works discussing the nature of human acts. He argues that the traditional evaluation of human acts, which was heavily influenced by Thomas Aquinas, was based on their physical structure.[14] But, as previously stated, he prefers a more holistic approach.[15] Thus, comparing the classicist view on the nature of reality, with the contemporary view, he contends that the former tends to concentrate on the individual substance and nature of things, whereas the latter tends to emphasize relationships. Regarding the classicist view, he writes: "Notice how such a view of reality affects morality. Human action depends upon the human nature. Human action is its intrinsic unfolding in the person. Nature, therefore, tells what actions are to be done and what actions are to be avoided. To determine the morality of an action, one must study its nature."[16] In contrast, he holds that: "A particular being can never be adequately considered in itself, apart from its relations with other beings and the fullness of being."[17]

Applying his anthropology to prenatal life and conflict situations, he would justify "assisted abortion" in the case of a pregnancy that cannot come to term: "Why should the doctor sit back and wait for nature to take its course when by interfering now he can avoid great harm to the mother?"[18] Hence, he proposes a resolution of such conflict situations similar to the one used in justifying killing an "unjust aggressor,"[19] a relational model which would overcome a mere physicalism: "I am not proposing that the fetus is an unjust aggressor but rather that the ethical model employed in solving problems of unjust aggression avoids some of the problems created by the model of direct and indirect effects when the direct effect is determined by the physical structure of the act itself."[20]

C. HOMINIZATION AT IMPLANTATION

Regarding hominization and personhood, Curran holds that, since individuality is a fundamental characteristic of human beings, and twinning and recombination can occur before implantation, then human life does not begin until after nidation.[21] Accordingly, he states: "In my judgment human life is present from very early in the pregnancy (the fourteenth to twenty-first day), and abortion after that time is justified only for the sake of another life or a value commensurate with life."[22]

Another article revelatory of his position on delayed hominization is the one he wrote on abortion in the first volume of the Encyclopedia of Bioethics.[23] Once more he declares that the core of the matter is the status of prenatal human life. Thus, he begins by noting the terminological distinction which some authors make between: human life and personal life; human being and human person; biological existence and fully human existence. He states that he will use the term "truly human being" or "truly human life" to mean a human person deserving of rights and value.[24] Then, he seeks to define his own holistic view by pointing out that, whereas our human existence is connected with our biological existence, biological data are not enough to solve the issue of when truly human life begins. Rather, such data need to be interpreted philosophically.[25] He then summarizes four different groups of criteria by which to determine when "truly human life" begins: individual-biological, relational, multiple and conferred rights.[26] He further subdivides the individual-biological criterion into five possible moments at which truly human life begins: at birth, at viability, at morphism-brain development, at conception or at implantation. Finding flaws in the first four,[27] he espouses the fifth one, implantation, since this is the earliest possibility for individual human life.[28] He also finds the other three sets of criteria (relational, multiple, and conferred rights) wanting.[29]

D. COMMENSURATE REASON

Curran's analysis of the moral act as applied to prenatal life and conflict situations may be seen best in his evaluation of abortion, where he distinguishes between two fundamental moral questions: "...when does individual human life begin, and how do we solve conflict situations involving the fetus and the mother or other values?"[30] As to the first question, his belief is that human life begins at cellular segmentation, but that one should not base this decision on mere biological or genetic data. However, he returns to biological arguments when rejecting other developmental theories based on the beginning of the brain activity of the fetus as analogous to cessation of brain waves at the end of life.[31] Regarding the second question, he restates the possibility of differing with traditional Catholic theology by interpreting the moral act in a way not exclusively physical. Applied to abortion, he would allow it to save human life or other values commensurate with human life: "This would obviously include grave but real threats to the psychological health of the woman and could also include other values of a socio-economic nature in extreme situations."[32]

Delving more deeply into his moral analysis of abortion, Curran asserts regarding the first question that the precise moment of animation is still debatable.[33] Yet he concedes that the official position of the church is that: "If there is doubt whether or not life is present, the benefit of the doubt must be given to the fact that there is human life present."[34] Regarding the second question, he notes that the church allows indirect abortion for proportionate reasons (typically, an ectopic pregnancy or a cancerous uterus), but he then points at some historical evidence of dissent from authentic, non-infallible teaching, and concludes: "In fact I argue there can be both dissent from and change in the accepted Catholic teaching denying direct abortion."[35] He bases his argument on the position that in complex moral matters (such as animation and conflict situations), one cannot exclude all fear of error, and on the fact that some contemporary Catholic theologians are still debating these issues: "Thus even in the question of the morality of abortion it is impossible to speak about *the* Roman Catholic position as if there cannot exist within Catholicism a legitimate dissent from that teaching."[36]

He discusses the solution of conflict situations, such as when the interests of the fetus vie against the interests of its mother. He contends that traditionally, such conflict situations were resolved by the principle of double effect, but rejects its application in the case of abortion because it does not meet the third criterion ("the good effect should not be produced by means of the evil effect"), since: "When applied to the question of abortion, this means that abortion cannot be the means by which the good effect is accomplished -for example, one cannot abort to save the life of the mother which might be endangered because her heart cannot take the pregnancy."[37] Instead he proposes a solution similar to that of an "unjust aggressor," even though the fetus may only be trying to obtain nourishment and protection from its mother.[38] He states that in conflict situations involving abortion, the mere physical causality of the act is not morally significant. Instead, all the human values must be considered, and asserts that: "In my judgment abortion can be justified for preserving the life of the mother and for other important values commensurate with life even though the action aims at abortion as a means to an end."[39] Yet he does seem to want to set limits to his position when he declares: "My own position does differ somewhat from the accepted Catholic position both about the beginning of human life and the solution of conflict situations, but I am adamantly opposed to any position which does not recognize some independent life in the fetus and which justifies abortion as just another form of contraception."[40]

It is significant to note, however, that in another article Curran recognizes the unborn to be a "third, innocent party,"[41] and concludes on this basis that: "If the doctor truly believes abortion to be the killing of innocent persons, I do not see how he could ever perform such an operation except in the most extreme cases."[42] Nonetheless, he fails to illustrate what those extreme cases might be.

E. THE ILLUSION OF PERFECT CONTROL

Regarding moral dilemmas in prenatal diagnosis, Curran maintains that Ramsey opposes diagnosis and screening on two counts: first, because false positives may lead to the destruction of innocents. Second, because qualitative factors of the defect or of the risks of diagnosis are unquantifiable and incomparable.[43] He disagrees on both counts: regarding the first, because he says that Ramsey's argument presupposes that the fetus is an individual human being.[44] Regarding the second, he notes that many medical decisions are in fact made by comparison of qualitatively different impairments.[45]

He then presents several other concerns which Ramsey seems to have regarding prenatal diagnosis and screening,[46] and concludes by stating his own similar position:

> Although I do not agree with all the reasons Ramsey offers, I am in general agreement about his position on screening. There is the danger that individuals might be sacrificed to the greatest net good of society. In the particular question of amniocentesis, the procedure must be for the good of the patient involved and proportionate to the risks of the procedure itself. Logically, I could justify aborting the fetus only in the comparatively few cases in which the dying process has already begun. There are also many other subtleties that arise in screening for particular diseases, especially when the disease is common to a particular race. Another important question is whether or not screening should ever become compulsory. I argue in favor of voluntary programs except in truly emergency situations or in cases of contagious diseases.[47]

In another work, Curran discusses the possible risks for the child-to-be, and points out that some justify such risk because they have no problem aborting a defective fetus, but that he does, since he believes that at this stage a human life is already present.[48] Thus, he surmises that such risk should be proportionate to that of normal childbearing.[49] He does not elaborate on what those normal risks might be, or how they could be adequately evaluated. However, he does provide his own cautious evaluation of reproductive technologies in general:

> An unbalanced quest for the goal of perfect control would have deleterious effects on our compassion for those who are suffering which has traditionally been called the hallmark of Judaeo-Christian civilization.
>
> There already exists a popularly accepted slogan that every child should be a wanted child. In many ways I agree with the sentiments behind such an adage, but I would have great difficulty in accepting the possibly broader indications that we can control everything about our offspring and our own lives. Experience reminds us there are many things that happen to us in life that we do not want. The reality and mystery of suffering will always accompany us in our living and in our dying. Human existence would be rather sterile if we were able to totally determine everything that happens to us.[50]

F. HUMANIZING BIO-MEDICAL TECHNOLOGY

Curran's understanding of the shift in medicine is in terms of a rapidly advancing medical technology which could tend to dehumanize us. Accordingly, he insists on medical technology being at the service of humanity and not vice-versa: "Briefly, technology is a limited good that must be guided and directed by the truly human perspective."[51] He then discusses various contemporary moral issues related to medical technology:

1) Regarding experimentation on children, he states that whereas he previously maintained a position of no discernible risk, he now justifies some degree of risk, discomfort, or inconvenience. He attributes his shift to a greater value of the social, relational dimension of human nature. And he proposes the

same criterion when commenting on the HEW[52] regulations for all incompetents: minors, fetuses, abortuses, prisoners and mentally handicapped.[53]

2) Regarding eugenics, he distinguishes between negative and positive eugenics,[54] but considers that even negative eugenics is practically impossible to attain due to heterozygosity.[55]

3) Regarding abortion as a means of population control, he rejects such a solution.[56]

G. A CLASSICIST VERSUS A HISTORICAL MODEL

In another book on moral theology,[57] Curran defends his dissent from official Catholic teaching in the area of sexual morality. He expands on his theory of two models of doing theology: classicist versus historical.[58] He maintains that, while the church now uses a historical model in developing its social teaching, it still employs a classicist model when it comes to its sexual teaching.[59] He criticizes *Dv* and the document on Sexual Ethics[60] for lacking historical consciousness, and affirms that this tends to give more importance to human faculties than to human persons.[61] He holds that, while in social issues the church admits to gray areas, it does not do so in sexual issues. Rather, something is either permitted or forbidden.[62] He concludes that there are three methodological differences between hierarchical Catholic social and sexual teaching: "Whereas the official social teaching has evolved so that it now employs historical consciousness, personalism, and a relationality-responsibility ethical model, the sexual teaching still emphasizes classicism, human nature and faculties, and a law model of ethics."[63]

Notes

[1]Curran CE, **Themes in Fundamental Moral Theology**. Notre Dame, IN: U. of Notre Dame Press 1977, 38-39.

[2]"Here and in subsequent usage 'human life' refers to truly human life, or that human life which constitutes one a being with all the rights of a human person. Some other authors distinguish between human life which might be present from the time of conception and truly, fully, or personal human life, which does not begin until later." Curran CE, **Issues in Sexual and Medical Ethics**. Notre Dame, IN: U. of Notre Dame Press 1978, 204. See also; Curran CE, **Transition and Tradition in Moral Theology**. Notre Dame, IN: U. of Notre Dame Press 1979, 207.

[3]Curran CE, **Catholic Moral Theology in Dialogue**. Notre Dame, IN: Fides 1972, 82; Curran CE, **Directions in Fundamental Moral Theology**. Notre Dame, IN: U. of Notre Dame Press 1985, 130-131; Curran, **Themes**, 72; Curran, **Transition**, 208.

[4]Curran, **Issues**, 203-204.

[5]Curran CE, **Moral Theology: A Continuing Journey**. Notre Dame, IN: U. of Notre Dame Press 1982, 132.

[6]Curran CE, **New Perspectives in Moral Theology**. Notre Dame, IN: Fides 1974, 191-192. He also states that: "In the case of abortion, for example, the story as reported about women in Bangladesh who were raped and would no longer be accepted in their communities if they bore a

child out of wedlock illustrates a concrete application of the theory of compromise." Curran, **New Perspectives**, 192.

[7]Curran CE, **Toward an American Catholic Moral Theology**. Notre Dame, IN: U. of Notre Dame Press 1987.

[8]Curran, **American Catholic Moral Theology**, 67.

[9]Curran, **American Catholic Moral Theology**, 65-70.

[10]"The traditional Catholic position maintaining that there is no obligation to use extraordinary means to preserve human life and existence recognizes that physical human existence is not an absolute for the believer." Curran, **American Catholic Moral Theology**, 73.

[11]Curran, **American Catholic Moral Theology**, 70-78.

[12]Curran, **American Catholic Moral Theology**, 80-81.

[13]Curran, **American Catholic Moral Theology**, 82-83; here 83.

[14]"I am not asserting that Thomas always identified human actions with animal processes or the physical structure of the act. In fact, the general outlines of the hylomorphic theory, by speaking of material and formal components of reality, try to avoid any physicalism or biologism. Nevertheless, the adoption of Ulpian's understanding of 'nature' and 'natural' logically leads to the identification of the human act itself with animal processes and with the mere physical structure of the act. Such a distorted view of the human act becomes especially prevalent in the area of medical morals, for in medical morality one can more easily conceive a moral human action solely in terms of the physical structure of that action." Curran, **Themes**, 39.

[15]"A better anthropology would see the distinctive in human beings as guiding and directing the totality of one's being." Curran, **Themes**, 38-39.

[16]Curran, **Themes**, 59. See also: Curran, **Directions**, 151.

[17]Curran, **Themes**, 60.

[18]Curran, **Themes**, 71.

[19]"In unjust aggression the various values at stake are weighed, and the person is permitted to kill an unjust aggressor not only to save one's life but also to protect other goods of comparable value, such as a serious threat to health, honor, chastity, or even material goods of great importance." Curran, **Themes**, 71.

[20]Curran, **Themes**, 72; Curran, **Directions**, 163-164.

[21]He cites high pregnancy wastage as confirmatory of this. See: Curran CE, "*In vitro* fertilization and embryo transfer: from a perspective of moral theology" in: U.S. Department of Health, Education, and Welfare; Ethics Advisory Board. Appendix: **HEW Support of Research Involving Human In Vitro Fertilization and Embryo Transfer**. Washington: Department of Health, Education, and Welfare: Ethics Advisory Board, May 4, 1979, 4.1-4.33; Curran, **Moral Theology**, 125-126; Curran, **New Perspectives**, 188; Curran CE, **Ongoing Revision in Moral Theology**. Notre Dame, IN: Fides 1975, 156; Curran, **Transition**, 212.

[22]Curran, **Issues**, 217-218. He also affirms that: "On the question of the beginning of human life I see great wisdom in the teaching of the hierarchical magisterium of the Catholic Church and modify it only to the extent of placing the beginning of truly individual human life at two to three weeks after conception." Curran, **Transition**, 227.

[23]Curran CE, "Abortion: contemporary debate in philosophical and religious ethics", in: Reich WT, **Encyclopedia of Bioethics 1**. New York: Macmillan 1978, 17-26.

[24]Curran, *Abortion*, 17.

[25]Curran, *Abortion*, 17-18.

[26]Curran, *Abortion*, 18.

[27]Not at birth, since: "...the fetus one day before birth and the child one day after birth are not that

significantly or qualitatively different in any respect." (18). Not at viability, since: "The fetus immediately before viability is not that qualitatively different from the viable fetus. In addition viability is a very inexact criterion because it is intimately connected with rapidly changing medical and scientific advances." (18). Not at morphism-brain, since: "...it seems difficult to maintain that such early development of these organs constitutes the qualitative difference between truly human life and no truly human life. Self-awareness and reason are not actually present at this time, and much more growth and development are necessary." (18). Not at conception, since twinning and recombination may still occur (19). Curran, *Abortion*, 18-19.

[28]Once more, the reasons being twinning and recombination before implantation, and confirmatory of this is a high rate of spontaneous abortions. Important to note, however, is his claim that: "Before this time there is no organizer that directs the differentiation of the pluripotential cells so that without this organizer hominization cannot occur." Curran, *Abortion*, 19.

[29]Not relational, because different people have very different relational capacities and opportunities throughout life. Not multiple, since psychological and cultural dimensions are not that present even at birth, but rather much later. Not conferred rights, for it still does not answer the question of when human life begins. Curran, *Abortion*, 20-22.

[30]Curran CE, **Politics, Medicine, and Christian Ethics: A Dialogue with Paul Ramsey**. Philadelphia: Fortress 1973, 114. See also: Curran, **Catholic Moral Theology**, 257.

[31]Curran, **Politics**, 130-131.

[32]Curran, **Politics**, 131. See also: Curran, **Catholic Moral Theology**, 257-258.

[33]Curran, **New Perspectives**, 173.

[34]Curran, **New Perspectives**, 173.

[35]Curran, **New Perspectives**, 178.

[36]Curran, **New Perspectives**, 179. He sustains that, the more complex the question, the less certain the answer will be. See: Curran, **Catholic Moral Theology**, 259.

[37]Curran, *Abortion*, 23. See also: Curran, **Ongoing Revision**, 157.

[38]Curran, *Abortion*, 23-24. See also: Curran, **New Perspectives**, 191.

[39]Curran, *Abortion*, 24. He further maintains that: "Thus abortion could be justified to save the life of the mother or to avert very grave psychological or physical harm to the mother with the realization that this must truly be grave harm that will perdure over some time and not just a temporary depression." Curran, **New Perspectives**, 191. See also: Curran, **Issues**, 204; Curran, **Ongoing Revision**, 203; Curran, **Transition**, 222.

[40]Curran, **New Perspectives**, 192.

[41]Curran CE, "Cooperation: toward a revision of the concept and its application" *LinacreQ* 41,3 (1974) 152-167; here, 162.

[42]Curran, *Cooperation*, 162. See also: Curran, **Ongoing Revision**, 223.

[43]Curran, **Politics**, 171-173.

[44]"If the fetus is not a human individual, then there is no great difficulty in sacrificing some healthy fetuses for the greater good of the human race." Curran, **Politics**, 171.

[45]"The decision not to use extraordinary means involves such a decision for one compares added life against the realities of pain, expense, or inconvenience." Curran, **Politics**, 171-172; here 172.

[46]First, making medical decisions based on non-medical grounds opens medicine to possible abuses. Second, whereas couples may have a right to desire children, they don't have a right to have children proper, much less to have only perfectly healthy ones. Society's present striving

exclusively for normal children may discriminate against those with some abnormality. Curran, **Politics**, 172.

[47]Curran, **Politics**, 172-173.

[48]"However, from my perspective I cannot accept the general solution of abortion of deformed fetuses, since a truly human life is already present. My ethical analysis must then deal somewhat differently with the question of the risks to the child-to-be." Curran, *In vitro*, 4.18. See also: Curran, **Moral Theology**, 127.

[49]Curran, *In vitro*, 4.18-4.19. See also: Curran, **Moral Theology**, 128.

[50]Curran, *In vitro*, 4.24.

[51]Curran, **Issues**, 75.

[52]U.S. Department of Health, Education and Welfare: Ethics Advisory Board, Washington, DC.

[53]Curran, **Issues**, 95-98.

[54]"Negative eugenics aims at removing the deleterious genes from the gene pool. Positive or progressive eugenics tries to improve the genes existing in the gene pool." Curran, **Issues**, 106.

[55]He does see a value of negative eugenics, however, at the personal level, wherein certain affected individuals may be counselled either not to marry, or not to have children: "If a couple knows that the chances are one out of four that their child will be mentally retarded and two out of four that the child will be a carrier of such retardation, there seems to be a strong moral argument not to have children." Curran, **Issues**, 106.

[56]Curran, **Issues**, 191.

[57]Curran CE, **Tensions in Moral Theology**. Notre Dame, IN: U. of Notre Dame Press 1988.

[58]"Historical consciousness is often contrasted with classicism. Classicism understands reality in terms of the eternal, the immutable, and the unchanging; whereas historical consciousness gives more importance to the particular, the contingent, the historical, and the individual." Curran, **Tensions**, 89.

[59]Curran, **Tensions**, 88-107.

[60]Sacred Congregation for the Doctrine of the Faith, *Declaration on Certain Questions Concerning Sexual Ethics* (Dec. 29, 1975) in: Flannery A, ed, **Vatican Council II: More Postconciliar Documents**, vol. 2. Northport, NY: Costello 1982, 486-499.

[61]Curran, **Tensions**, 102.

[62]"The contemporary official Catholic teaching on social issues with its relationality-responsibility model recognizes significant gray areas.... Thus the very way in which topics are treated--namely, either forbidden or permitted--indicates again that a legal model is at work in the hierarchical sexual teaching." Curran, **Tensions**, 106.

[63]Curran, **Tensions**, 87-109; here 107.

CHAPTER VII

WILLIAM E. MAY

A. THE MORAL WORTH OF HUMAN BEINGS

May already begins to reveal his basic value system regarding human life in an early article on prenatal life and conflict situations.[1] In it he recognizes that the issue of the status of prenatal life is central, and maintains that contemporary medicine affirms that it is human.[2] He then states that the core of the abortion argument is not necessarily when human life begins, but when one is willing to protect such life, which in turn is based on one's belief of the moral worth of human beings: are humans worth because of what they achieve, or because of what they are? He believes the latter,[3] and states: "Put another way, I think that the major area of disagreement between those who defend abortion and those who oppose abortion over the status of fetal life comes down to the question: Is humanity, in the sense of being an entity that is the subject of rights, an endowment or an achievement?"[4] He stands on the side of endowment.[5] Hence, the only abortion which he can ethically justify is an indirect one.[6]

In a subsequent article, he further explicates what he means by the moral worth of a human being.[7] He states that a human being is a moral being, one who distinguishes between *is* and *ought*, and a being of moral worth, one who is valuable, precious, irreplaceable, and a subject of inalienable rights. While fetuses are human beings and of moral worth, he argues that they are not moral beings, since they are as yet incapable of distinguishing between *is* and *ought*.[8]

Applying this anthropology to the ethical issues raised by the new biology, he rejects consequentialism and distinguishes between two different types of deontologisms. He rejects consequentialist deontologism as unconcerned with the meaning of our deeds, and instead proposes a deontologism of basic human goods. This latter finds the human identity expressed in human deeds such that a being of moral worth ought never to willingly desire to set her or himself against a real good (life, health, justice, peace, friendship) of another being of moral worth.[9]

B. THE PROCESS OF HUMANIZATION

Some of May's philosophical and anthropological presuppositions can be elucidated in an early book where he expresses his beliefs regarding what it is to be human.[10] In it he states that there are two ways of being human: at a mere animal level, and at a truly human level, which implies a progressive "becoming," a process of humanization: "To use the term in this second sense is to imply that there is a process of humanization; it is to imply that a human being has a destiny to which he is called and that he fulfills his being by his struggle to attain this destiny."[11] This process of becoming human, as expected, is ongoing, extending even before birth.[12]

He describes how: we gradually come to know our humanness in and through associations, in society[13]; as we do, we steadily form our consciences[14]; as we engage in truly human acts (as distinguished from mere physiological acts such as blinking and snoring)[15]; but always within the context of a very real-weakened world.[16] He concludes by stating that for the Christian, and indeed for all peoples, this process of becoming human is perfected and exemplified in the incarnate Word of God, Jesus Christ: "...because the incarnation of God's Word, his othering of himself in what is not himself, namely man, illumines the meaning of human existence."[17]

In a later work,[18] May returns to the subjects of God and man, wherein he provides an unquestionably theistic definition of human existence:

> We can summarize the understanding of God and of human existence, mediated by Christian faith, in the following way. God, the *summum bonum*, the good that is to be loved above all other goods, made us to share his very own life. Because he made us for this purpose, we are in truth his images; we are his created words, and his Uncreated Word became, like us, a created word, a human being. Because we are his living images we are beings of moral worth; and because we are radically capable, by virtue of being his images and words, of becoming conscious of ourselves and of the meaning of our actions, we are capable of becoming moral beings, moral agents. We are radically capable of determining our own lives and establishing our own identity through our own choices.[19]

C. HOMINIZATION AT FERTILIZATION

Once again, May frames his theory of hominization within his analysis of abortion. He acknowledges that at the heart of the matter is the status of human fetal life.[20] He refutes arguments that propose the fetus as "protoplasmic rubbish," "gametic materials," "a blueprint," and "part of the mother," as mere rhetoric unsubstantiated by biological facts. Regarding viability, he points to the fact that the fetus is viable at all stages, as long as it is provided with the proper environment for sustaining life. Likewise, the beginning of the development of a brain is not the determining moment because prior to it the fetus already has the capacity to develop such a human brain. He also rejects the notion that, even if a fetus is recognized to be a human being, it can be aborted when its continued existence is in conflict with the happiness or well-being of someone else who has already achieved "meaningful" human existence.[21]

He then addresses the proposal that human life begins at segmentation-implantation, which he notes is based on the emergence of individual life.

Individual life, he insists, can also be postulated from conception-fertilization. On the issue of twinning, he proposes two possible explanations: first, by asexual reproduction whereby one twin gives rise to the other. Second, by the pre-implanted fetus dying as it gives rise to two (or more) twin-siblings (he finds the first explanation more likely).[22]

Regarding the argument of recombination, he maintains that there is presently no evidence of it in humans, but that even if the possibility existed, it could be explained by a process similar to grafting in plants, where the individuality of each plant is not questioned prior to the grafting: "Similarly, the combining of two developing human embryos into one would simply mean that the two had ceased to be and that a new embryonic human being had come into existence."[23] He concludes from this analysis that conception-fertilization must be the moment when individual human life begins, because:

> This new living entity is not potentially a human being but is *a human being with potential*, a potential it will develop if it is allowed to continue to be. This entity does not, at some subsequent stage in its development, *acquire* human potential; it *already has* such potential, and it has this potential precisely because *it is the kind of being it is.* Its human potential is *real*, not an abstraction. From the time of conception-fertilization there is in our midst, though hidden from view, a new living entity that is identifiable as a member of the human species and will develop all the properties or capacities that adult members of the species possess, not because the powers and capacities have been added to it from the outside but because they have been developed from within [emphasis his].[24]

More recently, May returns to his theory of immediate hominization in two articles on the status of the human zygote:

In the first he sustains that the zygote can indeed be an individual.[25] He refutes arguments by Shannon and Wolter that the pre-embryo is not yet an individual.[26] He says that Shannon and Wolter base their conclusion in part on evidence that the zygote needs information from the mother to develop, and that both twinning and recombination can occur before implantation.[27] To counter the first argument he cites Suarez,[28] who states that, based on research on hydatidiform moles and teratomas, the embryo does not receive any information from the mother necessary for development control.[29]

To counter the second argument he affirms that totipotentiality has been addressed by a number of people, among whom is Huarte, who states that:

> They [preimplanted human blastocysts] can become embryos only if they are separated from the original embryo and become independent biological units or if they are artificially severed from it [the original embryo] and are surrounded with a new zona pellucida. It is thus false to say that 'the unicellular or pluricellular embryo is a *potential* individual or totipotent,' because an embryo is always already in itself an individual of an animal species [the human] from the earliest stages of its development.[30]

He also cites Grisez, Ashley and Lejeune, who explain twinning as a form of asexual reproduction, or cloning.[31]

In the second article he holds that such an individual is a human person.[32] Following traditional hylemorphic arguments, he concurs with Siebenthal that, if Aquinas knew then what is now known about human fertilization (namely, that both the mother and the father contribute equally to the genotype of the zygote, thus forming a new and unique entity), he would conclude that the human zygote is an informed, human body.[33] And, if so, then this new human body would have to be considered a human person.[34]

He then quotes Grisez and Moraczewski to critique those who uphold delayed hominization based on the appearance of the brain primordia by countering that the brain primordia must also have their primordia, and so on in regression to the fertilized ovum.[35] He concludes by stating that if society begins to view the human embryo as only biologically alive, but not personally alive, then it might also begin to deny personhood to other members of society.[36]

D. DEONTOLOGISM OF BASIC HUMAN GOODS

As stated earlier, May's analysis of the moral act follows a deontologism of basic human goods. An elaboration of his deontology may be seen in an article where he touches on some basic criteria when dealing with medical dilemmas.[37] In it he cites prenatal diagnosis as one such dilemma.[38] Assessing consequentialism as an invalid method of normative ethics in solving such medical ethical dilemmas because it fails to adequately evaluate one basic human good against another, he espouses a nonconsequentialistic ethic; good is to be done and pursued, and evil is to be avoided.[39] As an example of the application of this theory he proposes that those dedicated to health care ought not to be involved in killing human beings, as in the case of abortion, which does not mean that one cannot intervene when the life of the mother is in danger, for in this case the death of the fetus is not intended.[40]

E. THE FETUS AND MORAL AGENTS

From his discussion of human procreation and reproduction, it is evident that for May human life begins at conception.[41] With this in mind, he discusses the morality of attempts to protect the human genetic pool. While he accepts the possible benefits of screening for the detection of genetic defects of those who are already born, he contends that screening the unborn by prenatal diagnosis usually leads to "therapeutic" abortion of defectives, which poses serious ethical problems.[42]

He distances himself from a pragmatic, consequentialist ethics which justifies such means of alleviating human suffering, and notes that even screening with a view to abortion is morally objectionable. He finds three such objections: First, the willingness to kill healthy unborns in the case of "false positive;" second, direct risk of the procedure to the unborn;[43] third, abortion is never therapeutic for the fetus. The clear association in these three objections, of course, is that amniocentesis is being done exclusively with a view to abortion if the diagnosis is positive.[44]

In view of the aforesaid analysis, he justifies abortion only to save the life of the mother; when the death of the fetus is foreseen but not intended. When applied to "defective" fetuses, he points out that since the developing fetus is not a direct threat to the life of the mother, it cannot be targeted for abortion. Thus, the practice of "therapeutic" abortion, which intends the death of the fetus, cannot be morally justified, and to call it "treatment" is to misuse language. Likewise, he notes that even if one sought to justify "therapeutic" abortions because they minimize human suffering, the physical evidence points to the contrary since there seems to be a higher propensity of premature deliveries among women who have undergone abortions, which thus actually leads to greater suffering and expense.[45]

He then addresses the issues of genetic therapy, genetic counseling, and responsible family planning. Regarding gametic genetic therapy, he holds that since the present technology cannot guarantee proven effectiveness of treatment to the individual, and lack of harm to the individual, to his or her progeny, and to the population at large, it is not morally justifiable. Regarding genetic counseling, he claims that presently there seems to be a link between prenatal diagnosis and abortion, but that in principle proper genetic counseling should be geared toward helping mature persons who are contemplating marriage choose genetically compatible spouses. Regarding responsible family planning, he maintains that spouses who become aware of being carriers of serious genetic disorders may have a moral obligation not to procreate, and encourages them to practice licit methods to achieve this, such as natural family planning.[46]

Finally, he addresses the issue of proxy consent in human fetal experimentation.[47] He states his approval of proxy consent of therapeutic situations, and disapproval of nontherapeutic ones, since only moral agents can give proxy consent. He holds that, while children and other incompetents are beings of moral worth, and may have the capacity to become moral agents, they are not so in their present state.[48] He is consistent with his theory of *becoming* a human moral agent by interaction with a human community, which cannot imply a completed process, certainly in the earlier stages of human life. To support his thesis, he cites the example of feral children, who though fully human, do not seem to have any self-awareness due to the lack of such human interaction. Since infants are not moral agents, they may not be subjects of nontherapeutic experimentation as though they were able to "volunteer" in the true sense of the word. He concludes by saying that, unlike adults who are moral agents, children and other incompetents are not responsible for contributing to the general benefit of society, and that we, as moral agents, have an obligation to protect them from being forced into making such contributions.[49]

F. A STRICT INTERPRETATION

Though not explicitly addressed, it can be seen from May's discussion of a nonconsequentialist deontology, of proxy consent, of "therapeutic" abortion, and of genetic counseling, that he would be opposed to any shift in medicine away from a strict physical interpretation of the classical medical dictum *primum non nocere* when it comes to protecting fetal life. Proof of this may be observed when he counsels those involved in the health profession not to be involved in killing the unborn.[50]

G. AN OFFICIAL POSITION

Also, it seems safe to say that May seeks to uphold official magisterial teaching regarding prenatal life and conflict situations.[51] He summarizes the unambiguous position of the Catholic Church against procured abortion, though he admits that the issue of the moment of ensoulment is still open.[52] In spite of this theoretical openness, he holds that doubt should lead us at least to provisional protection, for not doing so may also endanger other inviolable human rights.[53]

Notes

[1]May WE, "The morality of abortion" *LinacreQ* 41,1 (1974) 66-77.

[2]May, *Morality*, 69-70.

[3]May WE, "What makes a human being to be a being of moral worth?" *Thom* 40 (1976) 416-443.

[4]May, *Morality*, 70-71; here 71.

[5]May, *Morality*, 71.

[6]"In sum, in instances when an act that results in the death of the fetus and is foreseen to issue in this consequence, the abortion is 'indirectly voluntary' and not directly so if, and *only* if, the agent does not want the fetus to die (his motive or the *finis operantis*) *and* the thrust of the action *-its* 'intention' or direction or what used to be called the *finis operis-* is itself targeted, not upon the life of the fetus, but upon countering the injurious effect that the fetus, simply by its presence, is causing its mother." May, *Morality*, 74-75.

[7]May WE, "Ethics and human identity: the challenge of the new biology" *Hor* 3,1 (1976) 17-37.

[8]May, *Human identity*, 18-20.

[9]May, *Human identity*, 21-37.

[10]May WE, **Becoming Human: An Invitation to Christian Ethics.** Dayton, OH: Pflaum 1975.

[11]May, **Becoming**, 2-3.

[12]May, **Becoming**, 44.

[13]May, **Becoming**, 25-49.

[14]May, **Becoming**, 53-75.

[15]May, **Becoming**, 79-107.

[16]May, **Becoming**, 113-138.

[17]May, **Becoming**, 137.

[18]May WE, **Human Existence, Medicine and Ethics: Reflections on Human Life.** Chicago: Franciscan Herald Press 1977.

[19]May, **Human Existence**, 8.

[20]He uses the term "fetus" to include the unborn from conception until birth. See: May, **Human Existence**, 93.

[21]May, **Human Existence**, 94-99.

[22]May, **Human Existence**, 99-103.

[23]May, **Human Existence**, 101-102; here 102.

[24]May, **Human Existence**, 102-103.

[25]May WE, "Zygotes, embryos, and persons: Part I" *EthMed* 16,10 (1991) 2-4.

[26]See: Shannon TA, Wolter A, "Reflections on the moral status of the pre-embryo" *TS* 51 (1990) 603-626.

[27]May, *Zygotes I*, 2.

[28]See: Suarez A, "Hydatidiform moles and teratomas confirm the human identity of the preimplantation embryo" *JMedPhil* 15 (1990) 627-635.

[29]May, *Zygotes I*, 2-4.

[30]Huarte J, "Concepts fondamentaux d'embryologie" *L'Embryon: Un Homme: Actes du Congrès de Lausanne* 1986, Premier Congrès de la Société Suisse de Bioéthique 8 et 9 novembre 1986, Lausanne: Centre de documentation civique 1987, 65-68; here 67-68.

[31]May, *Zygotes I*, 4.

[32]May WE, "Zygotes, embryos, and persons - Part II" *EthMed* 17,1 (1992) 1-3.

[33]See: de Siebenthal J, "L'animation selon Thomas d'Aquin" *L'Embryon: Un Homme: Actes du Congrès de Lausanne* 1986, Premier Congrès de la Société suisse de bioéthique 8 et 9 novembre 1986, Lausanne: Centre de documentation civique 1987, 91-97.

[34]May, *Zygotes II*, 2.

[35]May, *Zygotes II*, 2.

[36]May, *Zygotes II*, 2.

[37]May WE, "Meeting ethical dilemmas in health care: some basic criteria" *LinacreQ* 49,3 (1982) 248-265.

[38]May, *Ethical dilemmas*, 248-249.

[39]"For *good* means what is truly perfective of a being, what any being needs if that being is to be what it is meant to be, and *evil* means the deprivation of good." May, *Ethical dilemmas*, 249-156; here 256.

[40]May, *Ethical dilemmas*, 258.

[41]May, **Human Existence**, 39-61.

[42]May, **Human Existence**, 87-88.

[43]"Second, amniocentesis involves risks to the unborn child. Admittedly, the risks are statistically low -1 to 2 percent- but the damage that may be induced in the unborn child by amniocentesis is quite grave. In fact, we do not know, nor can we learn, the full range of harm that the procedure may entail. It must be argued, however, that a slight risk of grave damage is a grave risk. And the risk is in no way connected with helping the being who supposedly is in need of therapy." May, **Human Existence**, 89.

[44]May, **Human Existence**, 88-90.

[45]May, **Human Existence**, 104-106.

[46]May, **Human Existence**, 116-128.

[47]May WE, "Proxy consent to human experimentation" *LinacreQ* 43,2 (1976) 73-84. See also: May WE, "Experimenting on human subjects" *LinacreQ* 41,4 (1974) 238-252; May, **Human Existence**, 29-33.

[48]May, *Proxy consent*, 78-79.

[49]May, *Proxy consent*, 80-82.

[50]May, *Ethical dilemmas*, 258.

[51]"In sum, the Church clearly teaches (a) that every human life, from the moment of conception on, is priceless and endowed with sanctity, (b) that every direct attack on unborn human life or abortion is intrinsically gravely evil, (c) that civil law has an obligation to recognize and protect the right of unborn human beings to the security of their own lives, (d) that civil laws in principle approving of abortion are iniquitous and unjust, and (e) that the Catholic faithful have a serious obligation in conscience not to support or approve of civil laws promoting abortion and not to be party to the application of such laws." May WE, "Abortion, Catholic teaching, and public policy" *LinacreQ* 52,1 (1985), 38-44; here 40.

[52]May, *Abortion*, 40-41.

[53]"If the right of unborn human beings to the secure possession of their lives is made dependent on the choice of others, then the right of born human beings is similarly subject to such choices. We have already seen how easy it is to pass from an acceptance of abortion to the acceptance of infanticide or the 'benign neglect' of handicapped newborns. This makes it unmistakably clear that here we are dealing, not with an issue of private morality where immoral choices can at times be tolerated, but with a central issue of public morality, where basic and inviolable human rights are at stake." May, *Abortion*, 42.

CHAPTER VIII

DONALD G. McCARTHY and ALBERT S. MORACZEWSKI, OP

A. THE PERSONAL RELATION BETWEEN GOD AND HIS IMAGE

McCarthy's basic value system may be seen in his Christian analysis of human life issues.[1] He begins by following Ashley and O'Rourke's definition of the human person as "embodied intelligent freedom," also noting the communitarian dimension of human nature.[2] His anthropology develops along biblical lines whereby the human person, the living image of God, is capable of sin due to our radical freedom, and in fact has sinned, but is redeemed by the Person of Jesus Christ out of love, the same love which calls us to fulfill our personhood in being for one another.[3] Thus, he considers it natural for people to be health stewards, both of selves and of others, comprising the physiological, psychological and spiritual dimensions of the total person. Also according to these values, one may never seek to directly destroy an innocent human life (Principle of Inviolability).[4] He also points to the basic human experiences of pain and suffering, holding that these can have redeeming value if one is able to identify them with the redeeming sufferings of Christ.[5]

Further insights into McCarthy and Moraczewski's basic value system are gleaned from a co-authored book on the ethical evaluation of fetal experimentation.[6] Here one finds two fundamental reasons for respect owed to the fetus by the community within which he or she will grow and develop: The first is grounded in the personal relationship between God and his image.[7] The second is based on the principle of equality: If human fetuses are recognized by the medical community to be *subjects* of research or therapy,[8] they must be treated equally at equal stages of development --even if their "personhood" is questioned--, otherwise it would be discriminatory.[9]

Further hints of Moraczewski's value system may be gleaned from his work evaluating specific actions in the realm of genetic medicine, such as selective abortion and genetic screening.[10] He is opposed to selective abortion and cost/benefit analysis because, instead of upholding the fundamental moral equality of all human beings, it involves judging whether an individual's life has a positive net worth for society or not.[11] He also notes that the practices of selective abortion and cost/benefit analysis may lead to endanger the lives of "defective" members of society who are already born.[12]

He is likewise very cautious about genetic screening programs, since these could increase the expectations of detecting carriers and aborting affected fetuses.[13] Regarding couples who choose not to participate, he notes that: "If there exists a diagnostic program designed to test such cases, and if the program has been presented to the public as a means of reducing the social costs of caring for affected children, then there arises the question of what the social attitude would be toward a person who did not choose to avail herself of the proffered services and as a result produced an affected child who consequently must be a drain on the resources of the society."[14] The danger is that such programs may intimidate couples, stigmatize defective parents and children, and might even shift the decision to procreate from the family to the state.[15] Since even with the most sophisticated programs genetic defects will still occur, he fears that society may become less tolerant of the abnormal and the imperfect due to raised expectations. In addition, a national policy of genetic screening may tend to unjustly discriminate against certain groups, such as in the case of sickle-cell anemia in blacks, and raise issues of confidentiality, and proper distribution of scarce medical and economic resources.[16]

Finally, he describes what he believes is the proper Christian witness to genetic defects[17]: For a Christian couple who is affected with or carrier of defects, the responsible option might be not to procreate,[18] but if already pregnant, abortion should not be an option.[19] Regarding the Christian genetic counselor, he or she should imbue his or her profession with the Christian belief of the transcendent value and dignity of all human life and of the family, with the Christian meanings of suffering and grace, and with a special concern for weaker members of society.[20] Specifically, this should mean competence: in scientific knowledge and technical skills (including natural family planning); in providing full disclosure and maintaining confidentiality; and in seeking a type of nondirective counseling which respects the moral autonomy of the counselee, while allowing for the expression of the moral views of the counselor, and discussion of the moral significance of the different courses of action.[21]

Lastly, further basic values may be gathered from an article McCarthy wrote where he discusses some ethical principles involved in prenatal diagnosis.[22] He begins by stating that, while not all immoral acts can be prevented by law, certainly condoning acts which vie against protecting innocent human life should not be codified either; the U.S. Supreme Court condoned such acts by legalizing abortion in 1973.[23] He goes on to briefly describe several ethical systems which might be used in deciding the morality of abortion of genetically defective fetuses: emotivism, intuitionism, consequentialism, utilitarianism, voluntarism, and prudential personalism.[24] He espouses the latter, defining it as a system where human actions are evaluated on whether they advance or undermine well-being, and is based on the classical scholastic interpretation of natural moral law, which sustains that certain fundamental human rights are grounded in the natural order of creation established by God, according to which basically evil actions are never justified by good consequences.[25]

B. OBJECTIFICATION OF CAUSAL RELATIONSHIPS

McCarthy's philosophical and anthropological presuppositions are already evident from his epilogue to a symposium on the beginnings of personhood.[26] He commences by examining potentiality in the zygote:

> The DNA molecules at conception have an informational content equivalent to one thousand volumes of an encyclopedia. Obviously this informational content is real because it determines to a great extent the individual characteristics of the developing human life. Since these characteristics are not yet *actually* present, they are *really*, but only *potentially*, present. These potential characteristics are gradually actualized: this is the process of development. That these potentialities are realities is evident from the fact that a human zygote, for example, if allowed to develop, never becomes any other species.[27]

This potentiality is continuously being actualized throughout one's entire lifetime, but never exhausted. In retrospect, the reality of an (human) infant is caused by the existence of the potential of the previous developmental stage, namely, the (human) embryo; such potentiality he says belongs to a scheme of objectification of causal relationships where the real potential of a previous stage causes the real actuality of the following.[28] Thus, he holds that it is possible to affirm the existence of personhood before it is apparent if one views it as self-determination which, by definition, is in continuous development.[29]

Later on, McCarthy and Moraczewski co-authored a book where they delve more deeply into their philosophical and anthropological presuppositions regarding prenatal life. They begin by defining a fetus to be an individual "human being," genetically unique and already in the process of life-long development.[30] If the fetus is a "human subject," as opposed to an "object" or a "thing," then he or she must be protected by the community from stronger adults who might victimize its weaker members. Yet, the fetus should not be over-protected from research which would benefit it; here the same proxy consent is required as that for experimentation on children, the mentally retarded, unconscious people, etc.[31]

They lay the groundwork for their belief of human individuality from conception, pointing out that even monozygotic twins show some subtle--but real--individuation. In spite of the unique individuality of each person, human development necessarily occurs in community. However, they note the inadequacy of defining the human fetus in mere legal or psychological terms. Rather, they espouse an organic criterion: "Thus the human fetus shows itself as an organism with an inner dynamism which, apart from accident or defect, naturally leads it to full adulthood in a smooth progression."[32] They distinguish between the passive potencies of the fetus (the capacity of chemical materials to be organized into macro-molecules, tissues, organs), and its active potency as a living organism to develop itself, differentiate, and eventually arrive at full adulthood. Since this active potency is already present in the genetic code of the zygote: "Must it not be admitted therefore, that the zygote is actually in a very significant sense a human person, since it is in the process of self-actualization?"[33]

They hold this position to be a personalist philosophy,[34] which affirms that: "The fetus is a person-in-process who will not be able to carry on the uniquely human activities of intellection and free choice as a part of a human community, until, with the assistance of that community, it has reached the use of reason through a complex sequence of changes."[35] Yet these changes do not interrupt, but complete its continuous existence. Thus the fetus, as a developing person among developing persons, is entitled to moral protection from conception (the beginning of such development) by the community within which he or she lives.[36]

Moraczewski's philosophical and anthropological presuppositions may be further seen when he speaks of three main schools of thought seeking to define the human person: social,[37] developmental[38] and genetic.[39] He rejects the social school because no society seems to have a clear, objective way of determining who has a right to belong to it, which in the case of the unborn would translate into an other-conferred rather than a self-deserved right to life.[40] He also rejects the developmental school because, not unlike the social school, it too fails to have a universally accepted standard of what characteristic defines one as truly human.[41] Finally, he agrees with the genetic school,[42] but only after distinguishing between a genetic dimension (human organism) and a moral dimension (human being) of the word "human:" in a genetic sense it means to belong to the species *Homo sapiens*; in the moral sense it means a subject of rights.[43] Once this distinction made, the question becomes: How is the undeveloped human organism *in utero* capable of characteristically human activity? He deduces that the only possible answer is by being capable of that activity which is self-directed, and that such self-direction begins at fertilization.[44] Hence, only a genetic approach to human life is able to protect unborn human life--especially genetically defective children--from the arbitrary decisions of others.[45] This view of the human person he grounds in biblical,[46] magisterial,[47] and personalist roots.[48]

In another work dealing with ethical implications of genetic manipulation, Moraczewski again alludes to his vision of the human person.[49] He analyzes the morality of seeking to perfect human nature through technological interventions: he asks two related questions; may we, and must we. He notes that the answer to these two questions depends on one's vision of the human person, and proceeds with his own Christian anthropology:

> What is man (in the generic sense)? Christians can obtain insights from the sacred scriptures which instruct that the universe and humans did not evolve by chance. Rather, in the Judeo-Christian perspective, the universe is the result of a decision and act of an intelligent being, God, of a creation *ex nihilo* done with a purpose and, indeed, with love. Thus, from that perspective the human is necessarily not the highest pinnacle in existence. At the very least there is a being who transcends us and to whom we are responsible. That position contrasts to the prevalent perspective of the culture in which Christians live. Christians eat, drink, and breathe in a culture of secular humanism that places the human at the very top, the pinnacle of reality. Therefore, from that perspective, the human being alone is the measure of himself and of everything else. An additional difference is that Christians believe that humans are redeemed by the Man-God, Jesus Christ.[50]

He then quotes Genesis to show that God has given human beings dominion over nature, but not necessarily over human nature.[51] Confessing that human evolution has taken place under divine providence, he asks whether we may or even must directly intervene in the human, given that we now technically can.[52] Coupled with this is what he perceives to be a shift in viewing the human person, from passive spectator, to active participant in the evolution of the world.[53] One aspect of this participation is technological progress, which in principle ought to be viewed by Christians as good.[54] Specifically, reproductive technology is good when it helps persons become more truly human and when it does not impede attaining eternal life.[55] Thus, to the question whether we may intervene in the human, he states that if it does not interfere with our goal of union with God, we may.[56] In fact, given the capacity of technology to truly enhance our humanity and our care for each other, we even must.[57]

C. THE SUCCESSION OF PRIMARY ORGANIZERS

McCarthy and Moraczewski's processural approach to the human person is based on an epigenetic interpretation of human embryology,[58] which leads them to oppose any theory of delayed hominization. Regarding the objections of twinning and recombination, they claim that these stem from a dualistic vision of God infusing a soul on matter prepared for it, and counter with three arguments: First, epigenetic development (ontogenic) is not to be confused with the evolution of species (phylogenic), for the latter occurs by natural selection of genetic mutations in an entire population, whereas the former is the normal expression of an already existing genetic code within an individual zygote. Second, Aristotle's theory that "fertilization" occurred by the uninformed menstrual blood of the mother being informed by the semen of the father over time has today been biologically disclaimed. Third, delayed hominization fails to explain how development occurs before individuation, or what causes implantation.[59] By contrast, maintaining individuality from the zygote stage can account for twinning by one (unicellular) organism generating another through a process similar to asexual reproduction or cloning. Likewise, recombination could be explained as the death of a once living twin, with its organic remains now being reabsorbed by the surviving twin.[60]

In another work, McCarthy again specifically discusses the beginning of human life, espousing a radical teleology:[61] He holds that due to the organization found in the fertilized ovum, this first cell is already a unified human body undergoing directional development.[62] Such development is not directed by a single but by a succession of primary organizers, such as the zygote nucleus, the embryonic primitive streak, and the fetal brain.[63] To consolidate his argument he maintains that it is philosophically consistent to view a living human body as a human person, and that God follows such logic by conferring a personal soul upon human conception; to argue otherwise would also deny personhood to other human beings.[64]

Moraczewski further addresses his theory of hominization in two articles:

In the first he states that personhood is not *purely* a moral concept, and that whereas (biological) science cannot declare when human personhood begins, it can identify when: (1) a particular organism is alive; (2) that life begins, and; (3) that living organism is a member of the species *Homo sapiens*.[65] Thus, members of the National Academy of Sciences generate confusion when they testify that science cannot identify when human life begins.[66]

In the second he refutes Sass,[67] who proposes as a compromise the time when integrated brain functions appear--at about 70 days after fertilization.[68] Sass bases his argument in that at the end of life one may consider a person dead when such functions cease, thus, to be consistent, the same criterion should be applied at the beginning of life.[69] Moraczewski refutes this argument because scientific evidence shows that the zygote is a living organism even before integrated brain functions occur--although the "primary organizer" is as yet not clearly identifiable. Proof that a "primary organizer" is already present comes from the fact that, left on their own, the first conglomerate of cells derived from the zygote gradually organize and differentiate into a recognizable human being. He then briefly explains the embryonic development of an organism from fertilization, and proposes his interpretation of an integrating center during human embryology to be: at the zygote level, the nucleus; at the morula level, some inner cell mass; at the embryonic level, tissues leading to the formation of the brain.[70] He concludes by pointing out that to propose the beginning of brain functions as the beginning of human life is to misunderstand both the beginning of brain functions, and the beginning of human life, for it fails to explain what causes differentiation prior to brain development, and to take into account that even early brain integrating activity is probably mediated by non-neural means since nerve networks are not yet fully functional.[71]

D. THE BEST INTEREST OF THE INDIVIDUAL

In accord with prudential personalism, McCarthy's moral analysis rejects the argument of the fetus as an "unjust aggressor," for the fetus is only living according to the order and dignity proper to its stage of development.[72] Also, when evaluating risks and benefits, the risks to an individual fetus may only be justified by a corresponding benefit to itself, and not only a benefit to the community at large, since the latter would lead to justifying imposing risks on other individual members of the community for the supposed benefit of society as a whole.[73]

Moraczewski's analysis of the moral act also develops along traditional lines of the principle of double effect, as witnessed by his work on the ethical evaluation of antenatal diagnosis.[74] In it he briefly describes six diagnostic techniques: radiography, electrocardiography, sonography, fetoscopy, biopsies, and amniocentesis.[75] He states that the moral liceity of such techniques is mostly guided by the principle of double effect.[76] As long as the mother is adequately informed of the risks to herself, she might decide that the psychological benefit of knowing the condition of her baby justifies running those risks. The fetus, on the other hand, is incapable of giving informed consent, which means that if the parents consent for the fetus, they should have its best interest in mind. Due to the present lack of proportionate benefit to the fetus, he finds it difficult to justify such antenatal diagnostic procedures.[77]

E. PRENATAL DIAGNOSIS: A TAINTED PROCEDURE IN GENERAL

Within the context of human sexuality, McCarthy now turns to a moral analysis of prenatal diagnosis. While noting the relief it brings to women who are reassured of carrying a normal fetus, he states that--due to the limited possibilities of prenatal therapy--it can also lead to a very real temptation to abort defective ones.[78] Likewise, analyzing X-linked disorders, he writes that since amniocentesis can detect the sex of the fetus, some parents with a 50% risk may choose to abort any male fetus, thus automatically being willing to destroy healthy ones.[79] Similarly, he points to an average 10% false negatives and false positives when diagnosing neural tube defects prenatally, and asserts that: "Increased knowledge of genetic defects will eventually lead to better therapy and even to preventive treatment and the occurrence of these defects might actually diminish. *In the meantime, serious moral issues are raised by the use of abortion and contraception to prevent the birth of defective children* [emphasis theirs]."[80]

Defining genetic diagnosis as the procedures used to determine whether a fetus has a genetic disease, or whether a parent is a carrier of a disorder, he now deals more directly with specific prenatal diagnostic procedures such as amniocentesis (chorionic villi sampling) and fetoscopy.[81] He notes two moral problems with amniocentesis: it often leads to abortion after a positive diagnosis; it might induce miscarriage or might injure the fetus. In line with Catholic teaching he considers the former immoral. If the information obtained does not lead to any real benefit to the individual fetus, such as *in utero* treatment, he also finds the risks involved in the latter difficult to justify.[82] Since fetoscopy presents--to date--greater risks than amniocentesis, including a higher rate of miscarriages, he finds it difficult to justify "except in rather exceptional circumstances."[83] Therefore, whereas prenatal diagnosis may not be used to confirm a fetal defect in order to decide on abortion, it can be used to diagnose some benefit to the affected fetus, such as determining fetal maturity for possible early delivery and treatment (*i.e.*, in the case of Rh incompatibility).[84]

He points at two more dilemmas with prenatal diagnosis information. First, at times this information is of no use to the parent, but can endanger the life of the fetus; should a counselor convey such information? Second, if a person contemplating marriage discovers to be a carrier, and refuses to share that information with his or her intended spouse; should the counselor break the seal of confidentiality to protect the third party?[85]

Regarding treatment of genetic defects, again he asserts that, in view of the few treatments presently available, risks may not outweigh benefits, but he acknowledges the possibility of rapid development in this area.[86]

In another article, McCarthy returns to the theme of selective abortion after prenatal diagnosis, and now provides three ethical principles of prudential personalism which apply to its moral analysis: respect for life,[87] promotion of health and bodily integrity,[88] and the power to procreate.[89] Applying these principles to prenatal diagnosis and genetic counseling, he asserts when they can be used in truly therapeutic situations, but that selective abortion of defective fetuses is not true therapy.[90]

He acknowledges some benefits to be gained by amniocentesis in specific clinical situations, but also points to its dangers. If amniocentesis is competently used during the third trimester for some direct benefit to the fetus, he has no moral objection.[91] But, when used early in the second trimester--with no possibility of therapy--, then it is much more difficult to justify the risks involved.[92] Regarding cooperation, he points out that, since over 90% of women receiving a positive diagnosis opt for abortion, in order not to incur complicity, a Catholic facility should: secure some assurance from the mother before the testing that she will not pursue abortion; offer counseling and support whereby abortion is effectively discouraged.[93] The reason for this is that, unlike pregnancy testing, amniocentesis is able to provide the specific information about the fetus which is used as the basis for the decision to abort, making the testing agency a necessary collaborator.[94] He concludes thus:

> The testing process cannot be adequately justified on the grounds that otherwise a more widespread unjust killing would occur. Referring back to the transcultural exceptionless norm against killing the innocent, this norm does not become less binding on pro-life health care facilities, even if society at large were killing greater numbers of innocent individuals. I thus conclude with my initial comment: amniocentesis for genetic diagnosis raises special ethical problems that must be faced.[95]

Likewise, in his other work, McCarthy discusses and discounts a number of "indications" for abortion, holding that today none of these cases absolutely threaten the expectant mother to such an extent that it is the only way to save her life,[96] and concludes that: "Pregnancy is not a disease; even seriously ill women can get pregnant an deliver normal infants. There is no absolute medical or psychological reason to abort a pregnancy. In fact, abortions can have serious medical and psychiatric side effects."[97]

Moraczewski's moral analysis of prenatal diagnosis follows similar lines. He notes that because medicine can now diagnose *in utero* far more diseases than it can treat, it is difficult to justify risks. Yet he does recognize some benefits, such as early delivery for early treatment.[98] But he also notes that since these conditions are treated after birth, it is likewise less risky to test for them after birth. In addition, he points out that if one considers the mother the sole patient in antenatal diagnosis, then all genetic defects can be "treated" by abortion.[99] In fact, he believes that the increased use of antenatal diagnosis is closely linked to the legalization of abortion in the United States.[100]

Relating antenatal diagnosis to genetic screening and counseling again points to its limited moral use, in view of the present narrow capacity for *in utero* treatment combined with the legal right to abort. Granted that other advantages of antenatal diagnosis may be: reassuring the parents of a normal fetus (if indeed the case), and monitoring viability for a possible early delivery and treatment when applicable, he holds that most women undergoing testing today are not concerned about antenatal therapy,[101] rather they at least contemplate abortion as the solution to a positive diagnosis.[102] He explains: "This attitude is another reason why amniocentesis appears to be such a tainted procedure to those who are opposed to abortion: the major explanation for most women's wanting to know whether their child is affected seems to be that they plan to abort the child if it is shown to be 'defective.'"[103] He also acknowledges the possibility of using antenatal diagnosis followed by abortion for sex selection, but rejects it as immoral.[104]

In sum regarding amniocentesis,[105] even in the vast majority of cases where there is no direct therapy for the unborn, he mentions three instances where it might be approved: First, if parental anxiety over a birth defect is such that it might compromise the pregnancy, a negative diagnosis would actually be an indirect form of fetal therapy.[106] Second, a positive diagnosis may help parents and doctors plan and prepare for what is possible: early treatment if applicable, or emotional and other support if no treatment is available.[107] Third, possibly, if the parents testing for a particular defect would have no problem justifying their actions to the individual after he or she had reached a mature age.[108]

In another article,[109] Moraczewski further points out that genetic counselors, in addition to possessing adequate medical knowledge, should also be familiar with the ethical issues involved, and that Catholic counselors may not advocate certain options--such as selective abortion or contraceptive sterilization--, even though they may be forced to mention them by law. He likewise foresees occasions where information may be withheld from a client (pregnant mother) if conveying such information can cause harm but no benefit--though he admits that a patient has a basic right to pertinent information. Finally, he notes that a Catholic medical facility may indeed provide for prenatal diagnosis and counseling, as long as these activities are not associated in any way with the promotion of selective abortion or contraceptive sterilization.[110]

In a later work, Moraczewski again addresses prenatal diagnosis,[111] and the ethical implications therein.[112] He begins by briefly describing four main prenatal diagnostic tools: ultrasonography, amniography, fetoscopy, and amniocentesis.[113] He then discusses amniocentesis in greater detail, pointing out six indications for it: maternal age;[114] a couple with a previous child with a nondisjunctional chromosome abnormality;[115] when a parent is a carrier of a chromosome abnormality (such as translocations);[116] parents who are carriers of inborn errors of metabolism;[117] mothers who are carriers of X-linked diseases;[118] and a family with a history of neural tube defects.[119] He then considers three possible risks involving amniocentesis. First is the risk of miscarriage, which today has been proven to be no greater than natural ones. Second is the risk of fetal trauma, which today can be minimized by perfected techniques and concomitant use of ultrasound. Third is the risk of amnionitis, which is very rare today and can be avoided by using sterile techniques, but which is very serious when present.[120] He concludes by acknowledging that these techniques are becoming safer with time.[121]

In yet another article, Moraczewski evaluates the issue of a Trisomy 13 infant.[122] In it he asserts that prenatal diagnosis may better prepare the parents to accept such a child, but it may also lead them to choose abortion.[123] He affirms that, due to the many pressures on the pregnant mother of a child diagnosed with Trisomy 13, the Christian attitude of all those concerned for her (husband, siblings, other relatives, genetic counselor, and friends) should be to give her support and encouragement during and after her pregnancy.[124]

Finally, Moraczewski wrote another brief article where he opposes preimplantation diagnosis, since it presently involves too much risk to the embryo.[125]

F. A PRAGMATIC BIAS

McCarthy has addressed two shifts in medicine regarding prenatal life and conflict situations: both have led to a mentality of "eugenic abortion" whereby the direct killing of a fetus is considered "treatment."

The first shift is what he considers to be part of an ever greater social pragmatic bias when seeking to solve conflict situations.[126] When applied to prenatal diagnosis, he acknowledges the benefits of the procedure, yet--due to the present legal and cultural acceptance of abortion--he points to the danger of amniocentesis becoming a tool for eugenic abortions.[127] He concedes that some have justified the possibility of very early abortion if the conceptus is not yet ensouled, but asserts that by the time amniocentesis is done, there can be no question about the humanity of the fetus.[128] He also notes that some justify eugenic abortion of a defective fetus as a merciful release from suffering, but counters that killing is not a Catholic cure for suffering.[129] He concludes that, since eugenic abortion is not a valid option of genetic defect treatment: "Hence the technology of amniocentesis, when undertaken to discover genetic defects, offers a new and extremely grave temptation to succumb to the pragmatic bias of our culture."[130]

The second shift in medicine which he notices is an increasing tendency to accept killing as a type of "treatment."[131] When applied to prenatal life, he notes that some are considering eugenic abortion to be a type of "medical treatment,"[132] and points out that, traditionally, medicine has proposed options to treat or not to treat, but this new option is to treat or to kill. Again he rejects such new approach because the humanity of the fetus at this stage is no longer in question,[133] and concludes that: "Only through semantic gymnastics can one suppose that both alternatives in the option either to treat or to kill represent genuine care for an infant or fetus."[134]

Moraczewski, on his part, has already noted some possible dangers of national genetic screening programs,[135] and what should be the proper attitude of Christian genetic counselors,[136] which implies the rapid growth of a new medical field of genetic counseling. He is also concerned that the new shift toward nondirective counseling which seeks to respect the freedom of conscience of patients, might neglect to respect the conscience of the counselor who is opposed to abortion of defective fetuses. On the other hand, failing to mention abortion as one of the options may cause the counselor to incur in legal liability for "wrongful life" or "wrongful birth."[137]

G. AGAINST DISCRIMINATION OF THE WEAKER

One sees from the aforesaid that McCarthy and Moraczewski follow the official teaching of the Church regarding prenatal life and conflict situations. In fact, they exhort the Church's hierarchy and the Christian faithful to witness to their faith by showing a special concern for all those affected by genetic defects, and to actively work and pray towards upholding their dignity and opposing their discrimination, including legal protection. Their interest, then, is to be able to enter into significant dialogue on this topic, both with the medical profession and with society at large.[138]

Notes

[1]McCarthy DG, Bayer EJ, **Handbook of Critical Life Issues**. St. Louis, MO: Pope John XXIII Medical-Moral Research and Education Center 1982.

[2]McCarthy and Bayer, **Critical Life Issues**, 10-12.

[3]McCarthy and Bayer, **Critical Life Issues**, 15-24. See also: McCarthy DG, Bayer EJ, **Handbook on Critical Sexual Issues**. St. Louis, MO: Pope John XXIII Medical-Moral Research and Education Center 1983, 3-10.

[4]McCarthy and Bayer, **Critical Life Issues**, 27-40.

[5]McCarthy and Bayer, **Critical Life Issues**, 65-74.

[6]McCarthy DG, Moraczewski AS, **An Ethical Evaluation of Fetal Experimentation: An Interdisciplinary Study**. St. Louis, MO: Pope John XXIII Medical-Moral Research and Education Center 1976.

[7]McCarthy and Moraczewski, **Fetal Experimentation**, 41-63.

[8]Note that the National Commission discusses fetal experimentation within the topic of *human subjects* of biomedical and behavioral research. See: McCormick, *Experimentation*, 5.1-5.14.

[9]"For example, healthier fetuses do not have *more* developing humanness than the less healthy ones. Those with a more satisfactory genetic heritage do not have *more* developing humanness than those, for example, with a genetic predisposition for sickle cell anemia." McCarthy and Moraczewski, **Fetal Experimentation**, 71-74; here 74.

[10]Atkinson GM, Moraczewski AS, eds, **Genetic Counseling, The Church, and The Law**. St. Louis, MO: Pope John XXIII Medical-Moral Research and Education Center 1980.

[11]"...the cost of allowing him [the fetus] to live is assessed along with the projected social benefit of doing so; and unless the individual's net balance of benefit over cost is greater than a required minimum, his life is judged unworthy of preservation and his direct killing can be justified and even declared obligatory." Atkinson and Moraczewski, **Genetic Counseling**, 105-106; here 106.

[12]Atkinson and Moraczewski, **Genetic Counseling**, 106-107.

[13]Atkinson and Moraczewski, **Genetic Counseling**, 107-108.

[14]Atkinson and Moraczewski, **Genetic Counseling**, 108.

[15]Atkinson and Moraczewski, **Genetic Counseling**, 107-108.

[16]Atkinson and Moraczewski, **Genetic Counseling**, 108-110.

[17]Atkinson and Moraczewski, **Genetic Counseling**, 113-161.

[18]Atkinson and Moraczewski, **Genetic Counseling**, 115-131.

[19]This, they say, is due to the inherent dignity of each individual ("affected" or not), which comes from being created, known and loved by God. Atkinson and Moraczewski, **Genetic Counseling**, 122.

[20]Atkinson and Moraczewski, **Genetic Counseling**, 131-132.

[21]Atkinson and Moraczewski, **Genetic Counseling**, 133-138.

[22]McCarthy DG, "Ethical principles and genetic medicine" in: Moraczewski AS, ed, **Genetic Medicine and Engineering: Ethical and Social Dimensions**. St. Louis, MO: Pope John XXIII Medical-Moral Research and Education Center 1983, 87-99.

[23]McCarthy, *Ethical principles*, 88.

[24]McCarthy, *Ethical principles*, 88-92.

[25]McCarthy, *Ethical principles*, 92.

[26]McCarthy DG, ed, **Beginnings of Personhood: Inquiries into Medical Ethics I**. Houston, TX: Institute of Religion and Human Development 1973, 65-70.

[27]McCarthy, **Beginnings**, 65.

[28]McCarthy, **Beginnings**, 66.

[29]"The continuity discussed above appears in this context as the continuity of a self-determining activity. If personhood consists in self- determination, it comprehends at once an actual

achievement and the nature which provides the potential for this achievement... Even the mature person is never completely self-determining, but always in reciprocal relationship with his surroundings. And that dynamic process began with conception..." McCarthy, **Beginnings**, 67.

[30]They refrain from defining the fetus a "human person" for now to avoid the theological and philosophical commitment involved in such terminology. McCarthy and Moraczewski, **Fetal Experimentation**, 15.

[31]McCarthy and Moraczewski, **Fetal Experimentation**, 15.

[32]They call this organic criterion a processural approach to human personhood: the fetus is in development, just like any other stage of human life. McCarthy and Moraczewski, **Fetal Experimentation**, 22-26; here 26.

[33]McCarthy and Moraczewski, **Fetal Experimentation**, 29-30; here 29.

[34]"Personalist philosophers have balanced their belief in the dynamic process of human growth and development with an equally strong belief in the continuing identity of the person as the ontological basis for that same growth and development." McCarthy and Moraczewski, **Fetal Experimentation**, 34.

[35]McCarthy and Moraczewski, **Fetal Experimentation**, 34.

[36]McCarthy and Moraczewski, **Fetal Experimentation**, 34.

[37]"Personhood is a status conferred or bestowed upon a member of the human species by the society of human persons." Atkinson and Moraczewski, **Genetic Counseling**, 60.

[38]"The second alternative proposes that full humanhood is a state into which a human organism develops or grows at some time after the point of conception." Atkinson and Moraczewski, **Genetic Counseling**, 60.

[39]"According to this position, a human being or person begins to exist from the time of fertilization-conception and ceases to live only when the human body is no longer alive, when it ceases to function as a living unity." Atkinson and Moraczewski, **Genetic Counseling**, 60.

[40]Atkinson and Moraczewski, **Genetic Counseling**, 62-64.

[41]Atkinson and Moraczewski, **Genetic Counseling**, 66.

[42]Atkinson and Moraczewski, **Genetic Counseling**, 68-71.

[43]Atkinson and Moraczewski, **Genetic Counseling**, 60-61.

[44]"*i.e.*, an activity carried on from within the organism itself, ordered to its own completion, and based on the distinctive genetic component present from the time of fertilization." Atkinson and Moraczewski, **Genetic Counseling**, 70-71; here, 70.

[45]Atkinson and Moraczewski, **Genetic Counseling**, 75.

[46]Atkinson and Moraczewski, **Genetic Counseling**, 78-85.

[47]Atkinson and Moraczewski, **Genetic Counseling**, 85-92.

[48]Atkinson and Moraczewski, **Genetic Counseling**, 92-97.

[49]Moraczewski AS, ed, **Genetic Medicine and Engineering: Ethical and Social Dimensions**. St. Louis, MO: Pope John XXIII Medical-Moral Research and Education Center 1983, 101-119.

[50]Moraczewski, **Genetic Medicine**, 103.

[51]Moraczewski, **Genetic Medicine**, 104-105.

[52]Moraczewski, **Genetic Medicine**, 106-107.

[53]"On a cosmic scale, we are not merely passive observers, but we are--within divine providence--active participants responsible for shaping, directing, and influencing the world and the time frame of events." Moraczewski, **Genetic Medicine**, 109.

[54]Moraczewski, **Genetic Medicine**, 110-111.

[55]Moraczewski, **Genetic Medicine**, 112.

[56]Moraczewski, **Genetic Medicine**, 112.

[57]"Yet present and future technological endeavors in the field of genetics--or indeed technology generally--must be directed and tempered by an ethic inspired by the wisdom of the Gospel." Moraczewski, **Genetic Medicine**, 117.

[58]Epigenic development (ontogenic) is not to be confused with the evolution of species (philogenic), for the saying that "ontogeny recapitulates phylogeny" is known today to apply only in a very broad sense. McCarthy and Moraczewski, **Fetal Experimentation**, 30.

[59]McCarthy and Moraczewski, **Fetal Experimentation**, 32.

[60]McCarthy and Moraczewski, **Fetal Experimentation**, 30-33.

[61]"...the newly formed human embryo is, from its very first days, preparing itself to be a parent to another human embryo years later...*Within four days* of conception, the hardly more than microscopic new embryo has succeeded in producing certain cells which will eventually become sperm or ova...*Thus, along with building up its own structure, one of the first things a new embryo does is to provide cells for the future existence of yet another entirely* distinct human being [emphasis theirs]." McCarthy and Bayer, **Critical Life Issues**, 80-81. See also: McCarthy D, "Testimony for the Subcommittee on investigations and oversights" *LinacreQ* 51 (1984) 315-321.

[62]"Once begun, this newly fertilized ovum, like all others, immediately begins to organize itself into an orderly body all its own. Its 'right' and 'left' are immediately established on each side of the place where the sperm entered the ovum, and from that point grows all the symmetry with which we are so familiar in our own bodies. Its 'top' is established at the other end from the 'bottom.' These points of 'length' and 'width' being settled from the outset, the production of RNA and other chemicals increases at what will become the 'back' of the newly fertilized ovum, while such synthesis is somewhat notably sparser at the 'front.'" McCarthy and Bayer, **Critical Life Issues**, 82.

[63]McCarthy and Bayer, **Critical Life Issues**, 86-87.

[64]McCarthy and Bayer, **Critical Life Issues**, 88-90.

[65]Moraczewski AS, "Can science identify human beings?" *EthMed* 6,7 (1981) 2-3.

[66]See: "Senate commences hearings on 'human life'" *Science* 212,4495 (1981) 648-649.

[67]Moraczewski AS, "No brain and yet alive" *EthMed* 16,12 (1991) 1-2.

[68]Moraczewski, *No brain*, 1.

[69]Sass H-M, *National Catholic Reporter* (Dec. 14, 1990) 3, in: Moraczewski, *No brain*, 1.

[70]Moraczewski, *No brain*, 1-2.

[71]Moraczewski, *No brain*, 2.

[72]McCarthy, **Beginnings**, 69.

[73]McCarthy and Moraczewski, **Fetal Experimentation**, 16.

[74]Atkinson and Moraczewski, **Genetic Counseling**, 13-29.

[75]Atkinson and Moraczewski, **Genetic Counseling**, 13-15.

[76]"The required conditions, or presuppositions, are that the action itself under consideration is not morally evil, that the intention is good, and that the proportionately good effect is not obtained by means of evil effects." Atkinson and Moraczewski, **Genetic Counseling**, 19.

[77]Atkinson and Moraczewski, **Genetic Counseling**, 13-19.

[78]McCarthy and Bayer, **Critical Sexual Issues**, 145.

[79]McCarthy and Bayer, **Critical Sexual Issues**, 146.

[80]McCarthy and Bayer, **Critical Sexual Issues**, 147.

[81]Chorionic villi sampling is given the same moral evaluation as amniocentesis. McCarthy DG *et*

al, **Handbook on Critical Sexual Issues**. Revised Edition. Braintree, MA: Pope John XXIII Center 1989. 144. See also: Moraczewski AS, "Some moral dimensions in genetic counseling" *HospProgr* 61,10 (1980) 52-55.

[82]"The moral principle which is operative here is that the child may not be subjected to risks unless they are balanced by realistically estimated benefits, not for someone else, but for the infant." McCarthy *et al*, **Critical Sexual Issues** (1989), 156-157; here 157.

[83]McCarthy *et al*, **Critical Sexual Issues** (1989), 157.

[84]McCarthy *et al*, **Critical Sexual Issues** (1989), 158-159.

[85]He estimates that the counselor is not obliged to inform the other person, but that he or she should do everything possible to convince the carrier of conveying such information. McCarthy *et al*, **Critical Sexual Issues** (1989), 159.

[86]McCarthy *et al*, **Critical Sexual Issues** (1989), 160.

[87]"This means it is evil to kill any innocent members of the human family. Those who recognize the unborn to be members of the family would also prohibit their killing." McCarthy, *Ethical principles*, 93.

[88]Whereas therapeutic medicine promotes individual health, nontherapeutic experimentation does not. Therefore, it can only be justified if proper consent has been obtained from the individual. See: McCarthy, *Ethical principles*, 94.

[89]Which he subdivides into two principles: respect, and responsible use. Regarding respect, he holds that the exceptionless principle condemning the direct destruction of the procreative power parallels the one on directly destroying innocent human life. Regarding responsible use, he maintains that this includes the obligation which certain couples who are affected with genetic disorders may have to not procreate (*i.e.*, if chances are 25% or better that they would beget an abnormal child). McCarthy, *Ethical principles*, 94-95.

[90]"If genetic diagnosis is performed to prevent the birth of a defective child, it is not accurate to say that genetic medicine has prevented the defect. Physicians have prevented the birth but have not really dealt with the defect." McCarthy, *Ethical principles*, 95.

[91]McCarthy, *Ethical principles*, 97.

[92]One possible justification might be if a negative diagnosis will considerably reduce maternal anxiety, which might indirectly benefit the fetus. McCarthy, *Ethical principles*, 97.

[93]McCarthy, *Ethical principles*, 97.

[94]McCarthy, *Ethical principles*, 97-98.

[95]McCarthy, *Ethical principles*, 98.

[96]*i.e.*, kidney, heart and lung disease, diabetes, cancer, high blood pressure, hypertension, psychosis, rape, incest, and genetic disease of the fetus. McCarthy and Bayer, **Critical Life Issues**, 101-104.

[97]McCarthy and Bayer, **Critical Life Issues**, 104.

[98]"For example, the development of the fetus of a diabetic mother can be monitored in order that the child may be delivered prior to term, after it has become viable but before damage has occurred. Rh incompatibility provides a similar example. A few genetic conditions, such as PKU and galactosemia, may be treated by restricting the diet of the child." Atkinson and Moraczewski, **Genetic Counseling**, 19. See also: Moraczewski AS, "Some moral dimensions in genetic counseling" *HospProgr* 61,10 (1980) 52-55.

[99]Atkinson and Moraczewski, **Genetic Counseling**, 19-20.

[100]Atkinson and Moraczewski, **Genetic Counseling**, 20.

[101]"For example, the estimation has been made that ninety-five percent of all antenatal tests would be done for Down's syndrome alone if all pregnant women over the age of thirty-five were

tested." Moraczewski, **Genetic Counseling**, 22-23; here 23. It is well known, of course, that there is no (antenatal) treatment to correct Down's syndrome.

[102]"Indeed, one observer has suggested that prenatal diagnosis should not even be undertaken unless the family is already committed to an abortion if one is deemed 'appropriate'." Atkinson and Moraczewski, **Genetic Counseling**, 23.

[103]Atkinson and Moraczewski, **Genetic Counseling**, 23.

[104]Atkinson and Moraczewski, **Genetic Counseling**, 23-24.

[105]Note the percentage of risk at the time of their writing: "Here again, how the objective, quantitatively stated risk associated with amniocentesis, namely, 1.5% of increased rate of spontaneous abortion, is *perceived* by a couple will greatly influence a judgment." Atkinson and Moraczewski, **Genetic Counseling**, 129.

[106]Atkinson and Moraczewski, **Genetic Counseling**, 127.

[107]They acknowledge, however, that this might also have the opposite effect on parents of rejecting instead of accepting the affected child. Atkinson and Moraczewski, **Genetic Counseling**, 127.

[108]Atkinson and Moraczewski, **Genetic Counseling**, 128.

[109]Moraczewski, *Moral dimensions*, 52-55.

[110]Moraczewski, **Genetic Counseling**, 53-55.

[111]Moraczewski, **Genetic Medicine**, 15-29.

[112]Moraczewski, **Genetic Medicine**, 101-119.

[113]Moraczewski, **Genetic Medicine**, 16-19.

[114]Usually at age 35 or older. Moraczewski, **Genetic Medicine**, 19-20.

[115]This may result in too many or too few chromosomes. Moraczewski, **Genetic Medicine**, 20-21.

[116]Balanced translocations may produce normal offspring, whereas imbalanced ones may result in chromosomal abnormalities in future generations. Moraczewski, **Genetic Medicine**, 21-22.

[117]There are hundreds of these metabolic errors; most are enzyme deficiencies, and are autosomal recessive. Moraczewski, **Genetic Medicine**, 22-24.

[118]At his writing, about one hundred X-linked disorders have been identified; sons have a 50% chance of being affected, and daughters have a 50% chance of being carriers. Moraczewski, **Genetic Medicine**, 24-25.

[119]The fact that a parent has a history of NTD does not necessarily mean that he or she is a carrier. Also, the percentage of risk varies with the type and degree of defect. In addition, there is approximately a 10% false negative rating when testing for AFP. Moraczewski, **Genetic Medicine**, 25.

[120]Moraczewski, **Genetic Medicine**, 25-26.

[121]Moraczewski, **Genetic Medicine**, 26.

[122]Moraczewski AS, "Trisomy 13 -- a dilemma" *EthMed* 11,2 (1986) 1-2.

[123]Moraczewski, *Trisomy 13*, 1.

[124]Moraczewski, *Trisomy 13*, 2.

[125]Moraczewski AS, "Test tube embryo testing" *EthMed* 17,5 (1992) 3-4.

[126]McCarthy DG, "Amniocentesis and our pragmatic bias" *EthMed* 4,4 (1979) 2-3.

[127]McCarthy, *Amniocentesis*, 2.

[128]"The fetuses discovered defective by amniocentesis are usually four to five months old, far too developed to speculate about delayed ensoulment." McCarthy, *Amniocentesis*, 2.

[129]McCarthy, *Amniocentesis*, 2.

[130]McCarthy, *Amniocentesis*, 3.

[131]McCarthy DG, "The either/or of genetic defect" *EthMed* 8,3 (1983) 1-2.

[132]See: Langman J, **Medical Embryology**, 4th ed. Baltimore: Williams and Wilkins 1982, 117.

[133]"These fetuses can hardly be called 'potentially' human; they *are* human. They have fully formed organ systems, thriving brains, and complex central nervous systems. They respond readily to pain and pleasure, and appear fully human to the naked eye. Christian philosophers are generally agreed that such fetuses must be considered to be animated by a spiritual soul with the promise of immortal life. Yet, killing these little individuals (whom some wish to call 'fetuses') is now designated by Dr. Langman a valid 'medical approach' to their care." McCarthy, *Either/or*, 1.

[134]McCarthy, *Either/or*, 2.

[135]Atkinson and Moraczewski, **Genetic Counseling**, 107-108.

[136]Atkinson and Moraczewski, **Genetic Counseling**, 131-138.

[137]Atkinson and Moraczewski, **Genetic Counseling**, 25-29. See also: Moraczewski, **Genetic Counseling**, 52, where he notes that nondirective counseling need not be valueless.

[138]Atkinson and Moraczewski, **Genetic Counseling**, 141-161.

CHAPTER IX

RICHARD A. McCORMICK, SJ, and LISA SOWLE CAHILL

A. SOCIALITY, COMPROMISE, AND REASONABLE ASSUMPTIONS

At least three of McCormick's basic values on prenatal life and conflict situations can be gleaned from his literature over the past twenty years: his principle of intersubjectivity, his theory of compromise, and his understanding of what can be reasonably assumed.

The principle of intersubjectivity or sociality he uses to evaluate the morality of actions. This may be seen in two of his articles:

The first one is the Pere Marquette Theology Lecture, wherein McCormick analyzes direct and indirect voluntariety.[1] In doing so, he discusses the status of the human fetus in such a way as to imply that its capacity for intersubjectivity is the determining factor between a good or an evil act on the fetus.[2] Yet his language regarding fetal personhood is ambiguous. He states:

> For instance, to redescribe emptying the womb of a nonviable fetus as 'destroying or removing the effects of rape' could be a rather hasty way of depersonalizing the fetus. The intention is, indeed, removing the effects of rape. But the most immediate, obvious, irrevocable implication of this removing is the destruction of nascent life. The language of intention dare not disguise this fact and suffocate the full implications of our conduct. To be consistent intersubjectivity must include all the subjects and the fetus cannot be that easily verbalized out of significance. We may characterize the action as 'removing the effects of rape,' but the question remains: is this morally appropriate when these effects are a person, or nascent human life?[3]

From this writing, it is not yet clear what he means by "nonviable fetus." If it is not yet a person; how can it be depersonalized? If it is not a subject; why can't it be treated as an object? If it is nascent human life; how does it differ from nascent human person? Still further on, when weighing the life of the mother versus the life of the fetus, he equates the fetus with a child.[4]

The second article deals with the treatment or nontreatment of infants with birth defects,[5] where he again returns to the notion of intersubjectivity, suggesting that the difference between treatment and nontreatment ought to be the potential for human relationships, or lack thereof.[6] However, here he fails to specify who makes the decision whether the "grossly malformed infant" is capable of human relationships or not.

Similarly, Cahill addresses the morality of abortion as a social rather than an individualistic issue.[7] Acknowledging the present unpopularity of criticizing the "pro-choice" position, she begins her analysis by grounding it in the biblical theme of protecting the weakest, and in the Catholic tradition of social ethics. She then notes that the status of fetal life is fundamental, even if not the exclusive issue to the discussion, and describes her own position as "developmentalist," meaning that the fetus increases in value with time of gestation.[8] She accepts the language of rights, but in a communal rather than in an individual context, for to maintain that in a pregnancy only the mother has rights may be too individualistic. She believes that such individualism is rooted in a liberalism that considers communal life secondary. By contrast, Catholic tradition speaks of the interdependency of human life where working for the common good is normative.[9]

In a section on *Dualism and Corporeality*, she rejects a Greek-Cartesian dualism (which tends to define the body as "bad," and resisted by the spirit), in favor of a Christian body-spirit unity. Applied to pregnancy, this unity implies a normal fetal dependence on its mother such that the mother does not simply have freedom over her own and her child's body, but that: "The body makes peculiar demands, creates peculiar relationships, and grounds peculiar obligations."[10] Maintaining that our culture shows a dualistic denial of our corporeality when, for example, we demand "perfect" cures by the medical arts and when we deny any moral connection between sex and procreation, she nonetheless wants to avoid any biologism. She also wants to avoid reductionisms, such as conceding full "humanity" or "personhood" to fetuses simply because they belong to the species *Homo sapiens* or begin to look like human beings at some gestational stage.[11]

Some of her basic value system can again be seen when she turns to the theme of suffering, noting that our contemporary liberal ethos finds little or no value in it--thus seeking to avoid it at all cost.[12] Against this, she asserts the value of suffering and accepts it as part and parcel of the human condition. Applied to pregnant women, this might translate into carrying an abnormal fetus to term as the morally mature course, which includes communal support for both of its members.[13] She is also very critical of an individualistic culture that values human life according to achievement and thus pressures parents to abort abnormal fetuses.[14] Instead, being that children ("abnormal" or otherwise) naturally belong in families, and families in communities, she emphasizes the moral responsibility of the human community to support nascent (and any other weak) human life--an argument which goes beyond trying to narrowly determine who is or is not a person.[15] Thus, she concludes that while the value and rights of human fetal life remain open questions, tentative answers to break the present impasse may be sought in the community's life-enhancing bias and responsibility of the stronger protecting the weaker.[16]

McCormick's theory of compromise is also seen in relation to the abortion issue, which he acknowledges to be so grave in the United States today so as to warrant even a compromise solution. Two articles are illustrative of this position:

The first article is written after 5 years of legalized abortion in the United States.[17] He considers the topic to be vitally important,[18] yet is keenly aware of the deep divisions which this issue elicits in our contemporary society. He feels that its seriousness demands that we come to some agreement.[19] In his view: "The core issue is, therefore, the evaluation of nascent life."[20] But he admits to having difficulty regarding the traditional Christian position that human life is inviolable from conception, mainly due to the phenomena of twinning, recombination, and high pregnancy wastage before implantation.[21]

The second article is written sixteen years later.[22] In it he proposes 20 points to keep dialogue open, touching upon a wide variety of topics, such as: respect for human life; abortion for mere convenience; alternatives; causes; public policy; enforceable laws; the fact that contraception does not seem to reduce abortions; hospital policy; no shouting, etc. While none of his topics have a direct relationship with the moral dilemmas surrounding prenatal diagnosis, his argument is important insofar as it touches on the moral status of the fetus. He suggests that the racism of abortion has now become so pervasive in the United States (1.3 to 1.5 million annually), that even the option of a middle ground should be considered in order to keep dialoguing.[23]

Lastly, McCormick's understanding of what can be reasonably assumed is evident throughout his discussions of experimentation and proxy consent. Basically, he maintains that the parents of a child may grant consent for both therapeutic and nontherapeutic treatments as long as there is minimal or negligible risk since it is reasonable to assume that the child would choose what he ought to choose, and he ought to choose what is good for himself and for humanity at large.[24] This principle he later applies to experimentation involving prenatal life.[25]

B. VIABILITY AND DISCERNIBLE RISK OR DISCOMFORT

In 1975, the U.S. National Commission for the Protection of Human Subjects of Biomedical and Behavioral Research--of which McCormick was a member--, published an appendix on research on the fetus.[26] In it, McCormick begins to define his basic philosophical and anthropological presuppositions regarding the status of the human fetus. In this report he also acknowledges that one's particular view of the nonviable fetus will make a difference with regard to one's analysis of which experimentation is permissible and which is not.[27] He states that a viable fetus should be treated as a child,[28] and a non-viable fetus (as an experimental subject), as follows:

In Utero	*Extra Uterum*
- No abortion contemplated	- Spontaneous abortion
	- living
- Abortion planned	- dead
- prior to abortion	
- during abortion	- Induced abortion *
- after abortion *	- living
- living	- dead
- dead	(* Probably identical in all decisive respects)[29]

He then states that with regard to experimentation on children, there are two identifiable schools: one which does not allow the child to be submitted to any risk, harm, or "offensive touching;" the other which does, as long as the risk is negligible. He supports the latter,[30] again based on his earlier argument that one may reasonably assume that a child would choose what he or she ought to, could he or she do so.[31]

Regarding fetal experimentation, he believes there are also two schools: one that sees fetuses as nonpersons or as "potential human life," thus without any claims or rights, and another that considers them protectable humanity.[32] The second school he further subdivides into three: 1) "The fetus is protectable humanity but to be valued less than a viable fetus or a born infant."[33] 2) "The fetus is a fellow human being and must be treated, where experimentation is concerned, exactly as one treats the child."[34] 3) Is basically the same as 2), "However, experiments on children, where no discernible risk or discomfort is involved, are morally legitimate if appropriate consent is obtained and if the experiments are genuinely necessary (trials on animals being insufficient) for medical knowledge calculated to be of notable benefit to fetuses or children in general."[35] He espouses the third view.[36]

He is trying to differentiate between the morality of abortion and the morality of fetal experimentation. That is why he earlier sought to distinguish between a fetus *in utero* and a fetus *extra uterum*. Accordingly, the morality of abortion depends on whether the fetus is an individual person or not, while the morality of fetal experimentation is based on treating the fetus as one would a child: "In summary, then, within the parameters of my evaluation of fetal life, fetal experimentation would be clearly justified, with appropriate safeguard, distinctions and consent, where the abortion is spontaneous or has been justifiably (morally) induced."[37]

Concluding his report, he proposes the following conditions for fetal research:

- the experiment must be necessary;
- there must be no discernible risk to the fetus or the mother;
- the above must be secured by prior approval and review.[38]

Further philosophical and anthropological presuppositions show in another article where he continues to explore the relationship between fetus and child.[39] This time he draws an analogy between infanticide and abortion.[40] He proposes that moral consistency demands that those who accept abortion of fetuses with congenital defects should also accept euthanasia of infants afflicted with the same defects. Granted that the claims of the fetus are physically dependent claims, and that those of the infant are physically independent of the mother, yet neither claim is morally different, otherwise the claim for human existence would become relevant to subjective approval or disapproval by others.[41] Hence, he concludes that, as relevant as personal factors are to the quality-of-life argument, they are not normative when deciding existence and personhood.[42]

C. GENETIC UNIQUENESS AND DEVELOPMENTAL INDIVIDUALITY

McCormick's theory of delayed hominization is most clear in an article on human life before implantation.[43] He believes that personal human life can only occur after implantation. To support his thesis he cites biological evidence, which distinguishes between genetic uniqueness (at fertilization), and developmental individuality (at implantation).[44] Once more he cites as the evidence of the lack of developmental individuality before implantation, the possibility of twins, of chimeras, and the development of extraembryonic layers from the blastocyst.[45]

He then criticizes Ford's book[46] because, even though Ford distinguishes between genetic uniqueness and developmental individuality, he concludes that there is still reasonable doubt about this fact, and that when in doubt, one should abstain.[47] McCormick contends that reasonable doubt of fact may allow one to proceed or act if there is enough reason to act, since true certainty is rarely required for human action.[48] He holds that the preembryo's lack of developmental individuality before implantation is sufficient reason to doubt its personhood.[49] He concludes: "And if the preembryo is not yet a person, it cannot be the subject of human rights."[50] Yet he still calls for respect for preembryos on two counts: because they have the potential to become a human person in the full sense of the word; because trivializing preembryo research may lead to further trivialization of embryonic research, etc., especially if results are promising.[51]

Lastly, he affirms that nontherapeutic research on preembryos cannot be excluded in principle, but he offers two proposals regarding its regulation: First, in view of the uncertainties still surrounding the issue, the preembryo should be treated *prima facie* as a person. Second, in view of its importance, any exceptions from this *prima facie* duty should be based on nationally established criteria.[52]

D. LIFE AND VALUES PROPORTIONAL TO LIFE

McCormick's analysis of the moral act regarding prenatal life and conflict situations is again couched within his treatment of the issue of abortion.[53] He returns to the crucial theme of evaluating nascent life: "By 'human life' I mean human life from fertilization or at least from the time at or after which it is settled whether there will be one or two distinct human beings."[54] He continues to express doubt regarding twinning, high number of spontaneous abortions, and recombination, and asserts that: "In doubt one generally favors life--but I think not always."[55]

On the issue of social policy, he would allow abortion when the alternative is tragedy, but not when it is inconvenience: "Such a policy would prohibit abortion unless the life of the mother is at stake; there is a serious threat to her physical health and to the length of her life; the pregnancy is due to rape or incest; fetal deformity is of such magnitude that life-supporting efforts would not be considered obligatory after birth."[56] He then mentions other social factors which vie against a positive fetal evaluation, such as present sexual practices,[57] fascination with technology, a utilitarian attitude, influence of the media, and an "overpopulation" mentality.[58]

Later on, McCormick published his first Notes on Moral Theology, this time doing a survey of the literature on moral issues from 1965 to 1980.[59] In a section dealing with abortion,[60] he explains his position on the matter to be very similar to that of Curran: individual human life only after twinning and recombination are no longer possible: "Thereafter life may be taken only if necessary 'to protect life or other values proportionate to life.'"[61] Hence, fetal life should be taken only as a lesser of evils; where at stake is a value comparable to life (e.g., self-defense, just war, capital punishment, indirect killing).[62] He also notes that today's discussion about hominization parallels previous discussions about animation, which he finds somewhat strained.[63]

Then he gives both a pastoral opinion and a policy opinion. He states that pastoral opinion should not be confused with the ongoing theological discussion, and that in a culture saturated with unwanted pregnancies there is a prophetic need to critique and transcend cultural limitations.[64] His policy position is similar to the pastoral one in that it seeks to look at the common good. He does not want a law that is more restrictive than the Catholic position, yet, in a pluralistic society; why should the Catholic position be normative? He thus concludes that the debate must continue.[65]

In his section on bioethics,[66] he discusses the issue of fetal and infant experimentation, noting that the issues are different if one considers the fetus as human as opposed to non human ("only maternal tissue"). The latter presents no problem for experimentation, as long as maternal health is safeguarded, whereas the former requires restrictions.[67]

Finally, discussing *in vitro* fertilization,[68] he once more touches on the unborn, suggesting three guidelines regarding abortion and discarded zygotes: First, the focus should not be on the possible personhood of the zygote, since many theologians and philosophers doubt it. Second, it is different to fertilize *in vitro* for achieving a pregnancy, than for experimenting on the product of conception (respect for nascent life rules out the latter). Third, if a high number of spontaneous discards naturally occur before implantation, what is wrong with accepting a similar ratio in an artificial procedure intended for the same purpose, namely, to achieve pregnancy?[69]

E. PRENATAL DIAGNOSIS AND COOPERATION

McCormick's analysis of moral dilemmas in prenatal diagnosis proper may be best seen in his book dealing with issues in medical ethics.[70] In it he analyzes the ethical guidelines for Catholic health care institutions. Regarding the unborn, he notes that guideline #15 rejects abortion because it violates the respect due to individual human life.[71] Here he identifies three problem areas: first, the status of the preimplanted embryo;[72] second, whether or not anencephalic fetuses have a sufficient biological substratum to be included among the morally protectable against abortion;[73] third, whether or not a natural rupture of membranes may or may not be medically completed to avoid the possibility of serious maternal infection.[74] The last two conditions are presently easily detectable by prenatal diagnosis. As noted earlier, the vast majority of fetuses diagnosed to carry some defect are aborted. For this reason, the question has been raised whether Catholic hospitals should be associated with any kind of prenatal diagnosis.[75] He maintains that they should because counseling against abortion and in support of the pregnancy may actually save fetuses that would otherwise be killed. He also states that: "Technically, amniocentesis (where an indication of fetal defect is followed by abortion) is a form of cooperation in the wrongdoing of another. But this cooperation is material, remote, and unnecessary--conditions that make it easier to justify."[76] Hence, to justify prenatal diagnosis, a policy of supporting problem pregnancies must be in place, and should include: not recommending abortion; respecting handicapped nascent life; knowledge of services for the handicapped; medically up to date on lessening or correcting handicapping conditions; and supporting programs that help the handicapped.[77]

He then discusses *in utero* interventions, stating that: "There are many aspects of this procedure that have ethical dimensions: for instance, safety, cost, risk to the mother, risk to the fetus, locus of decision. At some point or other, these dimensions are all intertwined and it is difficult to consider such cases abstractly in terms of a single dimension."[78] Therefore, he concentrates on a single case: hydrocephalic shunt. After the analysis, he concludes that there are three possibilities: to do nothing, to abort or to perform *in utero* surgery. He proceeds: "From a Catholic moral point of view, the second option is no option. The first option (do nothing) would depend on the state of the art and the risks to mother and fetus. As a general statement--and that only--I would suggest that where effective treatment is available and the risks are acceptably low, treatment is the only morally defensible alternative."[79] Nonetheless, he notes that those who allow for abortion, logically would accept only a much lower maternal risk and a much higher surgery success rate. Either way, *in utero* surgery now provides a third option which cannot be ignored.[80]

Finally, he discusses fetal experimentation, especially nontherapeutic, reiterating his allowance of it so long as risk is minimal.[81]

F. AN EUGENIC MENTALITY

McCormick frames the current shift in the self-understanding of medicine within a broader social shift toward greater individual rights on the one hand, and greater technological control on the other. The sum of these tendencies may also lead to a greater intolerance of "defectives." This is apparent in an article wherein he reflects on what he considers to be the twelve most important ethical issues in a decade.[82] First is abortion, with a close second being what he calls an "eugenic mentality" whereby only the "perfect" child is acceptable, facilitated today by prenatal diagnosis techniques.[83] He concludes that we must seriously think about these issues and come to some social consensus, lest they rule us.[84]

Cahill also acknowledges the present shift in medicine, and calls for a renewed approach to medical ethics.[85] She maintains that Catholics theology today has expanded the "natural law" tradition to include also the social dimensions of the patient. Since abortion is now a complex social and economic issue, it means that today it is not sufficient to simply condemn unwanted pregnancies; rather social and economic alternatives are needed.[86] Overall, she calls for a renewal of Catholic medical ethics by incorporating biblical, social, and experiential dimensions.

Always seeking to uphold the social accountability of medical ethics, Cahill wrote another article in which she addresses the subject of prenatal life.[87] Therein she contends that, in addition to the already-known moral dilemmas in abortion, the RU 486 pill poses new questions for moral analysis due to its capacity to further privatize abortion.[88] This also lessens public accountability of all concerned:

mother, father, physician, and society at large. Yet she seems to espouse a "gradation" evaluation whereby contraception would be preferable to abortion, and an early abortion to a late one.[89] She notes that RU 486 was presented in France as an "antigestation" pill by its inventors, and that the French team views "fertilization" as encompassing both fusion of gametes and implantation (nidation, placentation). Thus, by preventing implantation, RU 486 is considered to be "contraceptive." But she describes how British bishops have opposed redefining fertilization, a basic biological process. She also describes how the American Fertility Society, the Ethics Advisory Board of the Department of Health, Education, and Welfare, the American College of Obstetrician and Gynecologists, the Warnock Report, and various Australian bioethics committees all give special status to the preembryo, even if not full personal status.[90]

She then analyzes the language used in the report of the American research team, language which may be misleading, for it portrays RU 486 as a "contraceptive" while actually accepting its use after first menses, that is, after implantation (14 days after fertilization). She criticizes such misleading language,[91] because she contends that, even if the preembryo has "less" status than the embryo-fetus, he or she should not be thoughtlessly destroyed: RU 486 may allow for that.[92] She estimates that, if introduced into the U.S., it would considerably diminish late abortions, thus forcing the pro-life movement to re-evaluate their emphasis/strategy away from the evil of late abortions toward the contemporary debate on the status of the preembryo. Overall, this might diminish the present impact of the pro-life movement. She concludes by restating that, while an early abortion is preferable to a late one, privatizing it to such a degree might further lessen the moral obligation to avoid unwanted pregnancy rather than ending it.[93]

G. AN EVALUATIVE QUESTION

McCormick takes issue with the magisterium regarding prenatal life and conflict situations. This may be seen, for instance, when he analyzes the moral status of nascent life, this time in reference to *in vitro* fertilization and experimentation.[94] He restates his position that contemporary embryology points to a lack of developmental individuality in the early days after fertilization.[95] Since the status of the preimplanted embryo is an evaluative question and not a scientific one, he concludes that: "Therefore, I do not believe that nascent life at this stage makes the same demands for protection that it does later."[96] Yet, due to lack of unanimity on the subject, he counsels prudence: "Specifically, I believe that there should be a policy presumption against experimentation on embryos and that exceptions to this should be allowed only after scrutiny and approval by an appropriate authority."[97]

In another work, he again discusses the moral status of the preembryo, noting that it is not a new issue.[98] Rather, it follows a centuries-old debate of immediate or delayed animation; the two most recent church documents to address it are the *Declaration on Procured Abortion* (1974) and *Donum vitae* (1987). Regarding the latter, he points to inconsistencies in the language: one section of the document states that the "zygote is a person"[99] and another section says that the zygote should be "treated as a person."[100] He claims that the inconsistencies occur because these documents fail to differentiate between genetic uniqueness and developmental individuation.[101]

Cahill also takes issue with the magisterium in an article which again touches on the subject of prenatal life and conflict situations.[102] In it she examines two issues regarding the beginning of human life: abortion and reproductive technologies. Regarding abortion, she expounds on Cardinal Joseph Bernardin's "seamless garment" metaphor, or "consistent ethic of life," including the following: that abortion is not only a religious, but also a moral and philosophical issue; that there is no consensus condoning permissive abortion policy in the United States; and that moral principles should have practical, social consequences.[103]

Discussing the beginning of human life, she cites both Cardinals O'Connor and Law, who maintain that based on medical-biological evidence, life begins at fertilization.[104] But she counters that physical constitution is not sufficiently convincing. What is needed is to present the arguments supporting such position, of which she detects three possibilities:

> (1) At conception there are present the characteristics necessary and sufficient to constitute 'a human life in the full sense,' 'a human being with equal right,' 'a person,' etc. (2) Even if it is not possible to establish the constituents and moment of 'full' humanity, the conceptus must always be regarded as *absolutely* immune from direct destruction. (3) Diverging from the recent magisterium: the fetus, whether a 'person' or not, may be destroyed directly in dire circumstances and/or before a certain stage of development, e.g., threat to maternal life, or evacuation of uterine contents immediately after rape.[105]

She goes on to review an article by Carol Tauer,[106] who claims a weakness in the magisterium's argument prohibiting abortion due to the fact that it does not allow for probabilism. Tauer says that the *Declaration on Abortion* treats doubt about the status of an embryo as a "doubt of fact," but she contends that whereas the biological origin and development of the embryo (facts) are not in doubt, what is in doubt is its ontological and moral standing --a "doubt of law"--, hence probabilism is applicable.[107] Based on this, Cahill suggests that some of the traditionally held principles of the magisterium regarding abortion need revision.[108]

Concerning reproductive technologies, she points out how these also touch on the status and rights of the human embryo. Her point of departure is the Warnock Report,[109] noting that a similar debate is presently developing in the United States. She cites Richard McCormick as representative of this debate, in his treatment of the reality of pluralism in American society today and in the need for more ecumenical dialogue on the subject. Nonetheless--in view of the potentiality of the embryo--it must be significantly respected, otherwise further "erosion of respect for human life" is risked.[110] She concludes by saying that McCormick calls for prudential judgment, and that: "His suggestion demonstrates that if any consensus about IVF (or abortion) is to be achieved before every ethical unclarity is resolved, then that consensus will of necessity be limited to the middle ground, probably provisional, and not susceptible of universally persuasive 'proof.'"[111]

Lastly, Cahill published another article in which she touches on nascent life, but only tangentially, within a treatment of the public policy of medical ethics issues.[112] She proposes that the moral positions of the Catholic Church can and should influence public policy, but that in order to do so the arguments must be intelligible even to those who do not espouse Roman Catholicism. Regarding medical ethics issues, she seeks to avert the individualism of both the right ("duty to treat every person equally") and the left ("right to privacy"), emphasizing instead human sociality and interdependence.[113] She concludes that it is appropriate for the

Church (hierarchy) to address specific issues of social policy, but that its effectiveness lies in its broad consultation and consensus.[114]

Notes

[1]McCormick RA, **Ambiguity in Moral Choice**. Washington: Georgetown 1973.

[2]"Removing a nonviable fetus from the womb can be intersubjectively abortion (murder), removal of the effects of rape, saving the life of the mother and so on." McCormick, **Ambiguity**, 15.

[3]McCormick, **Ambiguity**, 22-23.

[4]"For instance, the saving of the mother is an aspect of the abortifacient act equally immediate, morally speaking, as the death of the child." McCormick, **Ambiguity**, 43; "The matter can be urged in another way. Suppose we are faced with a situation (suggested by Philippa Foot) with the following alternatives: an operation which saves the mother but kills the child, versus one that kills the mother but saves the child." McCormick, **Ambiguity**, 50-51. See also: "A concrete vehicle for bringing these questions [direct/indirect killing] into clearer focus is the classic, even if rare, obstetrical case where the physician faces two options: either he aborts the fetus and thus saves the mother, or he does not abort and both mother and child die." McCormick RA, "Reflections on the literature" in: McCormick RA, Curran CE, eds, **Readings in Moral Theology No.1: Moral Norms and Catholic Tradition**. New York: Paulist 1979, 294-340; here 331.

[5]McCormick RA, "To save or let die: the dilemma of modern medicine" *JAMA* 229,2 (1974) 172-179. See also: McCormick RA, "Saving defective infants: options for life or death" *America* 148,16 (1983) 313-317; McCormick RA, **How Brave a New World? Dilemmas in Bioethics**. New York: Doubleday 1981, 339-351.

[6]"Life's potentiality for other values is dependent on two factors: those external to the individual, and the very condition of the individual. The former we can and must change to maximize individual potential. That is what social justice is all about. The latter we sometimes cannot alter. It is neither inhuman nor un-Christian to say that there comes a point where an individual's condition itself represents the negation of any truly human--*i.e.*, relational--potential. When that point is reached, is not the best treatment no treatment? I believe that the *implications* of the traditional distinction between ordinary and extraordinary means point in this direction [emphasis his]." McCormick, *To save*, 175.

[7]Cahill LS, "Abortion, autonomy, and community" in: Callahan S, Callahan D, eds, **Abortion: Understanding Differences**. New York: Plenum 1984, 261-276. See also: Cahill LS, "Abortion, autonomy, and community" in: Jung PB, Shannon TA, eds, **Abortion and Catholicism: The American Debate**. New York: Crossroad 1988, 85-97.

[8]"My position on fetal status might be characterized as 'developmentalist' insofar as I view its values as incremental throughout gestation." Cahill, *Abortion*, 85-86; here 86.

[9]Cahill, *Abortion*, 87-89.

[10]Cahill, *Abortion*, 89-91; here 89.

[11]Cahill, *Abortion*, 89-91.

[12]Cahill, *Abortion*, 91-92.

[13]Cahill, *Abortion*, 92.

[14]"Our culture tends to estimate the value of human life in direct proportion to its level of physical and intellectual perfection or achievement. This attitude leads to the inability of parents and others to envision creatively or positively the task of raising an abnormal child, and it creates widespread support of abortion for so-called fetal indications. A question that often could be pressed

more critically is whether the abortion is intended primarily to serve the interests of the family (in its 'freedom') or of the fetus (in a 'happy' life), and in either case, what criteria of evaluation are used.

"The liberal individualistic theory of moral responsibility comes into play not only in the moral weight usually given to freedom, but also because society often seems to see parents as responsible for avoiding the births of defective (and hence burdensome) children; social willingness to provide structures of assistance for severely handicapped individuals and their families decreases correspondingly." Cahill, *Abortion*, 92-93.

[15]Cahill, *Abortion*, 93-94.

[16]Cahill, *Abortion*, 94-95.

[17]McCormick RA, "Abortion: rules for debate" *America* 139,2 (1978) 26-30. See also: McCormick RA, Walters L, "Fetal research and public policy" *America* 132,24 (1975) 473-476; McCormick, **How Brave**, 176-188.

[18]"If this is what many people think it is (unjustified killing of human beings, in most cases), then it certainly constitutes the major moral tragedy of our country." McCormick, *Abortion: rules*, 26.

[19]McCormick, *Abortion: rules*, 26.

[20]McCormick, *Abortion: rules*, 28.

[21]McCormick, *Abortion: rules*, 28.

[22]McCormick RA, "Abortion: the unexplored middle ground" *SecondOp* 10 (1989) 41-50.

[23]"The idea of an unexplored middle ground and the invitation to explore it will please few. Yet the abortion problem is so serious that we must grasp at any straw. A nation that prides itself on its tradition of dignity and equality for all and the civil rights to protect that equality cannot tolerate a situation in which 1.3 to 1.5 million human fetuses are being denied this equality and these rights. We must at least continue to discuss the problem openly. Quite simply, the soul of the nation is at stake. Abortion's pervasiveness represents a horrendous racism of the adult world. When it is justified in terms of rights, all of our rights are endangered because their foundations have been eroded by arbitrary and capricious application.

"For this reason (and for many others) I think it important that abortion continue to occupy a prime place in public consciousness and conversation, even though we are bone-weary of the subject. If we settle for the status quo, we may be presiding unwittingly at the obsequies of some of our own most basic, most treasured freedoms. That possibility means that any strategy--even the modest one of keeping a genuine conversation alive by suggesting a middle ground as its subject--has something to recommend it." McCormick, *Abortion: unexplored*, 49.

[24]"...it is a reasonable presumption of the child's wishes, a construction of what the child would wish, if he could do so." McCormick RA, "Experimental subjects: who should they be?" *JAMA* 235,20 (1976) 2197.

[25]McCormick RA, "Experimentation in children: sharing in sociality" *HastingsCRep* 6,6 (1976) 41-46; McCormick, **How Brave**, 87-98; McCormick RA, "Proxy consent in the experimentation situation" *Perspectives in Biology and Medicine* 18,1 (1974) 2-20; McCormick and Walters, *Fetal research*, 473-476.

[26]McCormick RA, "Experimentation on the fetus: policy proposals" in: **U.S. National Commission for the Protection of Human Subjects of Biomedical and Behavioral Research. Appendix: Research on the Fetus.** Washington: Department of Health, Education, and Welfare 1975, 5.1-5.14. See also: McCormick, **How Brave**, 72-86.

[27]"If one regards the fetus as 'disposable maternal tissue' or as 'potential human life' only, then the questions are sharply different and will yield a different moral conclusion, and ultimately a different

public policy. If, however, the nonviable fetus is viewed as 'protectable humanity' or a 'person' with rights, then the problems are quite similar." McCormick, *Experimentation on the fetus*, 5.2.

[28]"By the term 'nonviable fetus' I understand a fetus incapable of extra-uterine survival. (Attention in this study will be restricted to the nonviable fetus because I shall suppose that in all decisively relevant moral and policy respects touching experimentation, the viable fetus should be treated as a child.)" McCormick, *Experimentation on the fetus*, 5.1-5.2.

[29]McCormick, *Experimentation on the fetus*, 5.2. See also: McCormick RA, "Fetal research, morality, and public policy" *HastingsCRep* 5,3 (1975) 26-31, where he further refines his position by omitting from the *in utero* scheme two categories from the planned abortion: before abortion, and living after abortion.

[30]"I have attempted to argue for a position that would allow experimentation on children where there is no discernible risk or undue discomfort." McCormick, *Experimentation on the fetus*, 5.3.

[31]"The heart of my argument is this: If we analyze proxy consent where it is accepted as legitimate (sc., in the therapeutic situation) we will see that parental consent is morally legitimate because, life and health being goods for the child, he would choose them because he ought to choose the good of life. In other words, proxy consent is morally valid precisely insofar as it is a reasonable presumption of the child's wishes, a construction of what the child would wish could he do so. The child would so choose because he ought to do so. Life and health being goods definitive of his flourishing." McCormick, *Experimentation on the fetus*, 5.3-5.4.

[32]McCormick, *Experimentation on the fetus*, 5.4.

[33]"This school would probably tolerate experiments if the benefits are great, but no literature has made this conclusion explicit." McCormick, *Experimentation on the fetus*, 5.4, both quotes.

[34]"Just as the child may not be exposed not only to harm and risk, but also to 'offensive touching,' so the fetus may not be exposed to any risk or even to 'offensive touching.'" McCormick, *Experimentation on the fetus*, 5.4 both quotes.

[35]McCormick, *Experimentation on the fetus*, 5.4-5.5.

[36]McCormick, *Experimentation on the fetus*, 5.5.

[37]He emphasizes that the legitimacy of such experimentation is based on obtaining the proper proxy consent, which is an extrapolation of that involving experimentation on children. McCormick, *Experimentation on the fetus*, 5.7.

[38]McCormick, *Experimentation on the fetus*, 5.14.

[39]McCormick RA, "Life-saving and life-taking: a comment" *LinacreQ* 42,2 (1975) 110-115.

[40]"... if one approves abortion for serious genetic defect, must he in moral consistency approve infanticide for those who have slipped though the amniocentesis screen?" McCormick, *Life-saving*, 111.

[41]"To accept these as establishing a 'morally relevant difference' between abortion and euthanasia of the newborn is to accept human perceptions as normative -which is, unless something further is added, to forfeit the capacity to criticize these perceptions." McCormick, *Life-saving*, 114.

[42]McCormick, *Life-saving*, 115.

[43]McCormick RA, "Who or What is the Preembryo?" *KennedyInstEthJ* 1,1 (1991) 1-15.

[44]"I contend in this paper that the moral status--and specifically the controversial issue of personhood--is related to attainment of developmental individuality (being the source of one individual). This contrasts with the view that holds that personhood occurs earlier, at the point of genetic uniqueness. I believe that an embryo that has developed to the point where it can be one individual and one individual only, differs in moral status from a preembryo that has not, even if in many cases we may choose to treat them similarly." McCormick, *Preembryo*, 2.

[45]"As the blastocyst is attaching to the uterine wall, the inner cell mass becomes more adherent

and organizes onto two layers that make up the embryonic disc or primitive body axis. The process is reflected in the appearance of the primitive streak. It is at this point that developmental individuality or singleness can be said to be established.

"From this discussion, I would underscore two particularly important facts. First, early events in mammalian development concern, above all, the formation of extraembryonic--rather than embryonic--structures....

"Second, genetic individuality and developmental individuality do not coincide." McCormick, *Preembryo*, 4. Here he is dependent on Grobstein C, **Science and the Unborn**. New York: Basic Books 1988, 25.

[46]Ford NM, **When Did I Begin? Conception of the Human Individual in History, Philosophy and Science**. Cambridge: Cambridge U. Press 1988.

[47]McCormick, *Preembryo*, 10-11. See also: Ford N, "Letters: ethics, science, and embryos" *Tablet* Feb 3 (1990) 141-142.

[48]McCormick, *Preembryo*, 11. See also: Mahoney J, **Bioethics and Belief**. London: Sheed and Ward 1984, 79.

[49]He also mentions the failure of the *Declaration on Procured Abortion* and of *Donum vitae* to distinguish between genetic uniqueness (which the preembryo has) and developmental individuality (which it lacks). McCormick, *Preembryo*, 11-12.

[50]McCormick, *Preembryo*, 12.

[51]McCormick, *Preembryo*, 12.

[52]McCormick, *Preembryo*, 13.

[53]McCormick RA, "Abortion: a changing morality and policy?" *HospProgr* 60,2 (1979) 36-44. He begins in a similar fashion as the previous article (noting that over a million abortions are performed annually in the United States), and adds the new compounding phenomenon of "test-tube babies." See also: McCormick, **How Brave**, 189-206. A summary of his general methodology regarding where to begin the moral analysis in bioethics, is found in: McCormick RA, "Bioethics in the public forum" *MilbankMemQ* 61,1 (1983) 113-116.

[54]McCormick, *Abortion: changing morality*, 39.

[55]McCormick, *Abortion: changing morality*, 39.

[56]He mentions the last one hesitantly because it is subject to abuse. McCormick, *Abortion: changing morality*, 41.

[57]"Unless a genuine cultural change occurs in regard to sexuality [pure pleasure, sex without marriage, separate eros from philia, etc], I have little hope for a shift in fetal evaluation." McCormick, *Abortion: changing morality*, 42.

[58]McCormick, *Abortion: changing morality*, 43-44.

[59]McCormick RA, **Notes on Moral Theology: 1965 through 1980**. Washington: University Press of America 1981.

[60]McCormick, **Notes**, 473-520.

[61]McCormick, **Notes**, 499. See also: Cahill LS, "Teleology, utilitarianism, and Christian ethics" *TS* 42 (1981) 601-629.

[62]McCormick, **Notes**, 515.

[63]McCormick, **Notes**, 516.

[64]McCormick, **Notes**, 516-517.

[65]McCormick, **Notes**, 517-520.

[66]McCormick, **Notes**, 561-573.

[67]McCormick, **Notes**, 569.

[68]McCormick, **Notes**, 785-800.

[69]McCormick, **Notes**, 796-597.
[70]McCormick RA, **Health and Medicine in the Catholic Tradition**. New York: Crossroad 1984.
[71]McCormick, **Health**, 12.
[72]Mostly due to the aforementioned doubts raised by twinning, recombination, spontaneous wastage, hydatidiform moles, extraembryonic layers. McCormick, **Health**, 134.
[73]McCormick, **Health**, 135.
[74]"If nature has started a process (with extremely low fetal survival expectation and rather high incidence of serious maternal infection in attempting to bring the fetus to term), does human completion of this process deserve the rejection implied in the term 'abortion'?" McCormick, **Health**, 135.
[75]Some maintain that performing prenatal diagnosis when the results are used for deciding to abort is cooperating in what is morally wrong. McCormick, **Health**, 140.
[76]McCormick, **Health**, 141. See also: McCormick RA, "Bioethical issues and the moral matrix of U.S. health care" *HospProgr* 60,5 (1979) 42-45.
[77]McCormick, **Health**, 141-142.
[78]McCormick, **Health**, 142.
[79]McCormick, **Health**, 142.
[80]McCormick, **Health**, 142-143.
[81]"I myself argued [in the 1970s] that the fetus and the child are members of the human community and may be expected to render minimal service to that community if there is not significant cost to themselves. In other words, the child or the fetus could not reasonably object to such research if it offered significant hope of benefit (unattainable in other ways) without discernible risk.

"While this may not be a Catholic idea as such, it is consistent with traditional Catholic concerns." McCormick, **Health**, 143-144.
[82]McCormick RA, "1973-1983: value impacts of a decade" *HospProgr* 63,12 (1982) 38-41.
[83]"The cultural acceptance of abortion plus the availability and increasing accuracy of prenatal diagnosis (amniocentesis, ultrasonography, maternal serum alpha fetoprotein testing) have given powerful support to what may be called a 'eugenic mentality.' This phrase is meant to summarize the attitude of many people toward the procreation of children. It is accurate to say that increasingly in the minds of many only the 'perfect' baby is an acceptable baby. Thus we frequently hear the phrase 'the right to a healthy child.' Furthermore, there is an increase in tort cases for wrongful life. Acceptance of contrived neglect of defective newborns is increasing.

"These are but symptoms of a massive new change in attitude. From caring for the deprived and dependent we increasingly plan them out of existence. They are seen as an unnecessary burden. It is not an exaggeration to say that the procreative process is becoming in some sense a shopping process, with the baby becoming a consumer item. This attitude is fertile soil for the growth of the 'eugenic mentality,' planned breeding. The ultimate form of this is what we call 'positive eugenics,' the preferential breeding of so-called superior individuals." McCormick, *Value impacts*, 38-39.
[84]McCormick, *Value impacts*, 40-41.
[85]Cahill LS, "A fresh approach to Catholic health care ethics" *HealthProgr* 68,1 (1987) 20-21.
[86]Cahill, *Fresh approach*, 21.
[87]Cahill LS, "'Abortion pill' RU 486: ethics, rhetoric, and social practice" *HastingsCRep* 17,5 (1987) 5-8.
[88]"RU 486 poses additional difficulties for moral analysis because it enables very early

termination of pregnancy, but potentially privatizes the abortion decision to such an extent that moral scrutiny could be evaded almost entirely." Cahill, *Abortion pill*, 5.

[89]Cahill, *Abortion pill*, 5.

[90]Cahill, *Abortion pill*, 5-6.

[91]"If the issues of whether a fertilized ovum has any greater moral significance than an unfertilized one, and whether that value increases at implantation, are ignored or concealed by language, the moral seriousness of chemical termination of early pregnancy has not been appreciated." Cahill, *Abortion pill*, 7.

[92]Cahill, *Abortion pill*, 7-8.

[93]Cahill, *Abortion pill*, 8.

[94]McCormick RA, "Therapy or tampering? The ethics of reproductive technology" *America* 153,17 (1985) 396-403. See also: McCormick RA, "Bioethics in the public forum" *MilbankMemQ* 61,1 (1983) 113-126.

[95]McCormick, *Therapy*, 402.

[96]This is based on the previously-mentioned phenomena which question the individuality of the preimplanted embryo. McCormick, *Therapy*, 403.

[97]Due to the gravity of the issue, the authoritative body should be national in character. McCormick, *Therapy*, 403.

[98]McCormick, *Preembryo*, 6-8.

[99]*Dv*, Introduction, 5.

[100]*Dv*, I, 1.

[101]McCormick, *Preembryo*, 6-8. See also: McCormick RA, **The Critical Calling: Reflections on Moral Dilemmas Since Vatican II**. Washington: Georgetown 1989, 329-352.

[102]Cahill LS, "The 'seamless garment': life in its beginnings" *TS* 46 (1985) 64-80.

[103]Cahill, *Seamless garment*, 65-66.

[104]Cahill, *Seamless garment*, 66-67.

[105]Cahill, *Seamless garment*, 70-71.

[106]See: Tauer CA, "The tradition of probabilism and the moral status of the early embryo" *TS* 45 (1984) 3-33.

[107]Cahill, *Seamless garment*, 73-74.

[108]Cahill, *Seamless garment*, 74.

[109]See: *Report of the Committee of Inquiry into Human Fertilisation and Embryology of the Department of Health and Social Security*, Chairman: Dame Mary Warnock DBE (London: Her Majesty's Stationery Office, 1984).

[110]Cahill, *Seamless garment*, 79-80.

[111]Cahill, *Seamless garment*, 80.

[112]Cahill LS, "Catholicism, ethics and health care policy" *CathLawyer* 32,1 (1988) 38-54.

[113]Cahill, *Catholicism*, 54.

[114]Cahill, *Catholicism*, 54.

CHAPTER X

THOMAS J. O'DONNELL, SJ

A. TWO SOURCES OF TRUTH

O'Donnell begins to expose his basic value system in his early work on medicine and Christian morality.[1] He opens by defining Ethics and Moral Theology:

> The study of Ethics is an investigation into the goodness or evil of human actions in the light of natural reason. Moral Theology, on the other hand, investigates the morality of human actions against the background of man's supernatural life and destiny, and with the added assistance of divine revelation.[2]

Ethics and Moral Theology are concerned with human conduct. For Catholics, and indeed for all Christians, such conduct is illumined by the teachings of Jesus Christ through his Church, which seeks to authoritatively elucidate God's will by interpreting natural and divine law.[3] Natural law is discernible by the human conscience illumined by Christ. Elucidation of Divine law, by contrast, requires an act of faith.[4]

Fifteen years later, O'Donnell published a second revised and updated edition of his work on medicine and Christian morality.[5] It is revealing to compare his new opening statement defining Ethics and Moral Theology:

> The subject matter of Ethics is generally understood to be the 'right' and 'wrong' of free human actions as indicated by natural human reason drawn from philosophical considerations. Moral Theology, on the other hand, goes beyond Ethics (although including its authentic considerations) by seeking the further light of divine revelation, as handed on and interpreted by the teaching of the Church, to enlighten questions of 'right' and 'wrong' ('moral good' and 'moral evil') in human conduct. These two sources of truth, although different in their point of origin, become one in their terminus, simply because truth is necessarily one. This study combines both, and hence is entitled 'Medicine and Christian Morality' rather than simply 'Medical Ethics.'[6]

He now states that the authentic Catholic law or norm of morality is authoritatively promulgated by the magisterium for the common good, comprises both natural and divine positive laws (accessible by natural reason and further illumined by revelation) and requires respectful internal assent.[7]

O'Donnell also edited an article where he explicates further some of his basic values regarding moral theology.[8] Seeking to address issues of sexual morality, he rejects utilitarian and proportionalistic systems. Instead, he focuses on the principles underlying *Donum vitae*: an ethic founded on the existence of a totally transcendent Supreme Being. Acknowledging that some moral norms may change from culture to culture and age to age, he maintains that certain human actions have always and everywhere been seen as either praiseworthy or blameworthy.[9] He then states what he believes to be a solid ethic: each human being is individually created; there is an observable order in nature; and we are capable of understanding such order.[10] He states that ethical Catholic medical practice is based on a twofold concept: "The two concepts are the harmonious fulfillment of redeemed human nature, and the divine will of the Creator as discernible in human affairs. These two concepts are *one* in reality because they are identical in practice. They are merely two sides of the same coin."[11] The first concept is derived from observing human nature with natural reason. This provides broad precepts, which are further illumined by divine revelation, and the teaching authority of the Church.[12] He goes on to recognize that, while there is not as yet any *de fide* definition in medical morality, certain authentic Catholic teachings deserve internal assent: pontifical decrees, instructions, encyclicals, and pontifical authorization of Sacred Congregation decisions. Remarking that *Donum Vitae* deserves such respect and acceptance by the faithful, he calls dissenting from it an error which the magisterium has rejected.[13]

B. PREROGATIVES

Some of O'Donnell's philosophical and anthropological presuppositions already emerge in his work on medicine and Christian morality, where he states that the principle of inviolability of human life is based on the existence of God and on the fundamental equality of all people.[14] Such equality resides in our common final destiny and our intrinsic dignity, which imply certain rights and duties he calls prerogatives.[15] Some prerogatives are absolute (essentially subordinated to one's final end), while others are merely of use (rights restricted by the higher rights of others).[16] Accordingly, humans only have prerogative of use over other humans; absolute prerogative belongs solely to God. Applying these principles to medicine, medical action should always be stewardship, not ownership. Hence, the physician exercises a prerogative of use delegated by the patient.[17]

His classical philosophical and anthropological systems are likewise seen in his review of Atkinson and Moraczewski's book on genetic counseling which touches, in part, on moral dilemmas in prenatal diagnosis.[18] He agrees with the two authors that maintaining the identity between "humanhood" and "personhood" is key to the discussion, and notes that these terms are related to "sanctity of life" and "quality of life," which he seeks to clarify.[19] The distinction between "humanhood" and "personhood" he holds to be like the one between "essential quality of life" (its sanctity) and "operational quality of life" (human relationships, etc.); a distinction without a difference, and therefore not substantial but accidental. Ultimately, he says that "person" is not so much being capable of knowing as of being known; a subject known by other persons, in our case by God.[20]

In a different article, he once again reveals some of his philosophical and anthropological presuppositions when doing moral theology.[21] He begins by defining law: "A law is understood to be norm or directive of free activity, enacted by legitimate authority and duly promulgated (published), and designed to safeguard and advance the common good. Thus a law must have a legislator, a method of promulgation, a specification of who is subject to the law, and some sanction for violations of the law."[22] "Moral goodness" is measured against the "norm of morality," which is formed by natural law, divine positive law and ecclesial magisterium. Natural law "is the divine design of creation insofar as we can recognize it by natural reason (by looking around us at things as they are),"[23] which is further enlightened by divine positive revelation (the Decalogue and the teachings of Christ).[24] He then distinguishes between natural and divine law (concerned with true doctrine), and the Code of Canon Law (concerned mainly with discipline), without though denying that there is much doctrine in the Code.[25]

O'Donnell also published four articles which reveal his radical belief in the fundamental equality of all human beings:

In the first article he points out present inconsistencies regarding due protection of prenatal life.[26] Such inconsistencies come by an almost-blanket acceptance of abortion on one hand, and recognizing the fetus as a patient on the other. He cites a recent case in the medical literature where two physicians "managed" a twin pregnancy, one fetus diagnosed as Down and the other normal, by killing the Down fetus *in utero* (with parental approval, of course).[27]

In the second article he very briefly addresses the issue of selective abortion after prenatal diagnosis.[28] He begins by citing cases where one or more siblings of multifetal gestation, at times resulting from infertility treatments, is prenatally diagnosed carrying some defect, subsequently to be selectively aborted. He then quotes medical opinion which maintains that proper medical infertility treatment should be able to avoid multifetal pregnancies, and that in any case these pregnancies do not necessarily indicate a high health risk condition. He concludes that the trend of selective abortion in multifetal pregnancy further erodes the principle of basic equality among all people.[29]

In the third article he petitions the medical profession for consistency when seeking to do no harm.[30] He begins by noting Archbishop Pilarczyk's recent observation that legalized abortion is inconsistent with upholding the basic principle of the U.S. constitutional right to "life, liberty, and the pursuit of happiness."[31] He then points out the incongruence of an American medical profession which seeks to disassociate itself from active euthanasia and executing the death penalty by lethal injection, but fails to disassociate itself from procured abortion. He concludes by citing correspondence of some medical doctors who are acknowledging the same contradiction.[32]

In the fourth article he begins by pointing out some inconsistencies in medical thinking when looking at prenatal life.[33] He cites a case where a mother carrying triplets gave birth (by cesarean section) to a normal child at 26.6 weeks gestation,[34] while having the other two destroyed *in utero* due to a possibly poor outcome. He notes that whereas some physicians call this "selective fetal reduction," he calls it "murder."[35] He also holds that feminists and animal-rights advocates veer away from objective truth when the former claim that abortion is part of a woman's right to do what she wants with her own body, and when the latter seek to uphold the right to life of (even pre-born) animals but not of humans.[36]

C. THE PROBABILITY OF HUMAN LIFE FROM CONCEPTION

O'Donnell never explicitly asserts immediate hominization. However, he implies it in four articles:

In the first he seeks to expose deceptive language used, in part, in early abortions.[37] He counters the pretense of the progesterone antagonist RU 486 of being promoted as a contraceptive when referred to as "menstrual regulator," or that "the drug's postovulatory actions may allow a retrospective decision not to become pregnant." It means to abort.[38]

In the second he addresses a new moral issue in the diagnosis of tubal pregnancy.[39] He notes that some physicians are questioning whether it might now be possible, with the present possibility of early diagnosis, to remove the nonviable embryo without removing the affected fallopian tube, but states that this is not licit.[40] He further clarifies, however, that removing the affected segment of tube (even containing an embryo), with anastomoses of the remaining tube if possible, is licit since: it is needed to accomplish a good end (saving the mother's life), and the destruction of the embryo is not directly intended.[41]

In the third he returns to the moral issues surrounding the RU 486 pill.[42] He criticizes its inventor, Dr. Etienne-Emile Baulieu of the University of Paris, for referring to it as a "menses-regulator" or "contragestive," and not as an abortifacient, while also claiming that such pill causes the "passage of products of conception."[43]

In the fourth he touches on the morality of preimplantation diagnosis.[44] Acknowledging the present possibility of such diagnosis leading to selective implantation of nondefective "preembryos," he notes that the concept "preembryo" is not a medical or scientific one, but one meant to avoid recognizing the presence of human life before implantation. If a "preembryo" in a petri dish is not human, how can it be subject to "trauma"?[45] He further asserts that even though for some, preimplantation diagnosis followed by selective implantation is no different than (post-implantation) prenatal diagnosis followed by elective abortion, the greater ethical concern is the ease with which some researchers seem to assume the role of human life quality controllers.[46]

Likewise, in his work on medicine and Christian morality, though holding that the Church has historically consistently condemned direct abortion, he acknowledges the speculation regarding ensoulment--noting that past judgments were based on limited scientific observation--, but finds it irrelevant at the practical level, "because the malice of abortion lies in the willingness to destroy intra-uterine life, although it is human or, in the very earliest stages of gestation, even if it is human."[47] Thus, for him the probability that there is human life from conception warrants its protection.[48]

He confirms this practical principle when he addresses the moral dilemmas of prenatal diagnosis of anencephalics.[49] Stating official Church teaching, he affirms that abortion is not an option even if the humanity of anencephalics was in doubt. The reason for this is that it would necessarily include the willingness to destroy the fetus even if he or she is human. He accepts, however, inducing labor for a legitimate medical indication.[50] Morally, he considers one legitimate reason to be lessening maternal trauma, given a confirmed diagnosis that it would not shorten the child's extra-uterine life.[51] A further possible moral benefit would be if induction of labor realistically gives the anencephalic a better chance at baptism, since many are stillborn.[52] Its moral liceity, however, presumes that inducing labor does not jeopardize the mother's health, a point which is still medically debatable.[53]

D. OBJECT, MOTIVE AND CIRCUMSTANCES OF THE MORAL ACT

O'Donnell's analysis of the moral act follows the classical lines of moral object ("What am I doing?"), motive ("Why am I doing it?") and circumstances (When? Where? How?).[54]

Also revelatory of his analysis of the moral act is his section defining some basic principles of medical ethics: law (a permanent rational norm for free activity), conscience (a judgement of the intellect about the goodness or badness of an action),[55] reflex principles (to solve doubts of conscience, such as probabilism), subjects of law (obliging all, though those without full use of reason cannot formally violate natural law), moral law (imposing an obligation directly in conscience), observance of law (thus an obligation to know the law), cessation of obligation of the law due to moral impossibility (except negative precepts of natural law), voluntary human acts,[56] the three determining elements of a voluntary act (moral object, motive and circumstance), a morally good act (whose moral object, motives and circumstances are in accord with right order), obstacles to voluntariety (ignorance, error, fear, concupiscence and habit), the principle of double effect, formal cooperation (adopting the evil intention), immediate material cooperation (which is also necessarily formal), mediate material cooperation (without evil intention), and negative cooperation (by omission; may be formal or material).[57]

Applying some of these principles mentioned above to cooperation in a therapeutic abortion, he maintains that it is difficult to see how a doctor could certify "medical" indications for abortion without formal cooperation.[58] He also analyzes three issues of cooperation in group practice involving abortions: division of funds (licit for his or her share of the work not involving abortions), abortion referrals (illicit), and scandal (morally questionable).[59]

He then seeks to clarify medical and moral terminology:

Medically, abortion is "the separation of a non-viable fetus from the uterus,"[60] which can be spontaneous (occurring naturally) or induced (precipitated artificially and purposely). An induced abortion can be "therapeutic" (to protect the life, health, or mental comfort of the mother) or "criminal" (in violation of civil law).[61]

Morally, he also distinguishes between spontaneous and induced abortion, but not between "therapeutic" and "criminal." He does distinguish, however, between "direct" (intended as an end or a means to an end) and "indirect" (foreseen but merely permitted; not intended).[62] Then he proceeds to apply these abortion categories in relation to the principle of inviolability of human life, concluding that: "Direct abortion, whether it be classified as therapeutic abortion or criminal abortion, is always and under all circumstances in direct violation of the natural law and the divine positive law. It is the usurpation of the uniquely divine prerogative of absolute dominion over human life."[63]

He goes on to describe and discount a number of "therapeutic" abortions, since today these are not truly medically indicated.[64] In ectopic pregnancies, the principle of double effect applies.[65] Finally, regarding hydatidiform moles he holds that while the embryo may have been a living human being before the neoplastic accretion began, he or she can now be presumed dead.[66] In true conflict situations, one life may not have prerogative over another, since both lives (that of the mother and that of the fetus) are of equal value; though life-saving treatment may be instituted on one, even with an unintended but foreseeable destruction of the other.[67]

E. MORAL ANALYSIS OF PRENATAL DIAGNOSIS

Early on, O'Donnell edited an article where he briefly discusses some moral dilemmas in prenatal diagnosis.[68] He begins by acknowledging the present possibility of amniocentesis for detecting some chromosomal abnormalities, and points to the results of a British study on the medical safety of this procedure (1-1.5% risk).[69] Based on these results, he counsels against general application of the technique due to over-kill of healthy fetuses ("false positives") and to the scarcity of skilled personnel. He also points at the practical impossibility of calculating possible benefits against definite risks.[70]

Somewhat later, he again addresses the morality of prenatal diagnosis.[71] Recognizing the rapid growth of the use of amniocentesis, he notes that most women who become aware of carrying a defective fetus choose to abort.[72] This presents certain moral dilemmas for physicians seeking to respect both the life of the mother and of the unborn; can he or she diagnose amniocentesis? If there is no connection to abortion, he or she can.[73] In fact, a favorable diagnosis may reassure the parents; an unfavorable one may help them and the doctors prepare better.[74] If the mother has expressed a conviction to abort a fetus found carrying defects, then the doctor should remove himself from performing the diagnosis, or from referring her to a colleague who will. Furthermore, in view of the fact that most women who find themselves carrying a defective fetus today choose abortion, a physician who regularly performs prenatal diagnosis may well require from his or her patient a pledge that she will not abort. Yet even here the procedures themselves are morally neutral.[75]

In another article, he discusses the moral implications for the Catholic physician of the intention to abort after information obtained by prenatal diagnosis.[76] Acknowledging the legal responsibility obstetricians now have to inform pregnant patients of the suspicion of birth defects, he notes that this might present a dilemma for Catholic physicians: if he knows the patient well enough to be assured that she will not abort given a negative fetal prognosis, he may proceed with the diagnosis. On the other hand, if the patient demonstrates either implicitly or explicitly a willingness to abort a defective fetus, the physician might have to remove himself from the case.[77] However, for a proportionate reason the doctor may still perform prenatal diagnosis on a woman contemplating abortion due to the principle of double effect, since the procedure is sufficiently removed from the abortion itself.[78] The Catholic doctor in this case is morally bound to identify due proportion between the intended good and the permitted evil effect before the diagnosis in order to avoid the possibility of scandal.[79]

In a later article, he seeks to clarify his position both regarding the morality of the techniques themselves, and the physician's possible cooperation in an immoral act.[80] He begins by noting that the morality of such techniques depends not on the moral object (they are not intrinsically evil), but on the circumstances[81] and the motive.[82] He then quotes John Paul II[83] and *Dv*[84] regarding the condemnation of prenatal diagnosis with a view to elective abortion, and concludes that in such a case a Catholic physician may not be involved.[85]

Lastly, in his revised book on medicine and Christian morality, within the medical-moral aspects of marriage, he briefly surmises his views on prenatal diagnosis in accordance with *Dv*:

> In addition to the strong reaffirmation of the immorality of procured abortion, the document points out that prenatal diagnostic procedures are immoral when done with the thought of possibly inducing subsequent abortion, depending upon the results of the diagnosis; that non-therapeutic research on the embryo is morally wrong while therapeutic experimental procedures which do not involve risk disproportionate to expected benefits are obviously acceptable.[86]

F. PATIENTS' WISHES AND PHYSICIANS' RIGHTS

Aware of a shift in medicine more and more toward complying with patients' rights and wishes, O'Donnell edited another article where he briefly addressed the morality of prenatal diagnosis in view of the fact that women in the United States have a legal right to abortion.[87] Affirming that there has been an increase in the number of physicians who use prenatal diagnosis with an option of abortion to accommodate patients who wish to select the sex of their offspring, he notes the Church's teaching on prenatal diagnosis.[88] He proceeds to quote the passage in *Dv* which disallows prenatal diagnosis used for inducing an abortion, and recognizes that this could mean loss of prestige and financial gain for some physicians. Commenting on an *amicus curiae* report, he also points out that viability is a bad term to use as a benchmark because it is subject to constant technological change.[89]

In another article he also asks whether legally forcing a physician to reveal fetal anomalies which might lead to abortion would not compromise the freedom of conscience of the doctor who disapproves of abortion, and states that such complex issues will eventually require the establishment of policies, which has already been done in Catholic hospitals.[90]

G. MAGISTERIAL AUTHORITY AND DISSENT

An understanding of O'Donnell's ecclesiology may be gained from his early work on medicine and Christian morality. In it he reminds the reader that the Church claims an authority which, in terms of faith and morals, is free of error. After briefly reviewing conditions of infallibility and noninfallibility, he concludes by noting that the validity of the Church's position does not rest on the credibility of the argument presented, but on its authority.[91]

A further understanding may be gained in an article where he rebuts Daniel Maguire's article on abortion and Catholic honesty.[92] He states that, contrary to Maguire's beliefs, Vatican II's condemnation of abortion is normative, the Bishops' disapproval of abortion, in union with the Roman Pontiff, is the mainstream of Catholic teaching, and that private dissent by some theologians is not sufficient ground for justifying direct abortions.[93] He concludes that Maguire has wrongly interpreted probabilism, authentic Magisterium, and even the revised Code of Canon Law.[94]

Applying this to prenatal diagnosis and genetic counseling, he addresses some difficulties which Catholic physicians might face when offering these medical services.[95] He begins by quoting literature which suggest that these procedures may lead to contraception, sterilization and abortion. He proceeds to state that the American College of Obstetrics and Gynecology may shortly be making prenatal diagnosis routinely available, which can pose moral dilemmas for the Catholic obstetrician. He then quotes the passage from *Dv* which approves of prenatal diagnosis, as long as it is not used toward inducing an abortion.[96] He also points out to Catholic physicians that dissent in this area is not an option, as stated by John Paul II on his second pastoral visit to the United States.[97] He concludes by noting that, in living the Gospel, the authentic Catholic physician may incur in financial and even legal martyrdom.

Lastly, he addresses the issue of freedom of conscience, stating that it does not mean that Catholics who do not agree with certain Church teachings are therefore free to "follow their own conscience."[98] He further takes issue with revisionists who seek to undermine the notion of intrinsic evil and the authority of the Church.[99]

Notes

[1]O'Donnell TJ, **Medicine and Christian Morality**. New York: Alba House 1976.

[2]O'Donnell, **Medicine** (1976), 6.

[3]To O'Donnell, natural law and positive law are one in their origin in God, and differ only in the method God uses to make His will known. O'Donnell, **Medicine** (1976), 11.

[4]O'Donnell, **Medicine** (1976), 6-13.

[5]O'Donnell TJ, **Medicine and Christian Morality**. Second Revised and Updated Ed. New York: Alba House 1991.

[6]O'Donnell, **Medicine** (1991), 1.

[7]O'Donnell, **Medicine** (1991), 1-7.

[8]O'Donnell TJ, "The roots of Catholic moral teaching" *MMNewsletter* 25,9 (1988) 33-36.

[9]O'Donnell, *Roots*, 33.

[10]"It all implies what we could describe in human terms as a purposeful creation rather than a random chance, and that translates into a divine design for human living that is not just of some importance, but all important. This is what the founding Fathers were saying when they wrote, 'We hold these truths to be self-evident; that all men are created...' Those words imply a rule or conduct and that is what Ethics is really all about." O'Donnell, *Roots*, 33-34.

[11]O'Donnell, *Roots*, 34.

[12]O'Donnell, *Roots*, 34.

[13]O'Donnell, *Roots*, 34-36.

[14]O'Donnell, **Medicine** (1991), 45-46.

[15]O'Donnell, **Medicine** (1991), 46-49.

[16]"A subordination of final ends implies absolute prerogative, whereas an equality of final ends admits of only a prerogative for use." O'Donnell, **Medicine** (1991), 46.

[17]O'Donnell, **Medicine** (1991), 47-49.

[18]O'Donnell TJ, "Genetic counseling, the church, and the law" *MMNewsletter* 17,6 (1980) 21-24. See also: Atkinson and Moraczewski, **Genetic Counseling.**

[19]"... the sanctity of life concept is rooted in the existence of God as Creator (a fact viewed as self-evident by the Founding Fathers of our American way of life) and the scriptural extrapolations of the absolute inviolability of human life simply because it is, in a unique way, of God.

"On the other hand, the usually accepted meaning of 'quality of life', looks rather to the operative potential of life at any given stage and condition." O'Donnell, *Genetic counseling*, 23.

[20]"The ultimate criterion of 'person' is not to be knowing, but to be known--a subject known by other persons in an I-Thou relationship rather than a subject knowing. This, we believe, is not only the common estimate of mankind but, much more importantly, the theological and scriptural data: 'The Lord called me from birth, from my mother's womb He gave me my name.' (Isaiah 49/1) How could one suppose that the earliest fetal form of the incarnate Son of God was not a person, the personal God who had entered human history in human form. Granted that His incarnation was unique, our personal biography must surely begin as His did." O'Donnell, *Genetic counseling*, 24.

[21]O'Donnell TJ, "*Beyond bioethics*" *MMNewsletter* 27,3 (1990) 9-11.

[22]O'Donnell, *Beyond*, 9.

[23]O'Donnell, *Beyond*, 9.

[24]Note that he considers natural law truly as divine law: "Thus, the natural law is not totally "natural." It is the divine design of the Creator (the eternal Law of God), imprinted in the **nature** of creation itself, and able to be recognized (and thus is promulgated) by **natural reason.** And this is why it is called the natural law, although it is properly **divine law**, *i.e.*, the Will of the Creator reflected in creation itself and promulgated by our natural reason." O'Donnell, *Beyond*, 10.

[25]O'Donnell, *Beyond*, 10.

[26]O'Donnell TJ, "Ambivalent current medical attitudes toward abortion" *MMNewsletter* 18,9 (1981) 33-34.

[27]He points out that these doctors, out of an "abundance of caution," obtained a court of law confirmation of the parents' right to consent to the "selective reduction" on behalf of the normal fetus, thus acknowledging that a "normal" human being has the right to kill another in equal developmental stage (fetal) who is affected with Down; according to this logic, some are more equal than others. O'Donnell, *Ambivalent*, 33-34.

[28]O'Donnell TJ, "Selective abortion In multiple pregnancy" *MMNewsletter* 26,2 (1989) 8.

[29]"Add to all this a survey recently reported in the *New York Times* indicating that abortions are being done with greater frequency merely on the score of sexual preference of offspring, and one sees how a civilization flounders when the basic ontology of human existence is abandoned and when the truth that 'all men are created equal' is jettisoned." O'Donnell, *Selective abortion*, 8.

[30]O'Donnell TJ, "Coherently consistent or morally meaningless?" *MMNewsletter* 28,3 (1991) 9-10.

[31]O'Donnell, *Coherently consistent*, 9.

[32]O'Donnell, *Coherently consistent*, 10.

[33]O'Donnell TJ, "Issues or objective truth?" *MMNewsletter* 29,5 (1992) 19-20.

[34]What may be the smallest recorded live infant delivered: Birth weight, 280 g; length, 25 cm; head circumference, 20 cm; gestational age at C-section, 26 weeks and 6 days; discharged at 120th day of life (44 weeks gestation); mother's age at delivery, 36, primapariens. See: Muraskas JK, Carlson NJ, Halsey C, Frederiksen MC, Sabbagha RE, "Survival of a 280-g infant" *NEJM* 324,22 (1991) 1598-1599.

[35]O'Donnell, *Objective truth*, 19-20.

[36]O'Donnell, *Objective truth*, 20.

[37]O'Donnell TJ, "Medical double-talk on abortion" *MMNewsletter* 24,1 (1986) 1-2.

[38]O'Donnell, *Double-talk*, 1.

[39]O'Donnell TJ, "Early diagnosis of tubal pregnancy: new issues" *MMNewsletter* 25,6 (1988) 23-24.

[40]He cites the Ethical and Religious Directives for Catholic Health Facilities, Directive 16: "In extrauterine pregnancy the dangerously affected part of the mother (e.g., cervix, ovary, or fallopian tube) may be removed, even though fetal death is foreseen, provided that (a) the affected part is presumed already to be so damaged and dangerously affected as to warrant its removal, and that (b) the operation is not just a separation of the embryo or fetus from its site within the part (which would be a direct abortion from a uterine appendage), and that (c) the operation cannot be postponed without notably increasing the danger to the mother." O'Donnell, *Tubal pregnancy*, 23-24; here 24.

[41]O'Donnell, *Tubal pregnancy*, 24.

[42]O'Donnell TJ, "Mifepristone: the new 'abortion pill'" *MMNewsletter* 26,2 (1989) 7.

[43]O'Donnell, *Abortion pill*, 7.

[44]O'Donnell TJ, "Ethics and production-line quality control of human life" *MMNewsletter* 28,4 (1991) 15-16.

[45]"There seems to be a strange inconsistency in the 'ethical' concerns voiced by the Jones Institute [for Reproductive Medicine, Norfolk, Virginia] and their consistent use of the term *preembryo* to designate the subject of the proposed research. If the 'preembryo' in the petri dish is viewed, however mistakenly, as some sort of not-yet-human thing, why the concern about damaging it by 'trauma' (medically defined as 'a wound or injury, whether physical or psychic')?" O'Donnell, *Quality control*, 16.

[46]O'Donnell, *Quality control*, 16.

[47]O'Donnell, **Medicine** (1991), 156.

[48]O'Donnell, **Medicine** (1991), 156-157.

[49]O'Donnell TJ, "Catholic doctors, Catholic hospitals and the prenatal diagnosis of anencephaly" *MMNewsletter* 18,10 (1981) 37-40. See also: O'Donnell, **Medicine** (1991), 177-178.

[50]O'Donnell, *Prenatal diagnosis of anencephaly*, 37-38.

[51]O'Donnell, *Prenatal diagnosis of anencephaly*, 38-39.

[52]"If induction of labor would be judged to not make any difference with regard to conferring the sacrament while the fetus was alive, it would seem that the shortening of the uterine occupancy would not be, in these circumstances, a real damage to any achievable good of the fetus." O'Donnell, *Prenatal diagnosis of anencephaly*, 39.

[53]O'Donnell, *Prenatal diagnosis of anencephaly*, 39.

[54]O'Donnell TJ, "The basic determinants of the morality of human action" *MMNewsletter* 27,6 (1990) 21-23. See also: O'Donnell, **Medicine** (1991), 20-24.

[55]The second edition contains the following clarification regarding "freedom of conscience:" "Thus, 'freedom of conscience' is not a freedom to adopt one's own moral principles independently

of the natural and divine positive law, or the norm of morality which one has recognized to be authentic. If an individual has come to accept the authenticity of the Catholic Church but decides that abortion, or contraception, or theft, or murder, or fornication or adultery are not sinful; such a one is not entitled to do these things under the rubric of 'freedom of conscience.' This would not be judging the morality of a particular action within an accepted norm, but rather changing the moral norm under the guise of 'conscience.' It is in this sense that conscience is not a *teacher* of morality." O'Donnell, **Medicine** (1991), 10-11.

[56]The second edition contains an explanation of *finis operis* and *finis operantis*: "A thing or action can have two distinct purposes, one of which is built into it (called the *finis operis*, or the purpose of the thing itself) and this may be different from the purpose of the agent, which is called the *finis operantis*." O'Donnell, **Medicine** (1991), 20-21; here 21. This section also contains his description of the "revisionist" movement: "During the 1970's there was a revisionist movement among some Catholic moral theologians both in Europe and in the United States which attempted to discredit any idea of an intrinsically evil moral object and sought to determine the morality of an action only by a simultaneous consideration of the physical action itself (devoid of any intentionality, moral formality, or *finis operis*) together with the *finis operantis* (the motive) for which it is done and the other circumstances of the act." O'Donnell, **Medicine** (1991), 23-24.

[57]O'Donnell, **Medicine** (1991), 9-43.

[58]O'Donnell, **Medicine** (1991), 40-42.

[59]O'Donnell, **Medicine** (1991), 42-43.

[60]O'Donnell, **Medicine** (1976), 137.

[61]O'Donnell, **Medicine** (1976), 137-138. In the second edition he omits the distinctions between therapeutic and criminal abortion, since he maintains that legalized abortion has now made them obsolete. O'Donnell, **Medicine** (1991), 147-148.

[62]O'Donnell, **Medicine** (1976), 138. In the second edition he adds a section explaining canonical terminology on abortion and excommunication. O'Donnell, **Medicine** (1991), 150-155.

[63]O'Donnell, **Medicine** (1976), 141-142. See also: O'Donnell, **Medicine** (1991), 154.

[64]Craniotomy, Addison's disease, breast and rectum cancer, cardiac disease, eclampsia, hyperemesis gravidarum, epilepsy, erythroblastosis fetalis, Gaucher's disease, Hansen's disease, hepatitis, Hodgkin's disease, idiopathic thrombocytopenic purpura, kyphoscoliosis, leukemia, lupus erythematosus, multiple sclerosis, myasthenia gravis, chronic polyarthritis, psychiatric illness, phocomelia, polyarteritis nodosa, pulmonary tuberculosis, renal disease and hypertension, maternal rubella, varicose veins, pregnancy hemorrhage, abruptio placentae, placenta previa, threatened, imminent and inevitable abortion. O'Donnell, **Medicine** (1976), 154-198.

[65]O'Donnell, **Medicine** (1976), 198-203. See also: O'Donnell, **Medicine** (1991), 162-168.

[66]O'Donnell, **Medicine** (1976), 175-176. See also: O'Donnell, **Medicine** (1991), 178-180.

[67]O'Donnell, **Medicine** (1976), 136. In the second edition he adds a clarification regarding cesarean sections: "Cesarean section for the removal of a viable fetus is permitted, even with risk to the life of the mother, when necessary for successful delivery. It is likewise permitted, even with risk for the child, when necessary for safety of the mother." O'Donnell, **Medicine** (1991), 146.

[68]O'Donnell TJ, "Amniocentesis and the defective child" *MMNewsletter* 16,3 (1979) 9-11.

[69] O'Donnell, *Amniocentesis*, 9-10.

[70]O'Donnell, *Amniocentesis*, 10-11.

[71]O'Donnell TJ, "Amniocentesis and abortion - the courts and the moral conscience" *MMNewsletter* 17,5 (1980) 17-20.

[72]O'Donnell, *Amniocentesis and abortion*, 17.

[73]O'Donnell, *Amniocentesis and abortion*, 18-19.
[74]O'Donnell, *Amniocentesis and abortion*, 19.
[75]O'Donnell, *Amniocentesis and abortion*, 19-20.
[76]O'Donnell TJ, "Wrongful pregnancy, wrongful birth, wrongful life" *MMNewsletter* 23,10 (1986) 37-40.
[77]O'Donnell, *Wrongful pregnancy*, 37-38.
[78]"Indeed, one could not even say that a subsequent abortion would be the evil effect of his action, albeit indirect. The evil effect would be the 'occasion,' at most, of the sinful act of abortion on the part of the patient. And if she is already determined to seek prenatal diagnosis and possible subsequent abortion, the physician's cooperation in the abortion instead could be judged to be somewhat remote as well as not-necessary." O'Donnell, *Wrongful pregnancy*, 38.
[79]O'Donnell, *Wrongful pregnancy*, 38.
[80]O'Donnell TJ, "Prenatal screening: some moral considerations" *MMNewsletter* 29,4 (1992) 13-14.
[81]"In regard to the circumstances, since the small but still significant risk is primarily to the life of the unborn child, it should be evident that prenatal screening should be performed only when there is expectation of some direct or indirect benefit to the fetus." O'Donnell, *Prenatal screening*, 13.
[82]"It is a deplorable fact that when there is a possibility that the fetus may not be completely normal in its development, the techniques of prenatal screening often become 'search and destroy missions.' In fact, some physicians prefer chorionic villi sampling over amniocentesis because the former can be done earlier in the pregnancy, thus offering the opportunity for earlier (and somewhat safer) abortion." O'Donnell, *Prenatal screening*, 13-14.
[83](*Discourse to Participants in the Pro-Life Movement Congress*, Dec. 3, 1982) O'Donnell, *Prenatal screening*, 14.
[84]*Dv* I,2; O'Donnell, *Prenatal screening*, 14.
[85]"In view of all this, it seems clear that a Catholic physician, faithful to the teachings of the Church, should have nothing to do with a case in which prenatal diagnosis might be followed by abortion. Indeed, the physician would do well to rule out this expectation before performing or making a referral for prenatal diagnosis. The Catholic physician whose advice was the determining element in a patient's decision to have an abortion would be a necessary cooperator in the crime of abortion and thus would automatically incur an excommunication (see Canons 1398 and 1329, no. 2). When there is a conflict of moral convictions in the physician-patient relationship, physicians have the option of withdrawing from the case rather than letting the patient impose her moral convictions upon the physician." O'Donnell, *Prenatal screening*, 14.
[86]O'Donnell, **Medicine** (1991), 242. Regarding fetal experimentation, he seems to undergo certain development: in his first edition he approves it as a last resort to save its life (in which case the "experiment" may be considered therapy), applying the same norms of research and consent as for other incompetent populations. See: O'Donnell, **Medicine** (1976), 98-99. However, in his second edition he holds that therapeutic research may be done when it offers greater hope than any other remedy available, but not non-therapeutic since one may not assume that the particular incompetent would consent to the specific procedure. See: O'Donnell, **Medicine** (1991), 112-113.
[87]O'Donnell TJ, "Roe vs. Wade: have the abuses helped turn the tide?" *MMNewsletter* 26,4 (1989) 15-16.
[88]"Reviewing the Church's teaching on prenatal diagnosis according to the classical fonts of morality (moral object, motive, and circumstances), we find that prenatal diagnosis in itself as a moral object offers no problem under the *circumstances* of parental consent and due safeguards for

both mother and fetus, without disproportionate risks. The procedure can become gravely immoral, however, because of an immoral motive or in morally unacceptable circumstances." O'Donnell, *Abuses*, 16.

[89]O'Donnell, *Abuses*, 16.

[90]O'Donnell, *Amniocentesis and abortion*, 20. See also: NCCB, *Ethical and Religious Directives for Catholic Health Facilities*, Washington, DC: USCC 1979.

[91]"The credibility of the conclusion rests on the teaching charism with which Christ has endowed His Church, not in the ideas proposed to illustrate the reasonableness of the conclusion." O'Donnell, *Beyond*, 10-11; here 11. See also: O'Donnell, **Medicine** (1991), 7.

[92]O'Donnell TJ, "'Abortion and Catholic honesty'" *MMNewsletter* 20,9 (1982) 33-36. See: Maguire DC, "Abortion: a question of Catholic honesty" *ChristCent* 100,26 (1983) 803-807.

[93]O'Donnell, *Catholic honesty*, 33-34.

[94]O'Donnell, *Catholic honesty*, 34.

[95]O'Donnell TJ, "Questions regarding genetic counseling" *MMNewsletter* 25,1 (1988) 3-4.

[96]See: *Dv*,I,2.

[97]See: *Origins* (Oct. 1, 1987) 261.

[98]O'Donnell, *Basic determinants*, 22.

[99]O'Donnell, *Basic determinants*, 22-23. See also: O'Donnell, **Medicine** (1991), 10-11; 23-25.

CHAPTER XI

THOMAS A. SHANNON and LISA SOWLE CAHILL

A. TWO DISTINCT WORLD VIEWS

Shannon's basic value system may be observed in a co-authored book on bioethics where he addresses, in part, the issue of prenatal life and conflict situations.[1] He begins by maintaining that, though based on different premises, a humanist and a theological perspective can complement each other in upholding the value and intrinsic dignity of human life.[2] Next, dealing with abortion, he notes that key to the issue is the definition of personhood. Following Daniel Callahan's general scheme, he describes three schools: Genetic school (from conception), developmental school (after some interaction with the environment), and the school of social consequences (social policy confers humanness); but he refrains from explicitly expressing a particular preference.[3] Also revelatory of his basic value system is his discussion of the sanctity of life, which he maintains involves at least five dimensions: Survival of the human species; survival of family lineage; respect for physical (bodily) life; respect for self-determination; and respect for bodily wholeness.[4] Contrasting the last two with the first three dimensions, he notes that at times the same motivation for respecting human life places people in opposite camps of the abortion controversy.[5] He states that the Catholic Church's abortion prohibition is based on the fetus' absolute right to life,[6] a principle he claims has been more strictly applied in abortion than in other life-and-death issues.[7]

Switching lines of argumentation, he declares that there are three basic positions concerning abortion: conservative (prohibiting abortion), liberal (allowing abortion), and moderate (allowing some). He further contends that these conflicting positions are based on two radically different worldviews: one views reproduction as a natural act not to be interfered with, while the other sees people responsibly acting on nature.[8]

Eight years later, Shannon revised and updated his book on bioethics.[9] The section on the sanctity of human life has been restated to include the inherent dignity and value of biological and personal life--with the human potencies of intellect and will reflecting the image of God--, which many hold to abide from the beginning of each one's existence, since the capacity for developing such potencies is already present then. Given the innocence and dependence of human life in its earliest stages, many insist that its absolute protection is the exclusive way of upholding its dignity and value.[10] He now also gives a more socially-based perspective of the five dimensions involved in the sanctity of life.[11] He concludes, however, with the same three positions on abortion: conservative, liberal, and moderate.[12] These three are still based on two different worldviews, which he has redefined somewhat: the first one seeing sexuality primarily for reproduction, rejecting contraception and abortion; the second one viewing sexuality as a personal, responsible act, accepting contraception and abortion.[13]

Further basic values may be observed in the section dealing with ethical analysis of medical interventions on incompetent individuals. He states that: "All decisions made on behalf of incompetent individuals are paternalistic. That is, they are either made on someone's behalf but not at that person's request, or they are refusals to cooperate with another's wishes."[14] Hence, he holds that when these decisions are necessary, they should at least be the most beneficial, and the least restrictive and insulting to the patient.[15] He ends this analysis contrasting two positions: "right to life,"[16] and "quality of life,"[17] concluding that the one could be a corrective to the other.[18]

Another basic value for Shannon seems to be the desire to reach social consensus on questions affecting prenatal life, as can be seen in his book on moral dilemmas related to medical technology.[19] He begins by again addressing the issue of abortion.[20] After a brief review of its history in the United States, he notes that one of the most compelling reasons for abortion seems to be, among others, "a strong chance of a serious defect in the baby,"[21] and attests that: "There is clearly a strong social consensus around the broadened concept of a therapeutic abortion."[22] He also notes that, at least as far as public policy is concerned, neither extreme in the abortion issue seems to have a proposal which can be endorsed by a national consensus. Therefore, he tends to advocate a compromise solution where some unwanted pregnancies will have to be carried to term and some fetuses will have to be aborted; which will be which, he does not say.[23]

Similarly, Cahill also proposes a compromise solution in an article where she considers the status of the embryo regarding public policy.[24] In it she contends that the Missouri *Webster* case (Webster v. Reproductive Health Services, 3 July 1989) is a perfect example of the intimate intricacy between morality, law and public policy, and that regarding abortion it might be practically impossible to separate the three. Maintaining that one key issue is the status of the developing fetus, she points at the difficulty of asserting when embryonic life is "personal," and questions: "Is it possibile [*sic*] or impossible to locate an 'all-or-nothing' point, before which abortion is entirely the mother's decision, and after which it is totally forbidden to her?"[25] She seems to favor a "compromise" solution (little or no restrictions of early abortion, but more significant ones later on), and to return the decision to individual States. This is for her a legal solution, not necessarily a moral one. Yet she hints at her belief that human life is involved, if not perhaps a human person, for she still maintains that abortion involves some sort of killing.[26] Thus, ethically, her ideal would be a climate of respect for the equality of women, and for the values of pregnancy, childbirth and parenthood: "In such a moral atmosphere, abortion might be discouraged among other options, seen not as a remedy of choice but only and rarely as a tragic necessity."[27] She ends by encouraging pro-life groups to expand their activities to include support (financial, emotional, etc.) for women with unwanted pregnancies.[28]

B. FORMAL AND MATERIAL DISTINCTIONS

Some insights into Shannon's philosophical and anthropological presuppositions may be gleaned from a co-authored article on the moral status of the pre-embryo.[29] In it he argues for delayed hominization, as will be more fully exposed in the subsequent section. Important to note, however, are the anthropological and philosophical criteria used therein. For instance: he distinguishes between genetic uniqueness (before implantation), and developmental singleness or individuality (after implantation), holding that only a human individual can be a human person.[30] Nonetheless, he believes that this genetic uniqueness yields the zygote "some" protection even before implantation.[31] Also, he accepts the definition of human personhood to be an individual substance of a rational nature, but asserts that a rational nature can only be present when the biological structures necessary to perform rational actions are themselves present--something which he estimates in human gestation to take place about the 20th week, when neural integration of the entire organism has occurred.[32] Likewise, he maintains that since the human soul ("principle of immaterial individuality or selfhood") is not necessarily responsible for human metabolism, biological development may well happen up to neural integration without the presence of such soul.[33]

Philosophically based on St. Bonaventure's Aristotelian interpretation of St. Augustine's theory of seminal reasons,[34] he holds that matter at each stage of formation needs only the corresponding form of each stage to be formed, suggesting that ensoulment is not needed in the early organic development of the pre-embryo, and concludes that: "The strong implication of these suggestions is that immaterial individuality comes into existence late in the development of the physical individual."[35]

Another hint at Shannon's anthropological and philosophical presuppositions may be obtained from his co-authored book on bioethics.[36] Within the discussion of genetic engineering, he asks the question; what is human nature? Dissatisfied with any number of current definitions,[37] he notes that genetics and psychology are now contributing to a better knowledge of ourselves, but that there is no cultural consensus on what human nature is, or on whether we should proceed slowly or quickly with genetic engineering.[38]

In a related work,[39] he briefly discusses the human genome project, and notes that these technological capacities to intervene in human evolution now challenge our assumptions about human nature and society, but he is skeptical about a mere genetic definition of the human.[40] He offers another brief glance at his own anthropology when he concludes that:

> The creation account in the book of Genesis tells us that we are created in the image of God. The rapidly developing capacities of genetic engineering will give us the power to create our descendants in another image. Whose image will that be, and what values will it embody? Such is the individual and social debate before us as we enter a new age of genetic discovery.[41]

C. VARIOUS POSSIBILITIES OF DELAYED HOMINIZATION

Shannon's theory of delayed hominization is most clearly stated in a sequence of three articles dealing with prenatal life:

The first one is his co-authored article on the status of the pre-embryo.[42] Detailing the process of human fertilization, he stresses the fact that it takes up to a day to complete, with another day for the two pronuclei to fuse. Passing on to describe the first cell divisions, he states the times required for the different stages, noting that at the morula stage: "Although the cells become compacted here, there is yet no pre-determination of any one cell to become a specific entity or part of an entity."[43] He also notes the possibilities of twinning and recombination before completion of implantation.[44] He further indicates that the zygote does not contain sufficient genetic information for self-formation, since he or she is also dependent on exogenous sources to develop into a human embryo.[45] He then describes embryogenesis from the third to the eight week after fertilization.[46]

Passing on to the theological interpretation of such data, he rejects magisterial language that speaks of "the moment of conception," preferring instead "the process of conception," possibly ending at implantation. Thus, he criticizes *Dv* for suggesting that the zygote is an individual human being, since it doesn't allow for the possibilities of twinning and recombination. He also points out that embryonic cells only lose their totipotentiality after restriction is completed with gastrulation. Hence, human singleness does not occur until after the first or third week, depending on the biological marker used: first week for implantation, and third for restriction. Translating this to philosophical language, he states that a human person cannot be such until after individuality has been established.[47] The issue, then, becomes once again the issue of ensoulment: immediate, or mediate; and if mediate, when so?

He traces the theory of immediate animation to the 17th century, but also points to an earlier tradition of delayed ensoulment.[48] Adding strength to the theory of delayed hominization he contends are the biological evidence of early pregnancy wastage, and twinning and recombination.[49] Commenting on this, he concurs with Häring[50] and Ford[51] that one cannot conclude that an individual human person is present from the moment of fertilization.[52] He then gives two further reasons against immediate animation: the need for the biological capacity for rationality, appearing rather late in fetal development, and the fact that the zygote's organic matter does not necessarily need a soul to inform its chemical behavior.[53]

His general conclusions cover biological data and moral implications. The biological data include true physical individuality, as distinct from genetic uniqueness, no earlier than two to three weeks after the onset of fertilization, the presence of at least one of three possible neural markers (gastrulation, organogenesis, or the development of the thalamus) for the capacity of rationality, and the developmental autonomy of the fully formed zygote (and embryo, and fetus) here due to its transcription capability.[54] The moral implications are explored in the subsequent section on the analysis of the moral act.

Shannon's second and third articles deal with fetal brain integration.[55] He now examines whether or not the beginning of a functional fetal brain can be considered an adequate criterion for determining the onset of personhood.[56] He briefly describes the gradual process of neural differentiation and development, starting with the formation of the primitive streak (week 3), to the physical integration of the nervous system (connection of the thalamus to the cortex, around week 20).[57]

Then he looks at the implications of these data, noting that some have proposed the concept of brain life (when fetal brain integration occurs) to be in symmetrical balance with brain death, wherein presence or absence of "consciousness" becomes the determining factor. He points to five current authors who, in one way or another, associate their demarcation of the beginning of personhood with the first functioning of the fetus' brain.[58] Yet he also points at some objections to using brain life as an analogous event to brain death for, unlike the former, the latter is a cessation of the organism as a whole. Also, no parallelism seems to emerge from the very gradual development of the embryonic brain, contrasted with the relatively spontaneous cessation of neurocortical activity at brain death.[59] But his main objection to defining personhood exclusively by brain life is that it is ultimately a biological reductionism.[60] Nonetheless, he maintains that certain benefits can be derived from the notion of brain life, namely, that human development is marked by processional stages and that each stage is morally differentiated, since each stage is necessary, but not sufficient, for personhood.[61]

D. A GRADATIONAL ARGUMENT

Moral implications of his theory of delayed hominization forbid calling a pre-three week abortion murder,[62] and regarding immaterial individuality proscribe the need of a soul for the pre-embryo to be and develop.[63] Summarizing his position, then, he holds that based on present biological data and corresponding philosophical interpretation, one cannot sustain an absolute prohibition of early abortion grounded on the pre-embryo's personhood.[64]

Expanding further on his moral analysis, he concludes that the preembryo (before implantation) can be sacrificed for another critical value due to its lack of individuality and of neural development; and the eight-week embryo, although already individuated and beginning to manifest neural activity, can be sacrificed to a more developed fetus or a more critical value, due to its lack of an integrated neural system.[65] Hence, his argument becomes one of gradation or priorities:

> Thus, should there be a conflict of values between the embryo prior to Brain Life I[66] and another individual past that stage or some other critical value, such as a duty to care for another or, in an extreme situation, the triaging of medical care, a decision in favor of the other person or other value could be made. That is, even though individuality has been established, the capacity for autobiography has not. Because of the lack of the biological presupposition necessary for autobiography, other persons or critical values could be given higher priority. Such conflicts must be significant and the values at stake serious. This means that the realities of individuality and possession of the human genome, when

combined with Brain Life I, have a developing but not ultimate claim for moral and legal standing within the human community. Because such claims are not total or full, other persons or values can be given priority.[67]

E. PRENATAL DIAGNOSTIC TECHNOLOGIES AND INFORMATION

Already in his early work on bioethics, Shannon addressed the issue of prenatal diagnosis.[68] He acknowledges the use of amniocentesis to detect birth defects, but also notes the present lack of therapy available. Thus arise the ethical questions: Why test? What to do with the knowledge gained?[69]

From an ethical analysis of birth defects, he identifies four issues to consider: the quality of life,[70] the values involved,[71] the right to make decisions,[72] and the interests of the child.[73] He is, of course, speaking of newborns; might similar arguments be used for the unborn?[74]

Concerning the issue of genetic screening, he opines that: programs should have well defined objectives, privacy must be safeguarded, and freedom to bear children should not be curtailed.[75]

More recently, Shannon wrote an article on ethical issues associated with genetic engineering.[76] In it, he evaluates some prenatal diagnostic techniques. Beginning with a brief description of amniocentesis, chorionic villi sampling, ultrasound and fetoscopy, he asserts that while several thousand genetic diseases are detectable, very few anomalies are actually treatable today.[77] He also notes that these techniques can detect the sex of the fetus, which may help determine certain sex-linked diseases, but can also lead to sexual discrimination by abortion of the "wrong sex" (a social rather than a medical reason).[78] Whereas these techniques are not immoral in themselves, he questions the morality of the prevalence of their use: "First, there is a 'guilty until proven innocent' assumption operating here. That is, the fetus is suspected of having a genetic disease until proven otherwise."[79] Yet only about three percent in fact show anomalies, therefore the assumption seems unfounded.[80] Second: "Screening assumes that those without genetic anomalies will incur lower health care costs or utilize fewer of the community's resources."[81] While this is true, it is also true that many other illnesses that are not genetically caused do account for tremendous health costs; should those individuals also be targeted for destruction? Finally, since genetic information about the fetus is typically known once the couple is already "emotionally invested in the pregnancy" (*i.e.*, second trimester), is the additional tension introduced by assuming there may be an anomaly justified?[82]

He likewise maintains that contemporary reproductive technologies are further clouding the status of the fetus by treating him or her more and more as a patient.[83] Does this mean that he or she should be granted the status of person? He does not answer, but overall, he counsels prudence.[84]

F. CONTEMPORARY SHIFTS IN DOCTOR-PATIENT RELATIONS

Shannon directly addresses the present shift in the self-understanding of medicine in an essay which touches on medico-technical advances in human genetics and some of its ethical implications, in part, on prenatal life.[85] He acknowledges the current possibility of prenatal diagnosis of birth defects, and notes that these and similar advances now allow for genetic screening of entire populations.[86] He points out that these new possibilities have caused at least two significant shifts in the medical world: from a rather detached and apolitical position, to one of advocacy of particular values; and from a more traditional stance of helping--but respecting--nature, to a more direct intervention in the course of human evolution.[87] Ultimately, these incredibly fast advances and discoveries are leading us to re-examine our self-identity, and our identity with the broader community, but he maintains that these lines of questioning remain presently open.[88]

In another essay within this same work, dealing with doctor-patient relations, he notes that the traditional authoritarian model whereby the patient passively accepted and unquestionably followed (or not followed) the physician's recommendations has been challenged by the "rights" movement, whereby patients now sought control of the whole healing process. Again seeking a compromise between these two extremes, he proposes a participatory or fiduciary model, where the patients' values and priorities can surface more clearly.[89]

In his earlier work on bioethics, he considers the issue of patient rights, holding that an increase public awareness has led to at least the following: the right to information; the right to refuse treatment to the extent permitted by law, and to be informed of the medical consequences of this action; the right to privacy; the restriction of access to hospital records; and the right to know about research and experimentation of benefit to the patient.[90]

G. NATURAL LAW AND THE MAGISTERIUM

Shannon and Cahill's dialogue with the magisterium regarding prenatal life and conflict situations may be seen in their co-authored book evaluating *Dv*.[91] Given the present ambivalence of prenatal diagnosis (it can lead to either saving the life of a fetus, or aborting it), they question its moral use.[92] After quoting the Instruction's conditional approval, they state:

> Thus the only valid purpose of prenatal diagnosis is to identify a problem and to help individuals begin to deal with it. The parents must be informed, give their consent, and there can be no disproportionate risks. One may not request or advise prenatal diagnosis if the results may lead to an abortion. Similarly, there should be no directives or programs of the state or of medical organizations that link prenatal diagnosis and abortion. The fetus has a right to life and this cannot be compromised.[93]

In view of this, they hold that when various Australian, British, and U.S. review committees (*i.e.*, the American Fertility Society, and the Ethics Advisory Board) are compared with *Dv*, the Instruction is at odds with their evaluations of reproductive technologies. Apart from differences in content, method, philosophy, and anthropology, these review committees tend to take for granted a positive evaluation of technology, bypassing social critique and confirming the technological imperative.[94]

Analyzing *Dv*, they maintain that it is based on the church's traditional interpretation of "natural law," but that such interpretation is framed within a personalist language: the special nature, dignity, inalienable rights, and integral good of the human person. This allows the church to appeal to values which go beyond credal differences because they concern society as a whole.[95]

Focusing their attention on prenatal life, they then discuss the present status of the embryo, but seem to distinguish between aborting fetuses which are already (naturally) implanted, and those which are a product of *in vitro* fertilization and have not yet been implanted, when they state that while individuals using reproductive technologies may act immorally, they are not endangering others.[96] Still, they are generally critical of disproportionate technological interventions in marriage, given their low success rate (said primarily of reproductive technologies, but applicable also to prenatal diagnosis). This notwithstanding, their overall conclusion is that perhaps *Dv* condemns more than is morally necessary, and that, from a practical standpoint, these condemnations are neither feasible nor enforceable. They would prefer to keep a more open dialogue.[97]

Notes

[1]Shannon TA, DiGiacomo JJ, **An Introduction to Bioethics**. New York: Paulist 1979.

[2]He holds that the humanist (philosophical) justification for the dignity of human life comes from within its own meaning, from human existence itself, whereas the theological one comes from being created by God, from being the image of God, but that both are complementary; "Again, the problem comes not in grounding but in applying the concept [of human life]." Shannon and DiGiacomo, **Introduction** (1979), 20.

[3]Shannon and DiGiacomo, **Introduction** (1979), 38-39.

[4]Shannon and DiGiacomo, **Introduction** (1979), 39-40.

[5]Shannon and DiGiacomo, **Introduction** (1979), 33-40.

[6]"Such a position is variously supported by a basic appeal to the genetic school, the defenselessness of the fetus, the right to life of each individual, and the authority of the Church." Shannon and DiGiacomo, **Introduction** (1979), 41.

[7]Shannon and DiGiacomo, **Introduction** (1979), 41.

[8]"The first sees sexuality and reproduction as a part of nature watched over by divine providence. In this perspective, sexuality is seen primarily as a biological function which, while having pleasure attached to it, has as one of its primary purposes the begetting of children. And since nature is watched over by God's providence, to practice birth control or to obtain an abortion is interfering with this order of nature and is therefore sinful. In the second world view, God's providence is seen not as expressed through nature but as a gracious action within human life which enables people to take greater responsibility for themselves and their environment. Sexuality is more than biology; it is a human reality with many meanings and purposes. Birth control for family planning is looked upon not as sinful but as an exercise of responsible parenthood. And abortion may be practiced as a means of taking responsibility for one's own destiny and for the future." Shannon and DiGiacomo, **Introduction** (1979), 41-43; here 43.

[9]Shannon TA, **An Introduction to Bioethics**. 2nd ed. New York: Paulist 1987.

[10]Shannon, **Introduction** (1987), 43-45.

[11]Shannon, **Introduction** (1987), 45-46.

[12]Shannon, **Introduction** (1987), 46-47.

[13]Shannon, **Introduction** (1987), 47.

[14]Shannon, **Introduction** (1987), 92.

[15]Shannon, **Introduction** (1987), 92.

[16]"The right to life position argues that life is the most important value, and that if that value is

not protected and defended against assaults, then all else stands to be lost." Shannon, **Introduction** (1987), 92-93.
[17]"How people live or the condition under which they live is often more important than whether they live." Shannon, **Introduction** (1987), 93.
[18]Shannon, **Introduction** (1987), 92-93.
[19]Shannon TA, **Twelve Problems in Health Care Ethics**. New York: Edwin Mellen 1984.

[20]Shannon, **Twelve Problems**, 1-35. See also: "Abortion: a challenge for ethics and public policy" in: Jung PB, Shannon TA, eds, **Abortion and Catholicism: The American Debate**. New York: Crossroad 1988, 185-201.
[21]Shannon, **Twelve Problems**, 9.
[22]Shannon, **Twelve Problems**, 9.
[23]Shannon, **Twelve Problems**, 13-30.
[24]Cahill LS, "Some ethical aspects of *Webster*" *BioLaw II (Update)* (1989) U:1525-U:1529.
[25]Cahill, *Webster*, 1525-1527; here 1527.
[26]"From a moral point of view, it is disturbing that the most politically visible and emotionally stirring symbol of women's equality and self-determination is a form of killing." Cahill, *Webster*, 1527.
[27]Cahill, *Webster*, 1528.
[28]Cahill, *Webster*, 1529.
[29]Shannon TA, Wolter AB, "Reflections of the moral status of the pre-embryo" *TS* 51 (1990) 603-626.
[30]"A human individual ... cannot be a human person until after individuality is established." Shannon and Wolter, *Pre-embryo*, 611-614; here 613.
[31]"Yet, since the pre-embryo is living and processes genetic uniqueness, some claims to protection are possible. But these may not be absolute and, if not, could yield to other moral claims." Shannon and Wolter, *Pre-embryo*, 624.
[32]"The presence of such a structure does not argue that the fetus is positing rational actions, only that the biological presupposition for such actions is present." Shannon and Wolter, *Pre-embryo*, 620.
[33]"...it means simply that the new substantial form is nothing more than that of the organic system itself, and that its new and unique dynamic properties stem from the complementary interaction of elements that make up the system. All that is needed is some external agent to bring the elements of that system together..." Shannon and Wolter, *Pre-embryo*, 620-621; here 621.
[34]"...he [St. Augustine] argued that if the potencies be understood as active rather than passive, then the Aristotelian formula that the new substantial *form is educed from the potency of matter* made sense." Shannon and Wolter, *Pre-embryo*, 621.
[35]Shannon and Wolter, *Pre-embryo*, 621-622; here 622.
[36]Shannon and DiGiacomo, **Introduction** (1979).
[37]"They fail to satisfy us, usually because they are so one-sided. Some focus only on capabilities or capacities, others on the potentials of individuals. Some stress the essential qualities of a person, others concentrate on emotions. Still others focus on rationality." Shannon and DiGiacomo, **Introduction** (1979), 136.
[38]Shannon and DiGiacomo, **Introduction** (1979), 136-137.
[39]Shannon TA, "Ethical issues in genetic engineering: a survey" *MidwestMedEth* 8,1 (1992) 26-29.

[40]Shannon, *A survey*, 28-29.

[41]Shannon, *A survey*, 29.

[42]Shannon and Wolter, *Pre-embryo*, 603-626.

[43]Shannon and Wolter, *Pre-embryo*, 607.

[44]Whereas twinning is abundantly documented in the scientific literature, they fail to cite any documentation on human recombination. Shannon and Wolter, *Pre-embryo*, 608.

[45]Shannon and Wolter, *Pre-embryo*, 608.

[46]Shannon and Wolter, *Pre-embryo*, 607-610.

[47]Shannon and Wolter, *Pre-embryo*, 611-613.

[48]The authors claim that two distinctions were used to support this dominant position: the distinction between active conception (physical union of egg and sperm) and passive (infusion of a rational soul) conception made by Pope Benedict XIV in *De festis* commenting on the doctrine of the Immaculate Conception, and the distinction between mediate and immediate animation held by several medieval theologians. Shannon and Wolter, *Pre-embryo*, 617.

[49]Again, no evidence for recombination is provided. Shannon and Wolter, *Pre-embryo*, 615-619.

[50]Häring B, "New Dimensions of Responsible Parenthood" *TS* 37 (1976) 120-132.

[51]Ford NM, **When Did I Begin? Conception of the Human Individual in History, Philosophy, and Science.** Cambridge: Cambridge University 1988, 171 ff.

[52]Shannon and Wolter, *Pre-embryo*, 619-620.

[53]Shannon and Wolter, *Pre-embryo*, 620-621.

[54]Shannon and Wolter, *Pre-embryo*, 622-623.

[55]Shannon TA, "The moral significance of brain integration in the fetus" in: Humber JM, Almeder RF, eds, **Biomedical Ethics Reviews: 1991. Bioethics and the Fetus; Medical, Moral and Legal Issues.** Totowa, NJ: Humana 1991. See also: Moussa M, Shannon TA, "The search for the new pineal gland: brain life and personhood" *HastingsCRep* 22,3 (1992) 30-37.

[56]Shannon, *Brain integration*, 124.

[57]Shannon, *Brain integration*, 124-128.

[58]Shannon, *Brain integration*, 129-133.

[59]Shannon, *Brain integration*, 128-135.

[60]"... such a perspective may be reductionist in that the position is open to an identification of the self with the brain." Shannon, *Brain integration*, 138. The 1992 article adds two further reasons for rejecting the "brain life" criterion: because it makes rationality the sole qualifying condition for humanhood, and because it subjects the pregnant woman to the fetus she carries: "One practical consequence of this metaphysical sleight of hand is to make pregnant women simply irrelevant to the issue of abortion. And women especially might worry about being treated as less than persons when fetuses *in utero* are treated as if they were fully persons. There are already some prepared to argue that women should be forced to undergo invasive medical procedures or incarceration for the supposed benefit of fetuses. And if 'brain alive' fetuses really are persons, then many would argue that women should not be allowed to have an abortion even if their lives would be threatened by bringing a pregnancy to term. Indeed, such an argument would make sense: after all, at the abstract level of 'personhood,' where the 'brain life' debate takes place, nothing justifies taking one innocent life over another; and, if the uterus is merely an intensive care unit,' as Goldenring [Goldenring JG, "The brain-life theory: towards a consistent biological definition of humanness" *JMedEth* 11 (1985) 198-204.] says, then preserving the new life seems at least reasonable." Moussa and Shannon, *New pineal gland*, 32-37; here 35.

[61]Shannon, *Brain integration*, 139-140.

62"We conclude that there is no individual and therefore no person present until either restriction or gastrulation is completed, about three weeks after fertilization. To abort at this time would end life and terminate genetic uniqueness, to be sure. But in a moral sense one is certainly not murdering, because there is no individual to be the personal referent of such an action." Shannon and Wolter, *Pre-embryo*, 623.

63Shannon and Wolter, *Pre-embryo*, 624.

64 "We thus affirm that any abortion is a premoral evil. That is, it is the ending of life. Consequently we do not want to be understood as proposing or supporting an 'abortion on demand' position or assuming that early abortions are amoral. Abortion is a serious issue, because life is involved and one needs always to respect life. We have made one major argument, however, in this essay. Given the findings of modern biology, there is no evidence for the presence of a separate ontological individual until the completion of either restriction or gastrulation, which occurs around three weeks after fertilization. Therefore there is no reasonable basis for arguing that the pre-embryo is morally equivalent to a person or is a person as a basis for prohibiting abortion. That is, there is no biological support for the position that the fertilized egg is from the beginning of the process of fertilization a distinct individual needing no outside agency to develop into a person. Neither is there good philosophical evidence that the principle of immaterial individuality [soul] need be present from the beginning to explain the physical development of the pre-embryo." Shannon and Wolter, *Pre-embryo*, 625.

65Shannon, *Brain integration*, 140-141.

66Brain Life I is defined by Sass as encompassing development from about the fifty-fourth day (the appearance of the cortical plate) to the seventieth day, when synapses begin to form; Brain Life II he defines from this point until birth. See: Sass H-M, "Brain life and brain death: a proposal for a normative agreement" *JMedPhil* 14,1 (1989) 45-59.

67Shannon, *Brain integration*, 141-142.

68Shannon and DiGiacomo, **Introduction** (1979), 80-82.

69"This failing creates a curious and ethically disturbing situation. In conventional medicine, diagnosis is aimed at treatment and cure, or at least at improving the patient's condition. But pre-natal diagnosis, while it aims to discover if the fetus will have a birth defect, offers little or no hope of effective treatment. Hence, many assume that the logical conclusion is abortion. Thus the question arises: If you ask for amniocentesis, are you indicating a willingness to resort to abortion? Or, to put the question another way, should amniocentesis be performed only if parents are willing to abort? When we can diagnose a condition but have no way of treating it except eliminating the patient, we face an ethical problem: What should we do with the knowledge that we have gained?" Shannon and DiGiacomo, **Introduction** (1979), 81-82.

70"Those who argue in favor of allowing children with birth defects to die, like those who argue in favor of abortion, base their stand on the importance of the quality of life. Right-to-life groups, which include many Catholics, oppose them and insist on the absolute sacredness of life. In their view, life itself, no matter what the condition, is better than no life at all. The problem with this argument, especially when used by Catholics, is that standard Roman Catholic theology and ethics have often used arguments based on the quality of life. The best example is the doctrine of the just war, first developed by Augustine." Shannon and DiGiacomo, **Introduction** (1979), 85.

71"A second ethical issue concerns the values on which we base decisions concerning infants with birth defects. The families of such children bring to the situation sets of values which are more or less conscious at the onset and which become more prominent as it develops. In a traumatic context, they are under severe pressure to make some kind of decision. They may not know how to express their value preferences, and they may even be ashamed to do so, but it is important for them to deal with their feelings and to face honestly the consequences of the choices open to them." Shannon and DiGiacomo, **Introduction** (1979), 87.

[72]They hold that, while doctors contribute with their medical expertise, the parents should decide: "It is to the parents that the child belongs, though not in the same way as property belongs to them. They are the ones who have the primary responsibility to care for the child. It is their life-style and quality of life that will be affected, and their values that will be put to the test. As such, they may be the ones who are entitled to make decisions in these cases." Shannon and DiGiacomo, **Introduction** (1979), 88.

[73]After analyzing how to determine the child's interests, they propose using "substitute judgment" (based on what a competent person would do in the child's place), again, most likely done by the parents. Shannon and DiGiacomo, **Introduction** (1979), 88-89.

[74]The second edition notes the ambiguity of prenatal diagnosis, which may lead to either aborting a defective fetus or sparing a healthy fetus from abortion, with the determining factor here being a possible birth defect. Shannon, **Introduction** (1987), 79-92.

[75]Shannon and DiGiacomo, **Introduction** (1979), 139-140.

[76]Shannon, *A survey*, 26-29. See also: Shannon TA, **What Are They Saying about Genetic Engineering**? New York: Paulist 1985.

[77]Shannon, *A survey*, 27.

[78]Shannon, *A survey*, 27-28; Shannon, **Genetic Engineering**, 58.

[79]Shannon, *A survey*, 27.

[80]Shannon, *A survey*, 27-28.

[81]Shannon, *A survey*, 27.

[82]"When indications call for it, prenatal diagnosis can be a helpful way of diagnosing problems. But we need to think carefully about the personal and social implications of routine screening." Shannon, *A survey*, 27-28; here 28.

[83]Shannon, **Genetic Engineering**, 67-68. See also: Shannon, **Introduction** (1987), 39-43.

[84]Shannon, **Genetic Engineering**, 79-94.

[85]"Ethical implications of developments in genetics" in Shannon, **Twelve Problems**, 37-74. See also: Shannon TA, "Ethical implications of developments in genetics" *CTSAProceeds* 34 (1979) 78-98.

[86]Shannon, **Twelve Problems**, 39-55.

[87]Shannon, **Twelve Problems**, 40-50.

[88]He points to the present exponential growth of information, to a shifting concept of health in a fuller sense, to a questioning of a static notion of personhood, and to certain possible insights of sociobiology--all factors which tend to affect our anthropology--, but he refrains from a strict ethical evaluation of each. Shannon, **Twelve Problems**, 50-72.

[89]Shannon, **Twelve Problems**, 99-112.

[90]Shannon and DiGiacomo, **Introduction** (1979), 145-153.

[91]Shannon TA, Cahill LS, **Religion and Artificial Reproduction: An Inquiry into the Vatican "Instruction on Respect for Human Life in Its Origin and on the Dignity of Human Reproduction"**. New York: Crossroad 1988. See also: Cahill LS, "Moral traditions, ethical language, and reproductive technologies" *JMedPhil* 14,5 (1989) 497-522.

[92]"Prenatal diagnosis permits the health status of the fetus to be evaluated. Thus it can help treatment begin earlier, can prepare the parents and health-care providers for the needs of the baby, and it can be the basis on which individuals request an abortion. While there are a large number of diseases that can be diagnosed *in utero*, unfortunately only a very small fraction can be treated then. Is its use moral?" Shannon and Cahill, **Religion and Artificial Reproduction**, 60.

[93]Shannon and Cahill, **Religion and Artificial Reproduction**, 60.

---

[94]Shannon and Cahill, **Religion and Artificial Reproduction**, 97-98.
[95]Shannon and Cahill, **Religion and Artificial Reproduction**, 103-107.
[96]Shannon and Cahill, **Religion and Artificial Reproduction**, 116.
[97]Shannon and Cahill, **Religion and Artificial Reproduction**, 132-139.

PART THREE

CRITICAL EVALUATION OF SEVEN RELEVANT THEMES

CHAPTER XII

BASIC VALUE SYSTEMS

Introduction

This chapter seeks to describe briefly the basic value systems found in the writings of the ten authors surveyed regarding prenatal life and conflict situations. Being Catholic moral theologians, all ten authors write within a theological value system. Even so, they all seek to express an understanding of the dignity of the human person that may appeal to a common humanity, hence their interest in exploring and developing as holistic a vision as possible. In doing so, the central theme of human nature comes immediately to the fore: no basic value system seeking to convey the intrinsic dignity of the human individual (at any stage of development) can afford to omit both the weakened and the graced dimensions of human nature. Likewise negligent would be to fail to address the social dimension of human nature.

Admittedly, human pregnancy affords one a very concrete and specific scenario for evaluating such basic value systems, for within those nine gestational months everything is in principle decided: viability, individuation, personhood, and the capacity for sociality; in a word, our humanity.

A. A THEOLOGICAL SYSTEM

It must be kept in mind at all times that the whole of the argument moves within the sphere of prenatal human life and conflict situations. Given this, all ten authors examined discourse within a Christian theological value system. This is said by way of contrast with a secular humanist system in its restricted contemporary sense. In this sense, secular humanism is not understood as a strategy of ever greater humanization, tending toward perfecting what is uniquely and universally human, but in its truncated meaning precisely of falling short of that goal by explicitly eliminating from human self-realization its origin, purpose, and ultimate end: union with God. In this sense, a secular humanist system moves diametrically opposed to a theological one.[1] Even so, it cannot be said that the one does not influence the other.[2]

It is precisely at the level of promoting certain values where possible points of contact between these two systems emerge. Specifically to be noted is that both seek to advocate the dignity and value of human life. That each one is established on radically different interpretations of the reason for what is and can be does not detract both of them from a valuable rendition of human life.[3]

B. THE DIGNITY OF HUMAN LIFE

Accordingly, fundamental to the ten authors is upholding the intrinsic dignity of human life. The grounding of this basic value is invariably to be found in the belief that individual human life is created by God, according to His image, out of an act of love.[4] This can be considered to be their shared structural principle.

This intrinsic dignity, therefore, is not dependent on either a particular achievement by any given individual, or on a bestowal or recognition by society at large. Rather, it is seen as an endowment from God. It is from here that its moral worth emerges: all human beings are beings of moral worth by virtue of being human.[5] Reflecting on one's being human presupposes a capacity to reflect, and to evaluate such reflection. This is a creative activity in the sense that prior to their occurrence, the reflection and the evaluation existed not: they are creatures of one's creative activity. Hence, human beings are creative creatures.[6] The terminus of being creative creatures involves the capacity to establish a personal relationship with God precisely in the creating act.[7]

The fact that human beings are creative creatures affords them a certain sanctity of life.[8] This is understood as a participation in the creative activity of God, a sacred activity. As such, this sanctity of human life can never be in true contraposition to the quality of life. For indeed, at its root, quality of human life speaks of what is proper to being human; it is its human quality.[9] If the fundamental quality of human life is its sacredness, then it cannot be compromised to lesser values without compromising its creative capacity.[10]

This sacred quality of human life must thus involve at least five aspects: survival of the human species, respect for family lineage, respect for physical (bodily) integrity, respect for self-determination, and respect for bodily wholeness.[11] If these five are fundamental to human dignity, then when in conflict among one another a resolution with the capacity to further humanize must be attainable. From here stems the challenge of a proper anthropology that can render justice to situations of moral dilemmas and value conflicts. For the believer, such justice springs from the recognition that human life is not only primarily God's gracious gift,[12] but absolutely so. For not to ground human life on absolute gratuity would imply that somehow any one of us may have actually asked or desired to have been created. Whereas we can assume that we may have been willed by God and by our natural parents, we cannot assume that we may have been willed by ourselves before we were: willing always presupposes a thinking willer. To sum: human dignity can only be God's absolute gratuity.[13]

C. A HOLISTIC SYSTEM

Thinking and willing in complex creatures also presupposes a body. We experience existing as bodies in a universe of bodies.[14] Hence, if one is to avoid falling hopelessly into past dualisms,[15] one must admit that human thinking and willing presuppose the existence of a body with certain basic needs, needs that require to be properly met in a genuine humanization.[16] Bodily experience, as the locus where these human needs exist, is integral to a truly holistic moral evaluation of human life; any theology considering the human body intrinsically "bad," to be resisted by the spirit, is immediately suspect.[17] To conclude, morality is what makes it possible for us to meet our basic human needs adequately.[18]

Conversely, to be avoided are simplistic biologisms. Mere genotypic or phenotypic human likeness does not a human person make.[19] The fact that at a particular gestational stage a human fetus begins to look like what one is used to recognizing as a human being does not mean that he or she becomes such then.[20] Hence, one needs to consider seriously the validity of the criticism that mere physical facts are not sufficient to evaluate the human moral act;[21] in this logic, there certainly is no immediate *ought* from *is*.

D. HUMAN NATURE

Granted that there is no immediate *ought* from *is*, a systematic observation of nature inevitably reveals certain dynamic patterns and sequences which, while remaining independent from the observer, are nonetheless understandable.[22] They allude to a natural order.[23] This understandableness of nature again points simultaneously to human reason and to human will. It does so because without these two faculties, the human person would be unaware of nature. She or he would be incapable of realizing that he or she is observing an understandable dynamic order. Because the understanding of this order did not exist prior to the person's conceiving it as such, its understanding is indeed a creative act. Hence, human rationality and volition are creative faculties: in this sense, they image God's creativity.[24]

This creative image of God, however, precisely because of its radical freedom, is also capable of sin.[25] Therefore, human perception of the goodness or badness of actions will necessarily always remain limited if evaluated exclusively by the light of natural reason.[26] This is why ethics needs to be complemented by revelation if it genuinely aspires to the fullest possible approximation of truth.[27] In the event of the incarnation, the mystery of man is completely revealed. In a single act of love, Christ has shown once and for all that to be human is to be for one another.[28] Thus, it is only natural for people to be health stewards, of selves and of others--including the physical, psychological and spiritual dimensions of the total person.[29] And this because, as a complex creature, the human person can also be very much aware of the times when she or he lacks health and wholeness.[30]

E. THE WEAKER

Integral to the human reality is the experience of weakness and suffering.[31]

While it is true that many in our contemporary liberal ethos find little or no value in human suffering--seeking to avoid it at all cost--,[32] it is likewise true that many others not only do not shun this reality but in fact seek ways to help those in greater need as an avenue of greater fulfillment of their humanness. This solidarity with the weaker is by no means the sole propriety of the Christian; indeed it appeals to the broadest possible spectrum of confessions. Even so, one particular dimension of it is the deep recognition of a "less-than-perfect" world, and therefore the acceptance of "less-than-perfect" people as fellow members of society.[33] It is also proper to the dignity of the human person to belong. It is then proper for groups and individuals within society to foster such belonging. Vigilance on behalf of the weaker demands and affords no less.[34]

Also, a theological value system cannot exclude grace from the discussion of sin and suffering. Granted that human life is a weakened life, it is also a graced life.[35] Protecting the weaker has both a strong scriptural and traditional backing in Catholic social ethics.[36]

F. SOCIALITY

Because of the connaturality of belonging, intersubjectivity and sociality are also proper to the human person.[37] In order to render justice to reality, these must be seen as capacities which are never fully exploited nor exhausted. Rather, they augment and diminish, wax and wane, in a complex dynamic of what can truly be called human living. Hence, to pretend to determine humanness by the attainment of any arbitrary level of sociality or intersubjectivity would be reductionistic. What is important by way of the dignity of human life is to uphold the capacity for intersubjectivity and sociality as intrinsically human, not any particular level of its actual development.[38]

Sociality also means that the individual be considered a member of society. This, however, is not seen in a relationship of a part to the whole whereby any part may be sacrificed for the good of the whole. In evaluating the sociality of individuals, one must keep in mind that the dignity of the individual forbids it from subjecting any one individual, either to another individual, or to the community at large.[39]

G. PREGNANCY

The consequences of the abovementioned values for the expectant mother and her pre-born need to be considered.[40] From the onset, one must acknowledge the complex, delicate, and mysterious dynamics of human pregnancy. If it is true that abortion must be shifted from a presently overly-individualistic, to a more socially-oriented concern,[41] then it is also true that society needs to render alternative support to mothers with problem pregnancies if it truly seeks to be consistent in upholding the sacred quality of human life.[42] In the case of a fetus diagnosed as carrying defects, it calls first for an open and vulnerable position of acceptance of the weaker.[43] It also calls for trying to elucidate what is the best interest to the fetus, given its condition of utter dependency. To this end, it is not sufficient to say that society has no authority to judge the positive or negative worth of an individual's life;[44] allowing a deformed fetus to live is already a statement of the positive worth of this individual's life. It is thus impossible to elude a risk-benefit analysis. Rather, what is needed is an expanded notion of this analysis, such that the fullest possible approximation is attempted, which can never exclude from its calculation the valuable theological contribution that weaker individuals need to be helped to belong.[45]

Given the drastic number of abortions currently performed in the United States,[46] in an effort to curtail this "racism,"[47] some of the authors examined are advocating a compromise solution,[48] while others are holding fast to an absolute prohibition of the direct killing of an innocent human person.[49] Since all ten authors researched move within a theological system which seeks to uphold the dignity of human life, the basis for their differing applications of these basic values lies rather in their varying interpretation of human life in general, and of nascent human life in particular. In other words, their disagreements stem from their contrasting anthropological and philosophical presuppositions.[50]

Notes

[1]See: Ashley, **Theologies**, 7-11.

[2]See: Ashley, *A child's rights*, 47-49; Shannon and DiGiacomo, **Introduction** (1979), 20. Integral to a humanist value system is the promotion of human rights. Holding that, since human rights are basic anthropological categories, they are also proper to a Christian theological anthropology, is: Demmer K, "Christliches Ethos und Menschenrechte. Einige Moraltheologische Erwägungen" *Greg* 60 (1979) 453-479. For a defense of the ethical basis of human rights within an Christian model, see also: Vidal M, **El Discernimiento Ético: Hacia Una Estimativa Moral Cristiana.** Madrid: Cristiandad 1980, 127-135. Sustaining that it is unrealistic today to pretend to engage in bioethics without entering into dialogue with secular humanism, is: Autiero A, "Il rapporto tra medicina e teologia per la prassi dell'etica medica" *RTMor* 79 (1988) 47-58.

[3]"Human life is perceived as sacred or having a certain dignity because human beings are basically valuable individuals. 'People are important.' As seen within the philosophy called humanism, the dignity of human existence rises from within itself, from within its own meaning, and has as its purpose and justification nothing other than itself. Similar and complementary to this point of view is a theological perspective which suggests that human dignity receives its sanctity from being created by God. Because individuals are made in the image and likeness of God, they are worthy of respect and receive the dignity that comes from being a special part of creation." Shannon and DiGiacomo, **Introduction** (1979), 20.

[4]See: Atkinson and Moraczewski, **Genetic Counseling**, 78-85; Ashley, **Theologies**, 258-259, 374, 693; Cahill, *Abortion*, 93-94; Curran, **Issues**, 203-204; May, **Human Existence**, 8; *Proxy consent*, 79; McCarthy and Moraczewski, **Fetal Experimentation**, 41-63; McCormick, **Ambiguity**, 22-23; Moraczewski, **Genetic Medicine**, 103; O'Donnell, **Medicine** (1976), 6, 41; *Genetic counseling*, 22-24; *Beyond*, 9-10; **Medicine** (1991), 45-47; O'Rourke, *Because*, 73-77; Shannon and DiGiacomo, **Introduction** (1979), 20; Shannon, **Introduction** (1987), 43-45.

[5]See: May, *Moral worth*, 416-443; *Human identity*, 17-37.

[6]See: Ashley, **Theologies**, 3-11; Gesché A, "L'homme créé créateur" *RTLv* 22 (1991) 153-184.

[7]See: O'Rourke, *Because*, 75. Since human life is fundamentally a gift and not a construction, its dignity is based on the human person as subject. Proposing a global vision of the human person--seeking to overcome every partiality--, leading to its protection and promotion at every stage of development, is: Lorenzetti L, "Trasmissione della vita umana da un'etica della natura ad un'etica

della persona" *RTMor* 71 (1986) 117-129. Also advancing a personalist model of bioethics, is: Possenti V, "La bioetica alla ricerca dei principi: la persona" *MedMor* 42,6 (1992) 1075-1094.

[8]The Christian claim that human life is sacred does not exempt one from exploring the reasons why this is so. See: O'Rourke, *Because*, 73-77.

[9]See: Herranz G, "Scienze biomediche e qualità della vita" in: CITM (Roma, 7-12 aprile 1986), **Persona, Verità e Morale**. Roma: Città Nuova 1987, 79-87.

[10]See: O'Rourke, *Because*, 74. Upholding the sacred quality and value of human life from conception, with its corresponding duty to protect it--thus allowing for that prenatal diagnosis intended to benefit the fetus, but not for the purpose of "eugenic" abortion--, is: Spinsanti S, "La tutela della vita" in: Goffi T, Piana G, eds, **Corso di Morale II: Diakonia (Etica della Persona)**. Brescia: Queriniana 1983, 198-219.

[11]Some find that, applied to prenatal life and conflict situations, upholding the first three aspects may at times conflict with upholding the last two. See: Shannon and DiGiacomo, **Introduction** (1979), 39-40.

[12]"Even in the womb the fetus is considered a human being with all the dignity and respect of human life, for such dignity depends primarily on God's gracious gift." Curran, **Issues**, 204.

[13]This dignity is most evident in the calling to live in the image of God--Jesus Christ. Sustaining that, precisely because of the believer's life lived in Christ, the human person is at the origin and center of all ethical decisions, is: Goffi T, Piana G, "La persona all'origine dell'etica" in: Goffi T, Piana G, eds, **Corso di Morale II: Diakonia (Etica della Persona)**. Brescia: Queriniana 1983, 9-15.

[14]See: Ashley, **Theologies**, 20-40.

[15]"... a Christian anthropology must retain the platonic defense of human spirituality and interior life, but it ought also to support Aristotle's criticism of Platonic dualism and accept the Aristotelian concept of the soul as the vital principle of the body and the body as the necessary instrument of the soul in thinking and willing." See: Ashley, **Theologies**, 238-239; here 238. Also rejecting a dualistic interpretation of the human person--in favor of a more personalistic one--, is: Sgreccia E, **Bioetica: Manuale per Medici e Biologi**. Milano: Vita e Pensiero 1986, 63-85.

[16]Ashley deduces six needs universally basic to human life: food, security, sex, information, society and creativity. See: Ashley, **Theologies**, 396.

[17]Traditionally, this negative connotation of the body has been most evident in the moral evaluation of human sexuality: "Twentieth-century philosophy and theology have been accustomed to repudiating the 'dualism' of ancient Greece and its remnants in Christianity or its facsimile in René Descartes. In sexual ethics, for example, we resist any attempts to define the body as 'bad' and the spirit as resistant to it, and instead, we insist on attention to bodily experience in definitions of moral obligation. The unity of body and spirit in human experience should also be taken into account seriously in discussions of pregnancy." Cahill, *Abortion*, 89.

[18]See: Ashley, **Theologies**, 458. A true holistic system of basic human goods ultimately seeks to promote the integral good. For an analysis of the ethical implications on the integral good of the human person, emanating from the present bio-medical capacity to manipulate human genes, see: Boné É, "Le génie génétique au prisme de l'éthique" *RTLv* 17 (1986) 156-191.

[19]It must be recognized that empirical science is immersed in a constant search of universals based on particular observations. Arguing that, in view of its great variety, the idea of the universality of the genetic code was perhaps established in a hasty and peremptory way, is: Ricard K, "Une révolution en biologie: a propos du code génétique" *Ét* 364,3 (1986) 355-366.

[20]See: Cahill, *Abortion*, 90-91.

---

[21]See: Curran, *Abortion*, 17-18; **Catholic Moral Theology**, 82; **Directions**, 130-131; **Themes**, 72; **Transition**, 208.

[22]This theory of dynamic patterns and sequences might begin to reconcile the perceived differences between the "classicist" and the "historical" views of nature and human nature. See: Curran, **American Catholic Moral Theology**, 65-73.

[23]See: McCarthy, *Ethical principles*, 92; O'Donnell, *Roots*, 33-34.

[24]See: Shannon, **Introduction** (1987) 44-45.

[25]Grounding the nature of human freedom specifically on the capacity for rationality and volition, is: Pinckaers S, **Les Sources de la Morale Chrétienne: sa Méthode, son Contenu, son Histoire**. Fribourg, Suisse: Éditions Universitaires Fribourg 1985, 380-399.

[26]See: O'Donnell, **Medicine** (1991), 1.

[27]To the extent that moral theology includes the datum of revelation, it seems appropriate to distinguish between it and ethics. See: O'Donnell, **Medicine** (1991), 1-4.

[28]See: McCarthy and Bayer, **Critical Life Issues**, 15-24. Also holding that the morality of contemporary human dilemmas must be seen under the guiding light of the gospel, is: Hamel E, "La morale cristiana e la cultura contemporanea" in: AA VV, **Attualità della Teologia Morale: Punti Fermi - Problemi Aperti**. Roma: Urbaniana 1987, 11-22.

[29]See: Ashley, *Constructing*, 501-520; McCarthy and Bayer, **Critical Life Issues**, 27-35; **Critical Sexual Issues**, 3-10.

[30]A sense of health or well-being is involved in our overall natural orientation to seek happiness. Holding that happiness for the human creature--the true goal of morality--lies precisely in respecting the laws of his or her nature, is: Bausola A, "Riflessione filosofica sulla fondazione della morale" in: CITM, **Persona, Verita e Morale**. Roma: Citta Nuova 1987, 37-48.

[31]See: McCarthy and Bayer, **Critical Life Issues**, 65-74.

[32]See: Cahill, *Abortion*, 91-92.

[33]See: Curran, **American Catholic Moral Theology**, 82-83.

[34]Also arguing in favor of protecting the unborn as the weaker in society, is: Lebacqz KA, "Prenatal diagnosis and selective abortion" *LinacreQ* 40 (1973) 109-127. Sustaining that with increased technological power comes a concomitant moral responsibility to use it properly, is: Jonas H, "Tecnica, libertà e dovere" *RTMor* 77 (1988) 25-35.

[35]See: McCarthy and Bayer, **Critical Life Issues**, 65-74.

[36]See: Cahill, *Abortion*, 85.

[37]See: Cahill, *Abortion*, 261-276; McCormick, **Ambiguity**, 22-23; *To save*, 175.

[38]It would seem that McCormick needs to answer to this criticism when he evaluates what may or may not be done to the fetus/newborn based on some demonstrable capacity for intersubjectivity: "Removing a nonviable fetus from the womb can be intersubjectively abortion (murder), removal of the effects of rape, saving the life of the mother and so on." McCormick, **Ambiguity**, 15. See also: McCormick, *Experimentation in children*, 41-46.

[39]"A utilitarian methodology which is willing to sacrifice one or another individual for the greatest good is opposed to such a Christian understanding [of human life]." Curran, **American Catholic Moral Theology**, 83.

[40]Pointing to the significant bio-technological possibility of intervening in human pregnancy today--with the ethical issues which this new power raises--, is: Autiero A, "Etica della vita prenatale: fatti, problemi, prospettive" *RTMor* 17,68 (1985) 31-44.

[41]The fact that the mother has certain inalienable rights is not questioned. But to pretend that she is the only bearer of rights stems from an individualistic liberalism where community is secondary. In contrast, Catholic tradition speaks of the interdependency of human life, where

working for the common good is normative. See: Cahill, *Abortion, autonomy, and community,* 261-276.

[42]See: O'Rourke, *Because*, 76.

[43]See: Curran, **American Catholic Moral Theology**, 82-83.

[44]See: Atkinson and Moraczewski, **Genetic Counseling**, 105-106.

[45]Calling attention to various contemporary socio-cultural conditions which together vie against a positive evaluation of pre-born human life, is: Elizari FJ, "Valoración de la vida humana antes de nacer -- condicionamientos sociales --" *Mor* 13 (1991) 187-204. For a personalistic analysis of human prenatal diagnosis, see: Tettamanzi D, **Bioetica: Nuove Frontiere per l'Uomo**, 2nda ed. Casale Monferrato, AL: Piemme 1990, 202-214. An appraisal of human prenatal disorders and diagnosis from a Catholic perspective is also found in: Wattiaux H, **Génétique et Fécondité humaines**. Louvain-la-Neuve: Cahiers de la Revue Théologique de Louvain 1986, 39-83.

[46]In 1990, there were 4,158,212 live births recorded in the United States. See: National Center for Health Statistics, *Advance Report of Final Natality Statistics,* **1991, Monthly Vital Statistics Report**, vol. 42,3 Supplement. Hyattsville, MD: Public Health Services 1993, 17. In that same year (the most recent statistic available), there were 1,429,577 procured abortions reported (with and estimated 16% under-reported). See: Center for Disease Control and Prevention, Dec. 18, 1992, **MMWR 1992**, vol. 41,50, Atlanta, GA: Department of Health and Human Services 1992, 936.

[47]"Abortion's pervasiveness represents a horrendous racism of the adult world. When it is justified in terms of rights, all of our rights are endangered because their foundations have been eroded by arbitrary and capricious application." McCormick, *Unexplored*, 49.

[48]See: Cahill, *Webster*, 1527; Shannon, **Twelve Problems**, 13-30; Curran, **New Perspectives**, 191-192; McCormick, *Fetal research*, 473-476; **How Brave**, 176-188; *Rules*, 26-30; *Unexplored*, 41-50.

[49]See: Ashley and O'Rourke, **Healthcare Ethics** (1989), 206-211; May, *Human identity*, 37; McCarthy and Bayer, **Critical Life Issues**, 40; McCarthy and Moraczewski, **Fetal Experimentation**, 71-74; O'Donnell, *Roots*, 33-36.

[50]Emphasizing the need for a contemporary theological anthropology which adequately serves the empirical scientist of today, especially in view of the tremendous advances in human genetics over the past thirty years, is: Serra A, "La 'nuova genetica': attualità, prospettive, problemi" in: Serra A, Santosuosso F, Bompiani A, Manni C, Cotta S, eds, **Medicina e Genetica Verso il Futuro**. L'Aquila-Roma: Japadre 1986, 5-23.

CHAPTER XIII

PHILOSOPHICAL AND ANTHROPOLOGICAL PRESUPPOSITIONS

Introduction

This chapter explores the ten authors' underlying presuppositions regarding the possibility of nature, of human nature, and of individual human life; all within the present historical context.

The area dealing with the possibility of nature is subdivided into the reality of nature and the nature of reality. Beginning, then, with the reality of nature, one universal experience is that of existing as bodily beings engaged in a multiplicity of relationships. But since this work is solely concerned with living bodily beings, then the organic criterion by which such are defined is a fundamental presupposition to explore in the writings of the ten authors studied. This leads to a discussion of the assumptions underlying the concepts of potentiality and actualization thereof, which, particularly in the case of the pre-born, necessarily leads to the presupposition behind the concept of pluripotentiality.

Given the observable reality of nature, to consider is also the nature of reality. Such nature is at its core regulated by certain fundamental natural forces. Yet, in order to avoid past determinisms as much as possible, a proper distinction between dualism and duality must be upheld. Once this is done, one may delve into the presuppositions beneath natural processes, circumscribed within natural systems. But again, because the whole of the argument moves within the notion of life as known on earth, then the objectification of causal relationships surfaces as the underlying criterion of the nature of living bodily beings.

A second area of presuppositions is the one on the possibility of human nature. Once more, beginning with the datum of being bodily, the process of becoming human is analyzed, together with its required minimal structures. Also, the dynamic between knowing and being known is explored, particularly with regards to the implications it may have within a theological system. Finally, the inviolability of human life comes to the fore precisely as the fundamental equality among all humans. This, then, bespeaks of the correct prerogatives one ought to have when dealing with prenatal life and conflict situations, prerogatives that can be maintained only if the argument of the inviolability of human life is upheld with consistency.

The third area addresses the presuppositions underlying the possibility of individual human life. First to be examined here is the concept of the self. It is noted that the different authors address in their writings various levels of the self, making the term anything but univocal. To this end, a clarification between moral beings and beings of moral worth is introduced. Also, the role of the principle of immaterial individuality is surveyed, especially regarding its relation to the beginning of individual human life. Lastly, the adequacy of postulating a difference between genetic uniqueness and developmental singleness is investigated.

The fourth area of presuppositions pertains to the present historical context. The first set of assumptions here have to do with the possibility of human history and of coexistence, with the necessary interaction between culture and the transcultural, and with the observed phenomena of information, terminology and interpretation. One assumption which is readily evident in the present historical context is choice; but choice can at times be radically differently interpreted related to the born or to the pre-born. Closely associated with choice, then, is the notion of viability, a term which is likewise not univocal among the ten authors examined. And this leads to the final consideration of this chapter: the anthropological and philosophical presuppositions underlying these authors' notion of consensus regarding prenatal life and conflict situations.

A. THE POSSIBILITY OF NATURE

1. The Reality of Nature

Bodily beings

When analyzing presuppositions, the analyzer cannot help working from within his or her own presuppositions. In this sense, the analysis is never new, but ongoing. Even so, reduction in analysis may allow for the possibility of discovery.[1] Because the analysis is ongoing, it presupposes a substrate of continuity: a time, place, and quality of residence. This residence is the body. It is impossible to deny bodily experience without denying experience itself. Since we experience, we are at least bodily beings.

Ashley proposes that bodily life as presently known seems to be a negentropic counter-eddy within and otherwise entropically evolving universe.[2] If so, he still needs to account how this countercurrent can be reconciled with the broader entropic current. Particularly to note is that bodily life as we know it does not seem to be independent, even for its very sustenance, from the broader forces of the universe.[3] Then, a necessary relationship of dependency is at work between bodily life and the broader universe of bodily beings, and his negentropic theory does not fully account for the reality of this natural relationship without certain presuppositions.[4]

Relationship

Regardless of one's explanation of the plausibility of the universal existence of bodily beings, it cannot be denied that one first bodily relationship is that between matter and energy.[5] This, however, implies a material pliability which cannot be unqualifiably accepted unless it also implies a limited pliability according to its nature. Even the dynamic interaction between matter and energy seems to occur only within certain limited possibilities.

Not unlike matter and energy, the possibility of interaction between bodies presupposes that they are influenceable, at least to the extent that they are agents and patients of such interaction. But, because we are here concerned with bodily life as we know it, we are only talking about the interaction between organic systems.[6] While it is true that in bodily life, interaction at the organic level happens between chemical molecules and elements, it is also true that such interaction in a living being is never totally random or disconnected from the teleology of a greater whole: what is known as the living organism.[7] Hence, when Shannon states that the dynamic properties of an organic system stem solely "from the complementary interaction of elements that make up the system,"[8] he still needs to explain how this dynamic process differs radically in a living or in a dead organism: molecules and elements in a dead organism are also dynamically interacting, and vigorously at that![9] Organic composition and decomposition do not seem explainable without the living principle, and he fails to account for such principle when he presupposes that early bodily life is solely dependent on biochemical interaction.[10]

Returning to the argument of the relationship between agency and patiency, if it points to the influenceability of bodily beings, in living bodily beings it also points to their unity and integrity: if a part of a living organism is affected, the whole organism is somehow also affected. Thus, when Curran contrasts a "classicist" view of reality with a "contemporary" view, rejecting the "classicist" view because it is based on individual substances and natures,[11] whereas the "contemporary" view includes the relational dimension,[12] he is interpreting "substance" and "nature" reductively by presupposing that they necessarily exclude the relational dimension of living beings. Conversely, to say that "a particular being can never be adequately considered in itself, apart from its relations with other beings and the fullness of being,"[13] denies particular beings their unity and integrity precisely as beings. Even individual living bodily beings are necessarily relational. Thus, his classification is artificial and partial;it fails to correspond adequately to the deeper reality of nature.[14]

Organic criterion

The unity and integrity of living bodily beings makes them natural units. Because these units are organic, if living they are in constant development. This development implies an inner dynamism which is directional.[15] And directionality presupposes the existence of a director, a "guiding system" as it were: in organic beings it is called the genome.[16] It must be acknowledged, however, that whereas a specific genome defines a particular species, a more-or-less ample variability is observed even within a specific genome.[17] Therefore, when McCarthy states that a human zygote never develops into any other species because of the specific information contained in its human genome (which he compares to a 1,000-volume encyclopedia), he must also adequately respond to the statement that no two human genotypes ever contain the exact same "encyclopedia."[18] The organic criterion of general bodily life can only hold true if it is interpreted as a system which remains permanently open to the selective actualization of potentialities by forces both internal and external to the system.[19]

Potentiality and actualization

A bodily being lives in an organic actualization of potentialities. Here, McCarthy and Moraczewski make a distinction between passive and active potentialities, restricting the former to biochemical capacities, but attributing to the latter the actual capability of a living organism to develop and differentiate itself as a whole.[20] The presupposition at the base of this distinction is a yet more subtle distinction between the physical and the meta-physical levels of living bodily beings, with the latter (the "active") controlling the former (the "passive").[21] One needs to question, however, the validity of distinguishing between different types of potentialities: if the distinction aims at describing different qualities of one and the same act, it seems valid enough. If, on the other hand, the distinction intends to grant certain potentialities involved in the development of living bodily beings a privileged existence and activity, independent from the organic substratum, then it must be admitted that this is suspect of an unacceptable dualism. Hence, potentiality is an ambiguous concept which cannot be used without further clarification.[22]

Pluripotentiality

Pluripotentiality is a more proper term than totipotentiality. Totipotentiality fails on two counts: it connotes an absolute openness to development; it denotes openness of developing into an absolute number of possibilities. Even the earliest stage of any living bodily being possesses neither. Pluripotentiality, by contrast, is a much more realistic term to apply for the rationale intended, indicating that there are somewhat different, but always limited, possible directions and outcomes in the development of any given living bodily system.[23] All ten authors examined are guilty of this improper usage.

This notwithstanding, they are all presupposing the same reality: the capacity of the earliest embryonic cells of living bodily beings to separate and develop into distinct individuals (of the same species). While none of the authors deny this reality, they do interpret the phenomenon in ways that inevitably places them into two radically different camps when it comes to the moral evaluation of earliest prenatal life and conflict situations: Ashley, May, McCarthy, Moraczewski, O'Donnell and O'Rourke maintain the possibility of individuality of pluripotential cells, whereas Cahill, Curran, McCormick and Shannon do not. The root presupposition of those who do maintain this possibility is the belief that if there already exists a metabolic gradient during this earliest stage, which in effect gives rise to all subsequent stages of development, then this development implies an individual, not a generic, event.[24] Given this biological reality, they still need to answer some very serious ontological questions regarding the possibilities of twinning, recombination, and high pregnancy wastage before implantation.
Conversely, those who don't sustain the view of ascribing individuality to

pluripotential cells have in fact failed to incorporate this biological datum of metabolic gradiency into their calculations. Therefore, their implicit presupposition is that development proper begins with nidation.

2. The Nature of Reality

Fundamental natural forces

If experience as we know it presupposes a bodily existence, since such body is necessarily subject to organic development, then it must also presuppose the existence of some fundamental natural forces under which this development takes place.[25] Still, the postulation of the universal existence of these forces must always be guarded against the danger of degenerating into a reductionistic determinism, lest one forget that human history can never be realistically proposed outside of universal history. And human history is by definition open-ended. An acceptable theory of fundamental natural forces must therefore leave sufficient space for human history, that is, for freedom and creativity. Hence, when Ashley states that universal history "exhibits the operation at every point of a few fundamental natural forces working with a beautiful, but not invariable, regularity,"[26] if he wishes to avoid determinism, he must limit his discourse of fundamental natural forces to the physical-organic dimension of universal history.

Dualism and duality

Another reductionism to be avoided when examining the nature of reality is that of dualism. When discussing dualism, however, one must guard against comparisons of elements which might actually belong to qualitatively different systems.[27] One dualism that is particularly insidious to the philosophical interpretation of physical reality is the recurring temptation to radically separate matter and form. If these two aspects of reality must be upheld, they must be upheld as a duality and not as a dualism: two qualities resident in a single reality.[28]

Ashley proposes that there is a degree of duality in all physical reality: not the dualism of mind and matter, but the polarity of matter and energy.[29] Yet, the difficulty with using this analogy resides in seeking to compare elements of two different systems: while both matter and energy (understood in this polarity) belong to a physical-quantifiable system, mind and matter either belong to two qualitatively different systems (such as "mind" as the cognitive activity of the brain, and "matter" as the neurological brain-matter itself), or they are intended in very specific ways (such as "mind" actually being the electro-chemical dimension of brain activity, and "matter" as the chemical structure where such activity takes place). In this sense, mind and matter are not unequivocal terms, and in order for his comparison to be valid, he is presupposing that they are.[30]

Natural processes

Granted the natural duality of matter and energy, all natural processes are observed to include minimally the following: a subject where the process is occurring; an agent causing the process; the new organization in the subject resulting from the process; and its teleology, that is, the directionality or orientation of the process itself.[31] This implies the existence of primary natural units (living bodily beings, in our discussion): subjects susceptible to change or process. So viewed, the subject is always a patient, that is, the receptor of some agent action. As such, the primary matter of primary natural units can be seen as pure potentiality.[32]

Natural systems

But the existence of natural processes alone is not sufficient to explain the nature of experienceable reality. They are not enough because, in themselves, natural processes may be seen as a continuum of dynamic relationships inherent in organic systems.[33] They only establish boundaries between agents and patients, not between different patients. Yet experience also detects the specific unity and integrity of the whole individual organism, as previously mentioned.[34] Therefore, natural processes must occur within certain natural systems. These systems serve the purpose, as it were, of "delimiting" the individual. At the same time, organic natural systems must remain sufficiently open to be influenceable by both, organic *and* inorganic agents, as is empirically demonstrable. Because natural systems are processural, they are teleological.[35]

Objectification of causal relationship

Natural organic systems are readily identifiable by their experienceability as natural units of reality. As such, they are always in dynamic development. It has already been mentioned that this development implies relationship. Because organic development is sequential (that is, it moves along a cause-and-effect trajectory), then it can rightly be said that it is the objectification of causal relationship.[36] Granted that this objectification in natural organic systems is seen as genetic self-determination, and that the real potentialities of a living bodily being are sufficiently open-ended that they can never be fully exhausted in a particular lifetime, when McCarthy asserts that on the basis of this self-determination the personhood of the human embryo can be "known to exist before it is fully apparent,"[37] he is again making a presupposition which is not without its ambiguity: self-determination at the bio-chemical level may indeed be seen as genetic directionality. Personal self-determination, on the other hand, involves a free act of the will, a quality which is lacking in DNA. In basing the possibility of the latter on the existence of the former, he has presupposed that these two qualitatively different levels of self-determination are in fact univocal.[38]

B. THE POSSIBILITY OF HUMAN NATURE

1. Being Bodily

Becoming

For humans, being bodily beings involves, not only a process of organic development, but also *becoming* gradually aware of our own humanness. No doubt this awareness happens in our association with other human beings.[39] This does not detract from the fact that humans are also subject to organic development. It is known today that organic development occurs in an epigenetic, not in a preformist, way.[40] And it is epigenesis which allows one to consider human organic development from the zygotic stage.[41] However, when Ashley and O'Rourke find in this epigenetic theory sufficient grounds for attributing personhood to the human embryo,[42] they might be presupposing that the development of personhood at certain stages of human life can be restricted to mere bio-chemical processes. This, in fact, would contradict their earlier statement that "our human self-awareness and freedom emerge only at high points of a very complex process, much of which is subconscious and part of the determination of nature."[43] If human self-awareness and freedom are what characterize the human person: are they present from the zygotic stage, or only at high points? Again, the ambiguity seems to rise from presupposing that organic and ontological development are coextensive in humans. Whereas this in fact might be the case, it cannot be stated without further clarification of what one means by "personhood," and what are the minimal structures which are needed to postulate its possibility.[44] Also, when they propose the human person to be one with the "need and capacity for intelligent freedom,"[45] they are obviously presupposing that this intelligent freedom does not occur in some abstract void, but in a body and, as such, that it is conditioned by the demands and limitations of that particular body.[46]

Minimal structures

If human development is epigenetic, then it involves the presence of a series of precursors which induce differentiation at various stages of development. Regarding the development of the capacity for human rationality, Shannon rightly acknowledges that certain minimal biological structures are necessary for the possibility of rational activity.[47] But when he states that "the presence of a rational nature would be around the 20th week, when neural integration of the entire organism has been established,"[48] he is presupposing that: first, neural integration is the sole biological criterion necessary for the possibility of rational activity. Second, that the possibility of rational activity is the sole philosophical criterion for establishing the possibility of human personhood.[49] Regarding the first, one may legitimately ask: might not the stage prior to neural integration also be biologically necessary for the possibility of rational activity, and so with the one prior to that one? Regarding the second, the question also arises: is rationality truly an all-or-nothing activity in humans, or rather does one here not intuit a broad range of possibilities?

2. Knowing and Being Known

Recognizing a range of rational possibilities is in itself a rational activity. Regardless of what minimal structures are required for it, or when they appeared, the existence of such activity cannot be experientially denied. Nor can it be denied that a human being who exhibits this activity, may be considered a person, even if one were willing to recognize personhood only in those human individuals who exhibit rationality. Minimally, rational human beings are human persons.[50]

Now, a person who is knowing, is also capable of knowing that he or she is knowing. And this, independent of whether she or he is recognized by another person precisely as capable of knowing. Hence, when O'Donnell asserts that "The ultimate criterion of 'person' is not to be knowing, but to be known--a subject known by other persons in an I-Thou relationship rather than a subject knowing,"[51] he is implicitly presupposing that the person is in fact knowing, for how could he otherwise know that to be a person is to be known, if not by a very act of knowing? Furthermore, he is also presupposing that God is knowing us, something which is exclusively proper to a theological system.[52]

3. Inviolability of Human Life

Fundamental equality

A theological view of human nature implies, not only the absolute gratuity of human life, but also a teleology common to all human beings.[53] This would complete the motion of issuing from God, by recognizing the possibility of a concomitant return. God is not only origin, God is also destiny. If this issuing-returning is the most common bond of human nature, then it is at the core of the fundamental equality of all human beings. This equality affords humans a generic dignity of equals, which is not necessarily contradicted by the experience of a myriad specific inequalities to be found in any given human population.[54]

O'Donnell rightly accuses those who uphold as valid the option of selective reduction in multifetal gestation to vie against the generic dignity of equals.[55] His presupposition, of course, is that the fundamental equality among all human beings carries through at every stage of development. The deeper presupposition here, however, is the belief that this fundamental equality is not due to any particular achievement--or capacity for achievement--on the part of the individual involved. Nor is it conferred by any other particular human individual (mother, father, medical doctor), or group of human individuals (society, Congress, the Supreme Court).[56] While perfectly justifiable, this deeper presupposition is not necessarily universally held by those outside of a theological system, and herein lies the challenge of the credibility of the argument.[57]

Prerogatives

O'Donnell's argument stems from the premise that to fulfill our destiny here on earth, we must use certain adequate means, which leads him to conclude that humans have corresponding rights and duties involved in the proper use of such means, which he calls prerogatives. One has absolute prerogative over something which is subordinated to one's final end, whereas one only has prerogative of use of something over which someone else has a higher right or claim.[58] Prerogative in human life is at most one of use, since all human beings have an equality of final ends.[59] Granted that for the medical situation this translates into stewardship, not ownership,[60] O'Donnell's presupposition here might be to assume that the belief that everyone has a right and a duty to preserve one's own health and bodily integrity is commonly held. And an even deeper presupposition might be that everyone would agree that all are called to a common finality.

Consistency

McCormick also argues from a position of fundamental equality among equals. Regarding the situation where a fetus is diagnosed to be a carrier of some birth defect, he sustains that, if this fetus is deemed expendable (*i.e.*, can be killed for carrying such defect), moral consistency requires that newborns with the same defect must also be deemed expendable.[61] Perhaps he fails to take the argument far enough: why stop with the neonate? If the consistency resides in the commonality of the disease at different stages of human development, that same consistency demands that all stages be included: childhood, adolescence, adulthood.[62] Perhaps the presupposition here lies in assuming that adult humans would have reservations about directly killing other humans who happen to carry a deformity.[63] As can be noted from the development of the euthanasia movement, at least some adults find this action totally legitimate: for these people, McCormick's argument is useless.[64]

C. THE POSSIBILITY OF INDIVIDUAL HUMAN LIFE

1. The Self

Levels of the self

The human self is not univocal. It may refer to self-development, self-awareness, or self-determination. Whereas these are all types of self-actualization, it must be admitted that they occur at different levels of being. Self-development may be seen merely at the physical-organic level; at this level, individuality strictly speaking is only bio-chemical. Self-awareness is a higher level, no doubt, but even if it involves an individual psyche, it is still inward-looking; it says nothing yet about establishing an intentional directionality. Self-determination implies taking a position, making an option; here the individual decides with the intention to act accordingly. In any moral theological discourse regarding prenatal life and conflict situations, it is imperative to distinguish between the different levels of self intended.[65]

Ashley speaks of the fact that individual human zygotes have the capacity for self-construction.[66] Whereas this cannot be empirically denied, nor can it be denied of *non-human* zygotes. The capacity for organic self-development does not necessarily point toward individuality in the personal sense. Therefore, if he sees a direct connection between the capacity of the zygote to process bio-chemical information, and the capacity of the individual human person to thoughtfully process information,[67] he is presupposing that these two qualitatively different levels of the self are in fact one and the same.[68]

When Moraczewski talks about the human individual, he distinguishes between the genetic dimension and the moral dimension.[69] Yet, in describing what is to be considered the characteristically human activity of the human fetus, he assumes that these two dimensions are coextensive when he states that it is a self-directed activity, an "activity carried on from within the organism itself, ordered to its own completion, and based on the distinctive genetic component present from the time of fertilization."[70] Might he not here be presupposing that genetic and embryonic teleology contain a certain moral imperative?

Moral beings and beings of moral worth

May makes a distinction between moral beings and beings of moral worth: human beings are beings of moral worth by reason of belonging to the human species, whereas they are moral beings because they can distinguish between *ought* and *is*. Hence, while all human beings are beings of moral worth, not all human beings are moral beings.[71] A human fetus is a being of moral worth, but not a moral being.[72] This presupposes a moral quality in human beings that is not found in other living bodily beings, which is consistent with a theological system of the human individual. But when he states that "a person (or an entity that possesses 'meaningful' human life) is indeed a minded entity, that is, a self-conscious and self-determinative entity,"[73] he is presupposing that self-awareness and self-determination are coextensive. Also, if only a person can undergo self-determination, then he is eliminating the possibility of the fetus being considered a person, unless he assumes it to be the *capacity* for self-determination.

2. The Principle of Immaterial Individuality

Shannon equates the principle of immaterial individuality or immaterial selfhood with the human soul.[74] He states that it is "the ultimate actualization of all the potencies contained within the forms or systems that constitute the organic life of the human being, [but that it] comes into existence late in the development of the physical individual."[75] This is the basis for his theory of delayed hominization. Yet, this statement cannot go unquestioned without certain presuppositions, for the organic life of the physical individual is a complex dynamic system containing at the start many potencies which are never fully actualized. In fact, epigenetic development works quite the opposite way: mostly by *restricting* or *inhibiting* potencies as differentiation occurs, so that cells, tissues and organs become more and more specialized along gestation. Furthermore, some of the organic potencies of human beings are not fully actualized even until years after birth (*i.e.*, sexual organs), which would proscribe the use of the principle of immaterial individuality as a valid principle for identifying the beginning of a human individual, unless certain assumptions are made. Hence, when he speaks of the actualization of *all* potencies, he is presupposing that these potencies include only those that will actually develop along a particular pregnancy, and this can have serious interpretative repercussions regarding the humanity of fetuses who are carriers of genetic defects.[76]

3. Genetic Uniqueness and Developmental Singleness

Likewise, Shannon makes a distinction between genetic uniqueness and developmental singleness or individuality, maintaining that whereas the former occurs from completed fertilization on, the latter can only occur after completed implantation (due to the possibility of twinning and recombination before nidation).[77] Again, this statement cannot be accepted without delving into its presuppositions.[78] Genetic uniqueness, in the organic-physical sense, implies a chromosomic makeup that is both phylogenetically and ontogenetically original. As such, it can be said that each living bodily being is the bearer of genetic uniqueness.[79] Human genetic uniqueness, then, is a characteristic proper to human individuals. And this genetic uniqueness is indeed observable from completed fertilization on. Conversely, it cannot be said that the human conceptus does not undergo organic development before implantation, for at this stage, the blastocyst is not only multicellular, but also exhibits minimal cellular differentiation. Thus, if Shannon insists that genetic uniqueness and developmental singleness are not coextensive, then he is either denying the existence of pre-implantation development, or he is at least presupposing that the term be applied in a non-organic sense.[80]

D. THE PRESENT HISTORICAL CONTEXT

1. Presuppositions

The possibility of human history and of coexistence

Humans are a product of evolution. To hold to the contrary would necessarily put humans outside of the influence of natural selection, a force that is confirmable in the simultaneous existence of distinct human races.[81] The interactions between and within these races have been, and continue to be, chronologically recorded in an increasing complexity of data which one calls human history. As such, human history is organic and, because of human creativity, it is also open-ended.

Now, while every natural living system seems to tend toward preserving itself, in view of the mixed review which human history merits so far, a legitimate question to ask is if human beings are also intended to preserve themselves. This query contains a double unfolding: are human beings capable of coexisting with one another?, are human beings capable of coexisting with the surrounding natural environment? When Ashley speaks of the harmonious coexistence of human beings with one another, and with our environment,[82] he is presupposing that this is a true and real possibility. However, this is something which history has yet to fully confirm.[83]

Culture and the transcultural

Similarly, when Ashley speaks of certain basic human needs as being transcultural,[84] and therefore deserving of respect by all cultures, he is presupposing that human culture somehow has a direct responsibility for guaranteeing the survival of the individuals within it by providing for the fulfillment of these needs. In fact, the phenomenon of culture is a much more complex, fluid and ambiguous one. Whereas one cannot deny its existence, one cannot deny the failure of all attempts to define culture in such narrow terms as to include its guaranteed responsibilities to its constituents (or, much less, as a pre-conceived system to be imposed).[85] In fact, culture properly understood can never exist outside, or independently of, the specific constituents who claim it--though it tends to transcend any one of its representatives.[86] This means that attempting to secure these transcultural needs remains always subject to interpretation through the filters operative in any particular culture. Indeed, whereas Ashley's six proposed basic human needs do have an overall universal appeal, one may not reasonably presuppose that these can be unequivocally interpreted.[87]

Information, terminology and interpretation

Also, interpretation of information is at the heart of the correct understanding of philosophical and anthropological presuppositions, even when they occur within a given historical and cultural context.[88] To this end, a proper terminology is of critical importance. This is the reason why Curran first seeks to clarify his terminology when discussing prenatal human life and conflict situations.[89] However, when he proposes "truly human being" or "truly human life" to be synonymous with "human person," he is not doing so without certain presuppositions. The adverb "truly" qualifies human life in such a way as to allow also for the possibility that there are times when human life can be "falsely" so; an "apparent" human life. This assumes that, either the apparent human life being observed is "truly" another specific type of life, or that it is not any particular type of life, simply "life." The contradiction with this reasoning in natural bodily systems is that, on the first count, one never observes specific life spontaneously "jumping" from one species to another as ontogenetic development occurs. On the second count, again in natural bodily systems, one never observes unqualified or unspecified life: bodily life always occurs in a specific organism, whatever the species may be.[90]

Ordinary/extraordinary is another term which deserves clarification, for as O'Rourke correctly points out, they do not necessarily mean the same to the moral theologian than to the healthcare professional. To the healthcare professional, it means the difference between standard and experimental procedures or practice. Hence, in this case the terms ordinary/extraordinary apply to the techniques themselves. To the moralist, on the other hand, the terms cannot be considered without considering the person of the patient, together with a host of conditions and circumstances which always surround him or her. But, when O'Rourke states that "the ethicist assumes that a person has a need or obligation to prolong human life, but that there are limits to this need or obligation,"[91] he is presupposing this obligation to be universally valid for all people at all times. Assuming this to be the case, he is also presupposing that the limits to this obligation likewise have a certain universal appeal, and that human persons can come to some common understanding as to what these limits are, otherwise he would have to admit to the possibility of arriving at different interpretations of the same limits. In the case of prenatal life, this may translate into one set of parents considering a particular handicap of their child to be a grave burden, while another set of parents considering the same handicap to be a lesser burden to them. In spite of the moral validity of their subjective evaluations, a certain underlying common standard would be needed if one is seeking to uphold the moral right to live which the handicap child has.[92]

2. Choice

Interpretation leads to choice. Given that the fetus cannot choose for himself or herself, the question then arises as to when and how does another choose for it? This question presupposes that, at some point in gestation, a particular choice has to be made on behalf of the fetus.[93] A particular situation might be when there is a suspicion that the fetus is the bearer of a handicap. While one may reasonably assume that the fetus would want what is beneficial to herself or himself in a therapeutic situation, may one assume the same in a non-therapeutic situation?

McCormick maintains that, in non-therapeutic situations, a parallel may be drawn between what one might assume of a born child and what one may assume of a (pre-born) fetus.[94] Following this line of argument, he holds that one may reasonably assume that the child would choose in favor of life and health because, these two being goods for the child, she or he ought to choose them. This, he says, is "a construction of what the child would wish could he do so."[95] There are several presuppositions contained within this line of reasoning that cannot go unexplored. First, it assumes that life and health are goods, and that a child ought to desire these goods; a Christian theological system must presuppose at least this much. Second, though, he presumes that a child would choose these goods *because* he or she ought to do so. Whereas it is easily observable that children seem to want to live, to assume that they do so because they intuit that they *ought* to do so posits a moral imperative on behavior that could nonetheless be adequately explainable by physiological and psychological stimuli alone. In other words, to impose a moral character on a child's innate desire for survival presupposes a particular anthropology which is not universally accepted without certain reservations.[96] Third, even assenting to the presupposition that the desire for survival contains some moral quality, since McCormick here is applying his analysis to non-therapeutic situations, he is supposing that the child has a moral obligation to consent to experimentation which is not directly beneficial to him- or herself, but rather based only on the possibility that the experimentation be of some benefit to others, which again is a presupposition that is not universally held.[97]

3. Viability

Related to choosing on behalf of the fetus is the issue of viability. McCormick grounds his criteria for what may or may not be done to the fetus on whether the fetus is viable or not.[98] Based on this distinction, he differentiates between a nonviable fetus *in utero*, and one *extra uterum*. The former he further subdivides into no abortion contemplated, or an abortion planned; the latter he subdivides into the product of a spontaneous abortion, or an induced abortion.[99] Once again, the presuppositions underlying this classification must be considered. First, beginning with the greater distinction, to ground one's evaluation of prenatal intervention on the difference whether the fetus is viable or nonviable carries with it certain implications. It must be recognized that viability is a technologically-conditioned state, not only with regard to the time of gestation, but also (and probably even more critically) with respect to the degree of availability of state-of-the-art technology that may or may not be accessible to a particular pregnant mother: what might be considered a viable fetus in a given medical facility, might not necessarily be considered so in another. Hence, this first distinction presupposes that the medical world can arrive at some commonly-held demarcation of human fetal viability which is available to all pregnant women. Second, whether a fetus is *in utero* or *extra uterum* seems to be a distinction merely of place, in itself without any moral significance. However, because he is here speaking only about the nonviable fetus, it implies that his or her normal place of residence is *in utero*, which means that these two categories might not actually be comparable without some further specifications. Third, classifying a nonviable fetus *in utero* according to whether an abortion is planned or not conditions the place of residence of such fetus to the decision of someone other than himself or herself. Whereas such decision in theory might seem to "merely" change the place of residence of the fetus, since he or she is a nonviable fetus, in practice this decision is lethal for the fetus: must one always assume that because the fetus is still at a nonviable stage, he or she may not wish to continue residing in the only place where he or she is likely to become viable? In conclusion, without certain presuppositions, McCormick's use of the concepts of fetal viability and nonviability shift back and forth, at times based on biological phenomena, at others on technological possibilities, and at others still, on the decisions made by moral agents.[100]

Notes

[1]Reductive analysis is based on syllogism, and therefore is dialectic. But dialogue admits of opinion by sacrificing a degree of certitude, counteracted by probability, hence allowing for the possibility of discovery. For a view on the possibility of discovery through analysis, see: Birch AC, "The dialectic of discovery" *NewSchol* 63 (1989) 295-312.

[2]He calls this a radical process interpretation of history. See: Ashley, **Theologies**, 259.

[3]One thinks of bodily life's vital need of light, gravity, heat, etc. For a re-evaluation of the theories of the existence of universal forces, see: Lachièze-Rey M, "Big bang et formation de l'universe" *Ét* 366,5 (1987) 627-648.

[4]An alternative review of the possibility of human existence in the universe is offered in: Lonchamp J-P, "Le principe anthropique" *Ét* 374,4 (1991) 493-502.

[5]This is why Ashley rightly speaks of matter being able to change and of energy being able to actualize matter by interacting on its primary units. See: Ashley, **Theologies**, 333-334.

[6]For a philosophical interpretation of biological life postulating its central constitutive to be operative recognition, a characteristic which can only occur in living forms, see: Crescini A, "La natura della vita: una indagine filosofica" **GMetaf** 14 (1992) 277-330.

[7]It must also be admitted that any living organism presents, at least by what can be observed, a degree of unity and integrity, both of which seem to reverse when the organism dies, that is, when it loses its life principle.

[8]See: Shannon and Wolter, *Pre-embryo*, 621.

[9]Note, for instance, the relatively large amount of heat which is released in the process of organic decomposition.

[10]Shannon and Wolter, *Pre-embryo*, 620-621.

[11]"A classicist worldview tends to see reality in terms of substances and natures which exist in themselves apart from any relations with other substances and natures." Curran, **Themes**, 59.

[12]"The contemporary worldview tends to see reality more in terms of relations than of substances and natures." Curran, **Themes**, 59.

[13]Curran, **Themes**, 60.

[14]The term "according to nature" is ambivalent. Arguing for a distinction between laws of nature (at a bio-physical level) and natural law (at a philosophical-theological level), is: Autiero A, "Natura e leggi di natura" in: Goffi T, Piana G, eds. **Corso di Morale II: Diakonia (Etica della Persona)**. Brescia: Queriniana 1983, 106-109.

[15] See: McCarthy and Moraczewski, **Fetal Experimentation**, 22-26.

[16]See: Weaver and Hedrick, **Genetics**, 86.

[17]For the variability in the human genome, see: Millard CE, "The effects of modern therapeutics on the human gene pool" *RIMJ* 63,11 (1980) 443-450.

[18]See: McCarthy, **Beginnings**, 65.

[19]On the provisionality of the theory of the universality of the genetic code, see: Ricard K, "Une révolution en biologie: a propos du code génétique" *Ét* 364,3 (1986) 355-366.

[20]See: McCarthy and Moraczewski, **Fetal Experimentation**, 29-30.

[21]For an analysis of how the actualization of potency provides substantial integrity to that which is real, see: Centore FF, "Potency, space, and time: three modern theories" *NewSchol* 63 (1989) 435-462.

[22]A convincing argument on the possibility of every natural agent tending to its end is found in: Makin S, "Aquinas, natural tendencies and natural kinds" *NewSchol* 63 (1989) 253-274.

[23]For example, the fact that monozygotic siblings develop from a single zygote does not mean that each sibling belongs to a different biological species: true zygotic *totipotentiality* implies that they could. See: Moore, **Developing Human**, 122-129.

[24]"The very existence of mosaic embryos, in which the position of a blastomere in the embryo determines absolutely the fate of that cell, suggests that determinants are present in the egg and that they are unequally distributed. The simplest form of unequal distribution of determinants would be a gradient from the top (**animal pole**) to the bottom (**vegetal pole**) of the egg. But a second gradient, from one side to the other, could coexist with the vertical one." Weaver and Hedrick, **Genetics**, 377-378.

[25]For a re-evaluation of the observation and measurement of natural forces, see: Klein E, "Introduction au débat quantique" *Ét* 375,6 (1991) 633-645.

[26]Ashley, **Theologies**, 259.

[27]Upholding the possibility of a fundamentally unitary interpretation of reality--without denying its inherent duality, but explainable as complementarity--, is: Rioja A, "La filosofía de la complementariedad y la descripción objetiva de la naturaleza" *RFil* 5,8 (1992) 257-282.

[28]But formal qualitative appreciation of matter is a typically human activity. For an anthropocentric proposal of universal matter, see: Mayaud P-N, "Une histoire de la matière" *Ét* 353,1 (1980) 5-21.

[29]See: Ashley, **Theologies**, 263.

[30]For an alternative view on the link between the psyche and genetics of the human fetus, see: Mattei J-F, "The use of prenatal diagnosis for psychiatric diseases" in: Srám RJ, Bulyzhenkov V, Prilipko L, Christen Y, eds, **Ethical Issues of Molecular Genetics in Psychiatry**. New York: Springer-Verlag 1991, 87-93.

[31]See: Ashley, **Theologies**, 287.

[32]This is consistent with the principle that "nothing causes itself." See: Ashley, **Theologies**, 285.

[33]To stay with the same example of living bodily beings, processurally, the passage of organic material from one level of a food chain to another may be seen as an organic continuum. Biologically, however, distinct individuals are involved.

[34]See: *Organic criterion*, under the section on **The Reality of Nature**, above.

[35]For an appeal in favor of the universal teleology of natural bodily systems, see: Engelman E, "Aristotelian teleology, presocratic hylozoism, and 20th century interpretation" *AmerCathPhilQ* 64 (1990) 297-312.

[36]"The notion of potentiality belongs within a schema of causality. To assume causal links between an embryo with human genetic programming and an infant embodying that programming is to admit an objectification of causal relationship." McCarthy, **Beginnings**, 66.

---

[37]McCarthy, **Beginnings**, 66.

[38]See: McCarthy, **Beginnings**, 67.

[39]May, **Becoming**, 25-49.

[40]The theory of epigenesis states that organisms develop embryonically from growth and differentiation of specialized cells, as opposed to the previously held preformist theories, which spoke of "miniature adults" that only needed to enlarge in size, without any differentiation involved (More on the theory of epigenesis below). See: Moore, **Developing Human**, 9.

[41]See: Johnson, **Human Developmental Anatomy**, 47-50.

[42]See: Ashley and O'Rourke, **Health Care Ethics** (1978), 221-226.

[43]Ashley and O'Rourke, **Health Care Ethics** (1978), 11. However, their 1989 edition reads instead: "....much of which is subconscious and dependent on bodily development and function." (p. 5)

[44]Similarly, May might be falling into the same ambiguity when he states that in order to become fully human, "we must go through a process that is variously called humanization, socialization, or simply human growth and development." May, **Becoming**, 44.

[45]Ashley and O'Rourke, **Healthcare Ethics** (1989), 4.

[46]For a description of the realization of the person as self-direction, see: López Azpitarte E, "El proyecto ético: la realización del hombre como persona" in: Rincón Orduña R, Mora Bartrés G, López Azpitarte E, eds, **Praxis Cristiana I: Fundamentación**. 5ta ed. Madrid: Paulinas 1980, 263-278.

[47]"One can speak of a rational nature in a philosophically significant sense only when the biological structures necessary to perform rational actions are present, as opposed to only reflex activities." Shannon and Wolter, *Pre-embryo*, 620.

[48]Shannon and Wolter, *Pre-embryo*, 620.

[49]A summary of the evolutionary interaction between the human mind and its necessary biological structures in: Boné E, "Paléontologie et reconnaissance de l'homme" *Ét* 352,1 (1980) 39-57.

[50]The extent of rationality needed to qualify as a human person has been theoretically debated, but this is an argument of degree which is irrelevant to the point at hand, as will be seen. See: Engelhardt, Jr. HT, "Some persons are humans, some humans are persons, and the world is what we persons make it" in: Spicker SC, Engelhardt, Jr. HT, eds, **Philosophical Medical Ethics**. Boston: Reidel 1977, 183-194.

[51]O'Donnell, *Genetic counseling*, 24.

[52]The sameness between knowing and being must not be taken for granted, for it is not an identity. For the possibility of viewing the I as both object and subject of knowledge, thus bridging the gap between knowing and being, see: Bigger CP, "St. Thomas on essence and participation" *NewSchol* 62 (1988) 319-348.

[53]A view on the compatibility of a non-theological and a theological approach to medical ethics in: Gillon R, "Ethics and clinical practice" *JInherMetabDis* 11,1 (1988) 120-124. For a contrasting view, see: O'Reilly S, "The ethics of genetic counseling" *AGenMedGem* 23 (1974) 207-210.

[54]In contrast with the generic dignity of equals, the justifiability or non-justifiability of these inequalities--physical, intellectual, social, etc.--inevitably depends on a wide range of factors to be balanced against goods, rights and duties due each member of the particular population. The fundamental equality of all human beings also points to the shared responsibility to collectively care for our humanness. See: Demmer K, "Man's appropriate stewardship of his biological nature" in: Malherbe J-F, ed, **Human Life: Its Beginnings and Development. Bioethical Reflections by Catholic Scholars** (International Federation of Catholic Universities). Paris:

L'Harmattan 1988, 259-271.

[55]See: O'Donnell, *Ambivalent*, 33-34; *Coherently consistent*, 9-10; *Objective truth*, 19-20; *Selective abortion*, 8.

[56]The popular opinion that parents should have a right to decide on selective reduction, can be seen in: Redwine FO, Hays PM, "Selective birth" *SemPer* 10,1 (1986) 73-81.

[57]For a further report of selective fetal reduction as a medical success, see: Still K, Kolatat T *et al*, "Early third trimester selective feticide of a compromising twin" *FetalTher* 4 (1989) 83-87.

[58]See: O'Donnell, **Medicine** (1991), 45-46.

[59]See: O'Donnell, **Medicine** (1991), 46.

[60]See: O'Donnell, **Medicine** (1991), 47.

[61]See: McCormick, *Life-saving*, 110-115.

[62]For a view arguing for consistency between selective abortion and infanticide, see: Santurri EN, "Prenatal diagnosis: some moral considerations" in: Schneider ED, ed, **Questions about the Beginning of Life: Christian Appraisals of Seven Bioethical Issues.** Minneapolis, MN: Augsburg 1985, 120-150.

[63]"It is not our sense of, experience of loyalty or acceptance that shapes our obligations. It is rather the objective reality of the fetus that ought to found our obligations and nurture our sense of loyalty." McCormick, *Life-saving*, 114.

[64]Seeking a more humane evaluation of euthanasia, and exploring its limits, is: Verspieren P, "Sur la pente de l'euthanasie" *Ét* 360,1 (1984) 43-54.

[65]For an account against determinism, and in favor of human freedom and self-determination, see: Boyle, Jr, JM, Grisez G, Tollefson O, "Determinism, freedom, and self referential arguments" *RMetaph* 26,1 (1972) 3-37.

[66]See: Ashley, *Constructing*, 507-508.

[67]See: Ashley, *Constructing*, 505-511.

[68]The question of individuated human matter cannot be avoided: an essay on individuated matter by a rational soul as the basis for human individuality, is in: Brown M, "St. Thomas Aquinas and the individuation of persons" *AmerCathPhilQ* 65 (1991) 29-44.

[69]See: Atkinson and Moraczewski, **Genetic Counseling**, 60-61.

[70]Atkinson and Moraczewski, **Genetic Counseling**, 70.

[71]See: May, *Moral worth*, 416-443.

[72]See: May, *Moral worth*, 425.

[73]May, *Moral worth*, 425.

[74]See: Shannon and Wolter, *Pre-embryo*, 614-615.

[75]Shannon and Wolter, *Pre-embryo*, 621-622.

[76]In other words, his requirement of actualizing *all* potencies may deny humanness to fetuses who are unable to do so due to some congenital abnormality; in this sense, his requirement would be morally unacceptable. An analysis of the topic is found in: Serra A, "La realtà biologica del neo-concepito" *CivCat* 126,3 (1975) 9-23.

[77]See: Shannon and Wolter, *Pre-embryo*, 611-614.

[78]For a view on the possible hidden agendas disguised behind distinguishing humanity before and after nidation, see: Sgreccia E, "A proposito del 'pre-embrione' umano" *MedMor* 36,1 (1986) 5-17.

[79]It is to be noted that even monozygotic twins develop subtle, but real differences between them. See: Watson *et al*, *Monozygotic twins*, 949-951.

[80]A contrasting analysis is given by: Zatti M, "Quando un 'pre-embrione' esiste, si tratta di un altro embrione" *MedMor* 5 (1991) 781-788.

[81]For a re-evaluation of the theory of evolution, see: Russo F, "L'evolution: une théorie en crise" *Ét* 370,3 (1989) 345-350.

[82]See: Ashley, *Constructing*, 505-511.

[83]For example, an analysis of the impact of humanity on the environment, can be seen in: Riou G, "Les défis de l'environnement: seuils, limites et irréversibilité" *Ét* 355,7 (1981) 43-58.

[84]He proposes six basic human needs: food, security, sex, information, society and creativity. See: Ashley, **Theologies**, 395-396.

[85]A description of the open-endedness of culture, and what Christianity can offer it today, can be appreciated in: Lustiger J-M, "L'homme sans fin: ou le redoutable paradoxe de la culture contemporaine" *Ét* 359,4 (1983) 293-301.

[86]Applied to the pre-born world, this issue compounds its complexity. For a review of specific cultural issues emerging from contemporary uses of prenatal diagnosis, see: Richards MPM, "Social and ethical problems of fetal diagnosis and screening" *JReprInfPsy* 7,3 (1989) 171-185.

[87]Pointing to the difficulty in arriving at a transcultural consensus regarding the practice of human medical genetics--in view of the fact that it touches upon the core of what it is to be human--, is: Serra A, "Transcultural problems in the use of medical genetics in clinical practice" in: Srám RJ, et al, eds, **Ethical Issues of Molecular Genetics in Psychiatry**. Berlin-Heidelberg: Springer-Verlag 1991, 120-130.

[88]Testimony on the applicability of human genetic information to today's historical context, is given by: Healy B, "Hearing on the possible uses and misuses of genetic information" *HGeneTher* 3 (1992) 51-56. And for a survey on interpretation ranges of genetic information, see: Wertz DC, Sorenson JR, Heeren TC, "Clients' interpretation of risks provided in genetic counseling" *AJHumGen* 39,2 (1986) 253-264. See also: Demmer K, "Theological argument and

[89]"A terminological problem exists in even framing the question [of abortion], for some authors make a distinction between human life and personal life, between human being and human person, between biological existence and fully human existence. To avoid confusion the term 'truly human being' or 'truly human life' will be used and understood as that human life deserving the value, rights, and protection due the human person as such." Curran, *Abortion*, 17.

[90]For a clarification of terminology regarding humanization, see: Fagone V, "Essere umano ed essere umanizzato: nuove prospettive antropologiche sul problema dell'aborto" *CivCat* 124,3 (1973) 20-36.

[91]O'Rourke and Brodeur, **Medical Ethics**, 70.

[92]A view on fetal right to self-development, even by those found to be carriers of handicaps, is described in: Serra A, "Aborto eugenico: diritto-dovere o delitto?" *CivCat* 124,4 (1973) 110-124.

[93]For a analysis of the role of choice in informed consent, see: Faden R, "Autonomy, choice, and the new reproductive technologies: the role of informed consent in prenatal genetic diagnosis" in: Rodin J, Collins A, eds, **Women and New Reproductive Technologies: Medical, Psychosocial, Legal, and Ethical Dilemmas**. Hillsdale, NJ: Lawrence Erlbaum 1991, 37-47.

[94]See: McCormick, *Experimentation*, 5.3-5.5.

[95]McCormick, *Experimentation*, 5.4.

[96]See, for instance, May's distinction between moral beings and beings of moral worth: May, *Moral worth*, 416-446.

[97]An exploration of possible consensus regarding experimental therapy can be seen in: Fletcher JC, "Ethics in experimental fetal therapy: is there an early consensus?" in: Evans MI *et al*, eds, **Fetal Diagnosis and Therapy: Science, Ethics and the Law**. Philadelphia: Lippincott 1989, 438-446.

---

[98]He has already stated that the viable fetus should be treated as one treats a child. See: McCormick, *Experimentation,* 5.1-5.2.

[99]For a full schematic classification, see *Viability and Discernible Risk or Discomfort* (Chapter IX), under Richard McCormick, in PART TWO of this work.

[100]For a review of alternatives to aborting a nonviable fetus, see: Watkins D, "An alternative to termination of pregnancy" *Practitioner* 233 (1989) 990,992.

CHAPTER XIV

HOMINIZATION AND PERSONHOOD

Introduction

This chapter investigates each of the ten authors' views on hominization and personhood during pregnancy, especially in light of the present possibility of earlier and earlier prenatal diagnosis in humans, and of the contemporary debate on the beginning of human individuality.

Accordingly, the ten authors researched line up into one of two main camps: those espousing delayed hominization, and those upholding immediate hominization. Some reasons for belonging to the former group are: the observed phenomenon of the process of conception, the possibility of referring to the conceptus before implantation as the pre-embryo, the various alternatives to human embryonic individuation, and the significance of brain integration as the beginning of such individuation.

Conversely, those authors upholding immediate hominization focus on: early zygotic differentiation, which is directed by a progressive sequence of primary organizers, thus allowing for the possibility of calling the conceptus before nidation a pre-implantation embryo. Within these early stages of development, the counterarguments of twinning, recombination, and hydatidiform moles and teratomas are addressed. In addition, a plausible interpretation is given to the observed phenomenon of high pregnancy wastage, and a probable argument is provided for the capacity for rationality in humans from the zygotic stage.

Finally, four presuppositions and interpretations are examined, namely: the meaning of a processural approach to (human) embryology, the validity of a distinction between genetic uniqueness and developmental individuality, at least two different possible interpretations of nonviability, and some precautions to maintain when accusing of biologism.

A. HUMAN PREGNANCY

1. Prenatal diagnosis

Standard prenatal diagnosis today is done once the human embryo has reached a certain stage of development, much after implantation has occurred.[1] However, because of the present possibility of pre-implantation diagnosis, it is also necessary to analyze the condition of prenatal human life before implantation.[2] The discussion of moral conflict situations involving pre-implantation human life centers mostly around whether it can be considered to be an individual human person or not.[3]

2. Individuality

Individuality and irrepeatability are no doubt constitutive of the human person.[4] Granted that the term "human person" is not univocal by any means,[5] it can still be maintained that, as created bodily beings, there was a time when each particular human person that has ever been, was not. This implies that there was also a time when each particular human person that has ever been, began. When does the individual human person begin to be such?[6]

Regarding the ten authors researched, two great camps appear on the horizon in answer to this question: those that hold for immediate hominization and personhood, and those that do not. To the former belong: B. Ashley, W. May, D. McCarthy, A. Moraczewski, T. O'Donnell, and K. O'Rourke. To the latter belong: L. Cahill, C. Curran, R. McCormick, and T. Shannon.

B. DELAYED HOMINIZATION

A case for the theory of delayed hominization and personhood could be built on a particular interpretation of human embryonic development. This theory is in fact a re-evaluation of the process of conception, the pre-embryo, individuation, and brain integration in light of contemporary biological data.[7]

1. The Process of Conception

Shannon correctly notes that human fertilization is a process that may take up to a day to complete, with the possibility of the male and female pronuclei taking up to another day to fuse.[8] Even after completed fusion of the two pronuclei, the resulting product of conception is not constricted to a single developmental fate, but can result in a number of biological entities. Since these possibilities generally seem to come to an end with the process of implantation, he prefers to extend the process of human conception up to the time of implantation.[9] There seems to be an ambiguity, however, in his usage of the term "conception," for whereas in one section he seeks to distinguish it from biological fertilization, in another section he seems to allot the same function to both.[10] Nonetheless, what he intends to emphasize here is the fact that human conception/fertilization is a process which involves the passage of time. To speak of the "moment of conception," then, is incorrect.[11]

In addition, he points out that "the zygote does not possess sufficient genetic information within its chromosomes to develop into an embryo that will be the precursor of an individual member of the human species. At this stage the zygote is neither self-contained nor self-sufficient for such further development, as was earlier believed."[12] The evidence cited here is from Bedate and Cefalo, who maintain that in order for the human zygote to further develop, it needs extra-nuclear genetic material contained in its cytoplasm.[13] Because this genetic material is not the product of the fusion of the two parental pronuclei, but rather originates from the paternal and the maternal cytoplasms, then it is not derived from the zygotic genome. However, to conclude from this biological fact that the zygote is not self-sufficient, seems to imply that this material continues to "belong" to the parents even after completed fertilization. If this reasoning is true, then one could also hold that the genetic material within the zygotic *nucleus* in not the zygote's either, for it too "belongs" to the parental gametes. This not withstanding, one fact that cannot be denied is the necessary interaction of the zygotic nucleus with its cytoplasmic organelles in order to further develop.[14]

2. The Pre-embryo

The authors espousing delayed hominization and personhood refer to prenatal life before implantation as the pre-embryo.[15] This is because they see in nidation the marker-moment for true individual embryonic development. Pre-embryo, however, is an ambiguous term which is not universally accepted in the scientific literature.[16] The main reason for this is that the various stages which it seeks to describe already have generic names which are also used for comparable developmental stages in other mammalian and vertebrate systems in general.[17] Still, the difference between a pre-embryo and an embryo is that the former can result in a number of possibilities, whereas the latter is individuated. Therefore, while genetic uniqueness may be said to occur from completed fertilization, developmental individuality proper does not occur until implantation has taken place. As McCormick states: "genetic individuality and developmental individuality do not coincide."[18]

3. Individuation

The evidence which these authors point to when upholding the lack of individuality in the pre-embryo is the possibility that a single human zygote may actually result in a number of different entities, such as: monozygotic twins, recombination, extraembryonic layers of the blastocyst, or a hydatidiform mole.[19] Given that individuality is one of the necessary, but not sufficient, conditions for the possibility of the existence of a human person, the fact that a single human zygote can result in or from several different entities vies against positing it with true human personhood.[20] Confirmatory of this lack of individual personhood before implantation these authors hold to be the observed phenomenon of high early pregnancy wastage in humans.[21]

4. Brain Integration

In addition to physiological individuality, some of these authors propose that true human personhood requires at least the capacity for rationality, even though there is no unanimity on what should be the minimum required capacity.[22] Note that what is argued here is not the presence of the actual physiological structure where human rationality is believed to occur, but rather the presence of at least that structure which actually allows for the capacity of the rational structure to develop.[23]

Taking the classical definition of personhood, then, to be *an individual substance of a rational nature*, one may argue that, based on present embryological evidence, the first half of the definition may not be fulfilled until completed implantation, and the second half, until well into fetal development.[24]

C. IMMEDIATE HOMINIZATION

It is precisely because human gestation is a gradual process, that those authors who hold for immediate hominization and personhood see as the only possible time when personhood begins to be the "moment" of conception.[25] In their reasoning, they point to zygotic organization from fertilization, the existence of a series of primary organizers along different stages of development, and a proper understanding of the phenomenon of spontaneous abortion or high pregnancy wastage.[26]

1. Zygotic Differentiation

McCarthy rightly points out that from completed fertilization, the zygote is already undergoing directional development, such that a metabolic gradient is established beginning at the area where the sperm penetrates the ovum.[27] Therefore, first and second cleavage will already involve protoplasmic bilaterality, and third cleavage will exhibit definite bipolarity.[28] This means that from its earliest stages of development, the human zygote is undergoing gradual differentiation. Because this differentiation is directional (*i.e.*, the overall growth of the organism happens by progressive mitosis of daughter cells. As it does so, the original cytoplasm of the zygote is further subdivided into smaller units.), there must be some center of organization which contains the minimal information necessary to control such directional activity. This center of information is what these authors call the "primary organizer."[29]

2. Primary Organizers

At the zygote level, the primary organizer seems to be the nucleus. It is understood that, in any organic system, the nucleus is incapable of functioning without interacting with the macromolecules and organelles that are found in the cytoplasm of its cell.[30] In addition, the proper physical conditions must be present in order for replication, transcription and translation to occur.[31] However, to conclude from this that "the zygote is neither self-contained nor self-sufficient for such further development,"[32] is to misunderstand organic development altogether, for it pretends a certain autonomy of the chromatic material which does not exist in natural systems as we know them.[33] In fact, what is crucial here is to maintain the discussion within the proper level of complexification: it is one thing to talk about the bio-chemical interaction between DNA, RNA and polypeptides; another is to speak of the relationship among the nucleus and its various organelles; another yet is to look at the rapport of the zygote with its surrounding environment. Taken as a whole, if a normal human zygote is provided with the proper environment, it is fully capable of self-development.[34]

At the morula stage, though each cell retains a certain "totipotentiality," the organism as a whole continues to follow a development of gradual "cytoplasmic compartmentalization" by progressive mitosis.[35] Evidence of organizational directionality may come from the fact that all blastomeres within the morula are evenly dividing in normal growth (as opposed to a cancerous growth, where some cells seem to divide in disproportion to their neighboring cells[36]). Hence, even though the exact centers of information have not yet been clearly identified, it can be deduced from these observations that a certain primary organizer is also present here to coordinate the overall differentiation of the morula into the blastocyst, the following stage.[37]

If the morula is differentiated from the zygote, the blastocyst is even more so, with an inner cell mass (forming the embryoblast), an outer cell mass (forming the trophoblast), and a hollow cavity.[38] The blastocyst is now ready to implant into the endometrium, and it does so by further differentiation of the cell layer at the embryonic pole, while the embryoblast continues to differentiate into two distinct cell layers.[39] Hence, from completed fusion of the two gametic pronuclei, to implantation, one observes a gradual, complex, organized cellular differentiation, a differentiation which could not take place without the presence of some "primary organizer" at each stage of development. Furthermore, this pre-implantation teleology is observed to follow normally the same pattern in all human fertilizations, something which seems to point to the universality of these "primary organizers."[40]

3. The Pre-Implanted Embryo

If there is indeed a directional teleology from fertilization to implantation, how is one to address the unquestionable evidence of the various possible outcomes from a single zygote? For the sake of clarity, each item is individually evaluated: twinning, recombination, hydatidiform moles, and high pregnancy wastage.[41]

Twinning

Dizygotic twins derive from two fertilized eggs and, as such, may be considered distinct individuals from conception.[42] Monozygotic twins, on the other hand, derive from a single zygote, whence the question: how can this zygote be considered an individual? To explore the answer, it must be noted that: first, separation does not necessarily happen at first cleavage (though it seems to be restricted to the very early stages of the morula); second, separation may not necessarily be complete (which might give rise to conjoined twins); third, in either case, separation seems to be an exception to normal development.[43] Given this, it must also be admitted that separation (whether complete or not) is a further development from the original zygote, since discrete redistribution of protoplasm necessarily occurs. The first conclusion, then, is that the appearance of monozygotic twins actually implies early differentiation.[44]

Can this differentiation be considered individualized? Yes, if by individuality one means singleness, uniqueness. Each monozygotic twin is unique at least in this sense: in that the specific chromatic material within its cells belongs to it and not to its twin, though this material is almost identical in chemical composition.[45] In other words, its matter is singularly its own. Secondly, can this matter be informed? Again, in so far as it is living matter, it *is* informed.[46]

Now the question: how can an individual human zygote give rise to two (or more) individual human beings? As McCormick rightly points out, this is an evaluative question,[47] and the evaluation of this group of authors upholding immediate hominization is that this is plausible by some mode of asexual reproduction, budding or cloning (a mode of reproduction which is commonly observed in other organic living systems).[48] If so, what prevents God from creating a soul for the new twin just as God did for the original twin at completed fertilization?[49]

Recombination

The authors proposing the possibility of recombination as an impediment to recognizing individuality in the human zygote fail to cite any confirmed cases of such phenomenon ever observed in human systems. Nonetheless, recombination having been experimentally achieved in other vertebrate systems,[50] one must remain at least open to the theoretical possibility of recombination in the human species. The question then arises: how can two individual human beings become one? Here again, the group of authors espousing immediate hominization propose the following plausible scenario:

A human ovum completes fertilization: an individual exists. Then, the zygote separates completely: now two individuals exist (see *twinning*, above). These two individual morulae subsequently re-unite into one: one individual dies and its matter is bio-chemically re-absorbed by the other individual's matter.[51] Biologically, this scenario is at least theoretically plausible. Theologically, it implies, first, that God creates each human soul *ex nihilo* (though not on matter incapable of sustaining such in-formation: for instance, on a zygote of a non-human species); second, that there is no pre-determined minimal time of human bodily existence, or of achieved level of development, to qualify as "human" (other than having at least been created); third, as far as Christian theology is concerned, that even this minimal bodily existence is no impediment for the possibility of the individual soul to establish union with God (a point which could be upheld if one is willing to accept that Jesus Christ began his own human existence as a zygote, *i.e.*, that the mystery of the Incarnation includes the zygotic stage).[52]

Hydatidiform moles and teratomas

These may come about from incomplete fertilization or from severe genetic abnormalities developing in early stages of cellular differentiation, giving rise to tissue growths of various types and sizes.[53] Because of their origin, it can be questioned whether such pathologic tissues ever were (or are any longer) true human beings. In the extreme case that fertilization was fully completed, and that the zygote had indeed begun to differentiate normally, with the pathology developing only after some discrete gestational time, it can still be theologically maintained that the human individual created at completed fertilization died when the pathology became so aberrant as to be unable to result in a living human individual.[54]

In fact, some authors point to the very existence of human hydatidiform moles and teratomas as confirmatory that the human embryo does not receive any information from its mother which is vitally necessary for developmental control.[55]

4. High Pregnancy Wastage

Along these same lines, the observed phenomenon of spontaneous abortion or high pregnancy wastage must be properly interpreted.[56] First, it can be maintained that not all these spontaneous abortions are completed or normal fertilizations,[57] thus allowing for the possibility that the resulting entity is not ensouled. Second, even in the most improbable event that all these spontaneous abortions are in effect ensouled human beings, there have been other historical times and places when infant mortality has also been as high as 50%, yet this mere fact is not sufficient to doubt that those children who died were indeed human beings.[58]

5. The Capacity for Rationality

In humans, rationality requires the presence of a physiological substratum. Further, the capacity for rationality is closely associated with a properly functioning brain. Yet, brain development is very slow and gradual in humans, even at the embryonic level.[59] This is believed to be so because of its high degree of complexification. Hence, the proper integration of the human brain (and indeed of the entire nervous system) requires the presence of certain specific precursors in prior embryonic stages.[60] The argument then becomes one of gradation: the presence of what precursor is considered sufficient to warrant the possibility of the capacity for rationality? Shannon, contending that one can only speak of a rational nature when the "biological structures necessary to perform rational actions are present,"[61] is arguing in favor of a proximate precursor, as opposed to a remote one, such as a normal human zygotic nucleus. However, because development of the capacity for human rationality is also epigenetic and not preformist,[62] it can be argued that this capacity could never exist in the proximate precursor if it did not already exist in the remote. To conclude, if the human capacity for rationality did not exist at the earliest possible stage of development (*i.e.*, the zygote), it cannot spontaneously appear at some later stage, no matter how integrated the brain becomes.[63]

D. PRESUPPOSITIONS AND INTERPRETATIONS

1. Processural Approach

A processural approach to the human person is based on an epigenetic interpretation of embryology, that is, that the development of specialized organ systems arises over time by the gradual differentiation of less specialized tissues and cells.[64] This ontogenetic development, though it may afford a certain limited range of vitally non-consequential variabilities, is fairly constant for each individual of the same biological species. As such, it is not to be confused with phylogenetic evolution,[65] where change occurs in an entire population over a more-or-less prolonged period of time due to spontaneous mutations arising within that same population, mutations that are discrete enough so as not to impede the continuous possibility of interbreeding.[66]

At the core of ontogenetic development is precisely the idea that, though the individual may undergo several gradual physiological and morphological changes within its lifetime, it nonetheless remains always the same ontological entity from the time that it first appears as an organic individual: a living bodily unit.[67]

2. The Validity of a Distinction

It is thus appropriate to question the validity of distinguishing between genetic uniqueness and developmental individuality.[68] Given that human embryonic development, like any other living embryonic development, is a dynamic system in constant interaction with the surrounding environment and transformation from within, there is no one stage at which it can be considered to be static or arrested (unless artificially induced), not even at the earliest possible stage. This dynamic directionality cannot occur were it not for the presence of specific genes within the genome of the individual zygotic nucleus which serve the function precisely of regulating the particular development of the individual in question and none other. Hence, genetic uniqueness necessarily implies developmental individuality: no other individual entity may arise from its particular genome except the one it codes for, whether normal *or* abnormal.[69]

3. Nonviability

In a processural approach to human embryology, nonviability can also be understood in two ways: either in the sense that an embryo is so immature that it cannot yet survive outside the uterus (but given sufficient gestational development, it can),[70] or in the sense that the embryo is so abnormal that it will die before full gestation (even if it remains *in utero* all this time).[71] In the first sense, it is not hard to see that nonviability is heavily dependent on the present technological state of the art. Indeed, it is conceivable that some day biomedical technology may arrive at sustaining extrauterine life throughout the entire nine months of gestation. In the second sense, it can be said that the embryonic genome carries within it a teleology such that, either it was never a "true human being" (due to such radical genetic transformations), or the human being that was, died when the pathology arose.[72]

In either of the two senses, however, nonviability does not pose a difficulty in maintaining the possibility of human life from the time of completed fertilization, since in order for these two possibilities to occur, either technological or chromosomal nonviability, the genomic teleology must be such that it is either human or not.[73] The fact that biomedical technology is presently unable to reverse either of these two nonviabilities only points at the possibility of further development in the field.

4. Biologism

Associated with a processural approach to human embryology is also the correct understanding of biology. Delayed hominization authors accuse immediate hominization authors of biologism,[74] yet in doing so, the very arguments used in refuting the possibility of immediate hominization are based on biological data.[75] The fact is that a proper understanding of the human person cannot leave out its corresponding biological data, for, as stated earlier, human beings are necessarily bodily beings. Given this, any theologizing about the ontological status of prenatal life, or any speculation about the possible beginning of human individuality and personhood, cannot prescind from the biological data known today.[76] Hence, as Moraczewski points out, whereas human personhood cannot be defined in biological terms, biological science *can* state when a particular organism is alive; when that life began; and whether or not the particular organism in question is or is not a member of the human species.[77]

Acknowledging this, the only other possibility for sustaining delayed hominization today is to hold that human being and human person are not coextensive, that is, that at least *some* human beings are not human persons. Of course, the inherent danger in this argument is that once personhood is denied to some group of human beings (*i.e.*, the pre-implanted embryo), what is there to prevent one from denying it to other groups of human beings (*i.e.*, the severely handicapped, or the deeply comatose)?[78] Whereas it must be admitted that all the typically human characteristics that are associated with being a human person can admit of an infinite variety of intensity, colouring and expression (no two human personalities are ever the same, either diachronically or synchronically), it must also be admitted that human personhood is an all-or-none quality which can only be properly attributed to certain living bodily beings: those belonging to the species *Homo sapiens.*[79]

Notes

[1]See: *Prenatal Diagnosis Techniques*, in Chapter IV of PART ONE of this work.

[2]Descriptions are found in: Coutelle et al, *Preimplantation diagnosis*, 22-24; Handyside et al, *Preimplantation diagnostic testing*, 905-909; McBride, *Preimplantation genetic diagnosis*, 894-895; Read and Donnai, *Preimplantation diagnosis*, 3.

[3]For a summary of the various evaluations of the status of prenatal life, see: Paoletti RA, "Developmental-genetic and psycho-social positions regarding the ontological status of the fetus" *LinacreQ* 44 (1977) 243-261. See also: Lizotte A, Reflexions philosophiques sur l'âme et la personne de l'embryon" *Anthr* 3 (1987) 155-195; Marra B, "L'embrione e la sua natura" *Sap* 46 (1993) 87-89; Serra A, "La sperimentazione sull'embrione umano: una nuova esigenza della

scienza e della medicina?" *MedMor* 43 (1993) 97-116.

[4]An analysis of the necessarily material individuality of human personhood, is in: Brown M, "St. Thomas Aquinas and the individuation of persons" *AmerCathPhilQ* 65 (1991) 29-44. Upholding the developmental nature of individual human persons, is: Barry R, "Personhood: the conditions of identification and description" *LinacreQ* 45 (1978) 64-81.

[5]An evaluation of ontological, ethical and juridical embryonic "personhood," is found in: Bondolfi A, "Statuto dell'embrione. Considerazioni di metodo" *RTMor* 90 (1991) 223-241. See also: Serra A, "Per un'analisi integrata dello 'status' dell'embrione umano. Alcuni dati della genetica e dell'embriologia" in: Biolo S, ed, **Nascita e Morte dell'Uomo**. Atti del 46 Convegno del Centro Studi Filosofici di Gallarate, Genova: Marietti 1993, 55-106.

[6]For an appeal to consistency when speaking both of the biological and of the ontological reality of the beginning of human life, see: Fagone V, "Essere umano ed essere umanizzato: Nuove prospettive antropologiche sul problema dell'aborto" *CivCat* 124,3 (1973) 20-36; "Vita prenatale e soggetto umano" *CivCat* 126,1 (1975) 441-460. See also: Ford NM, **When Did I Begin? Conception of the Human Individual in History, Philosophy, and Science**. Cambridge: Cambridge University 1988, 55-101; with a critique, in: Tonti-Filippini N, "A critical note" *LinacreQ* 56,3 (1989) 36-50, and a rebuttal, in: Ford NM, "**When Did I Begin?** A reply to Nicholas Tonti-Filippini" *LinacreQ* 57 (1990) 59-66.

[7]An argument in favor of delayed hominization on the basis of twinning before implantation also in: Bedate CA, "Reflections concerning questions of life and death: towards a new paradigm for understanding the ethical value of the biological human entity" in: Malherbe J-F, ed, **Human Life: Its Beginnings and Development**. Paris: L'Harmattan 1988, 67-97. See also: Smith PA, "The beginning of personhood: a thomistic perspective" *LavalPhilT* 39,2 (1983) 195-214; Tauer CA, "Personhood and human embryos and fetuses" *JMedPhil* 10 (1985) 253-266.

[8]See: Shannon and Wolter, *Pre-embryo*, 607. See also: Glass, *Sperm and egg transport*, 108-115.

[9]"Biologically understood, conception occurs only after a lengthy process has been completed and is more closely identified with implantation than fertilization." Shannon and Wolter, *Pre-embryo*, 611.

[10]"A critical finding of modern biology is that conception biologically speaking is a process beginning with the penetration of the outer layer of the egg by a sperm and concluding with the formation of the diploid set of chromosomes. This process takes at least a day." Shannon and Wolter, *Pre-embryo*, 610.

[11]Also speaking of the process of conception, is: Attard M, "Dimensioni etiche della medicina genetica: la moralità dei bambini in provetta" *RTMor* 43 (1979) 367-384.

[12]Shannon and Wolter, *Pre-embryo*, 608.

[13]That is, "the genetic material from maternal mitochondria, and the maternal or paternal genetic messages in the form of messenger RNA or proteins." Bedate CA, Cefalo RC, "The zygote: to be or not to be a person" *JMedPhil*, 14 (1989) 642.

[14]Summarized in: Weaver and Hedrick, **Genetics**, 410-434.

[15]See: McCormick, *Preembryo*, 1-15; Shannon and Wolter, *Pre-embryo*, 603-626.

[16]A review of the historical and semantic origin of the various terms used in describing prenatal stages of development in: Biggers JD, "Arbitrary partitions of prenatal life" *HumanRepr* 5,1 (1990) 1-6.

[17]From whence zygote, morula, blastocyst and gastrula. See: Johnson, **Human Developmental Anatomy**, 33-40. For a possible hidden agenda behind the attempt to change conventional prenatal terminology, see: Sgreccia E, "A proposito del 'pre-embrione' umano" *MedMor* 36,1 (1986) 5-17.

[18]McCormick, *Preembryo*, 4. See also: Shannon and Wolter, *Pre-embryo*, 606-610.

[19]See: Curran, *Abortion*, 19; *In vitro*, 4.15-4.16; **Moral Theology**, 125-126; **New Perspectives**, 188; **Ongoing Revision**, 156; Transitions, 212; McCormick, *Abortion: rules*, 28; *Bioethics*, 124; *Changing morality* , 39; **Health**, 134-135; **Notes**, 797; *Preembryo*, 4; Shannon and Cahill, **Religion and Artificial Reproduction**, 116; Shannon and Wolter, *Pre-embryo*, 608, 615-619.

[20]An argument in favor of human life before implantation, but not yet individuated, is also given by: Lacadena JR, "Status of the embryo prior to implantation" in: Malherbe J-F, ed, **Human Life: Its Beginnings and Development**. Paris: L'Harmattan 1988, 39-45.

[21]An in-depth study of the phenomenon, is found in: Campos L, Tejedo A, Abel F, Cefalo RC, "Genetics and scope of spontaneous abortion and fetal wastage" in: Malherbe J-F, ed, **Human Life: Its Beginnings and Development**. Paris: L'Harmattan 1988, 125-146; Cinque B, Pelagalli M, Daini S, Dell'Acqua S, Spagnolo AG, "Aborto ripetuto spontaneo: aspetti scientifici e obbligazioni morali" *MedMor* 42,5 (1992) 889-908; Glass and Golbus, *Habitual abortion*, 437-446.

[22]See: McCormick, *Abortion: changing morality*, 37; Moussa and Shannon, *Pineal gland*, 30-37; Shannon, *Brain integration*, 123-144; Shannon and Wolter, *Pre-embryo*, 620-622.

[23]"One can speak of a rational nature in a philosophically significant sense only when the biological structures necessary to perform rational actions are present, as opposed to only reflex activities. The biological data suggest that the minimal time of the presence of a rational nature would be around the 20th week, when neural integration of the entire organism has been established. The presence of such a structure does not argue that the fetus is positing rational actions, only that the biological presupposition for such actions is present." Shannon and Wolter, *Pre-embryo*, 620.

[24]For a contrasting interpretation of Boethius' definition of the pre-embryonic human person, see: Doran K, "Person - a key concept for ethics" *LinacreQ* 56 (1989) 38-49; Possenti V, "La bioetica alla ricerca dei principi: la persona" *MedMor* 42,6 (1992) 1075-1094; Zatti M, "Quando un 'pre-embrione' esiste, si tratta di un altro embrione" *MedMor* 5 (1991) 781-788.

[25]An analysis in favor of the beginning of individual human life from conception, is also given by: Daly TV, 'The personhood of the human embryo" *LinacreQ* 57,1 (1990) 83-88; Guinchedi F, "Considerazioni sullo statuto embrionario" *RasT* 34 (1993) 62-76. Lee P, "Personhood, the moral standing of the unborn, and abortion" *LinacreQ* 57,2 (1990) 80-89; Privitera S, "Riflessioni sullo status morale e giuridico dell'embrione" *RTMor* 89 (1991) 93-100; Serra A, "Quando comincia un essre umano. In margine ad un recente documento" *MedMor* 37,3 (1987) 387-401.

[26]See: Ashley, *Critique*, 1113-133; *Constructing*, 507-508; Ashley and O'Rourke, **Healthcare Ethics** (1989), 211-213; May, **Human Existence**, 93-103; *Zygotes I*, 2-4; *Zygotes II*, 1-3; McCarthy and Bayer, **Critical Life Issues**, 80-90; McCarthy and Moraczewski, *Fetal experimentation*, 30-33; Moraczewski, *No brain*, 1-2; *Science*, 2-3; O'Donnell, *Anencephaly*, 37-40; *Double-talk*, 1-4; *Mifepristone*, 7; *Tubal pregnancy*, 23-24; *Quality control*, 15-16.

[27]See: McCarthy and Bayer, **Critical Life Issues**, 82.

[28]A summary is found in: Moore, **Developing Human**, 31-32.

[29]See: Ashley, *Critique*, 114-117; May, **Human Existence**, 93-103; McCarthy and Bayer, **Critical Life Issues**, 86-87; Moraczewski, *No brain*, 1-2.

[30]See: Weaver and Hedrick, **Genetics**, 162-188.

[31]See: Weaver and Hedrick, **Genetics**, 264-285.

[32]Shannon and Wolter, *Pre-embryo*, 608.

[33]See: Weaver and Hedrick, **Genetics**, 226-259.

[34]For a theory on the capacity of a natural entity to effect its characteristic end, provided the proper conditions germane to the development of that entity exist, see: Makin S, "Aquinas, natural tendencies and natural kinds" *NewSchol* 63 (1989) 253-274.

[35]See: Moore, **Developing Human**, 32-33.

[36]Narrated in: Weaver and Hedrick, **Genetics**, 472-489.

[37]Ashley suggests that the aggregate of cells at the superior pole of the morula may have an overall regulatory function. See: Ashley, *Critique*, 123-124.

[38]Diagrams are found in: Moore, **Developing Human**, 33-35.

[39]See: Moore, **Developing Human**, 38-43.

[40]The proposed sequence of "primary organizers" would be: the nucleus of the zygote; the cluster of blastomeres at the animal pole of the morula; the embryoblast of the blastocyst; the primitive streak of the gastrula; the neural plate of the embryo; the brain of the fetus. See: Ashley, *Constructing*, 507-508; McCarthy and Bayer, **Critical Life Issues**, 86-87; Moraczewski, *No brain*, 1-2.

[41]An excellent synopsis of various possible outcomes stemming from a human zygote in: Filice FP, "Twinning and recombination: a review of the data" *LinacreQ* 48 (1981) 40-51.

[42]See: Moore, **Developing Human**, 124.

[43]See: Moore, **Developing Human**, 124-126.

[44]See: Yanguas JM, "Experimentación con embriones humanos" in: CITM, **Persona**, 109-121.

[45]It has been found that some chromatic variation may be evident even in monozygotic twins. See: Watson *et al*, *Monozygotic twins*, 949-951.

[46]Recall that in natural bodily systems, life is never observed to exist in the abstract, but rather as existing in the specific body of the particular individual being observed.

[47]See: McCormick, *Bioethics*, 124; **Critical Calling**, 344; **Health**, 134-135; *Therapy*, 402-403.

[48]See: Weaver and Hedrick, **Genetics**, 67. See also: Tonti-Filippini, *Critical note*, 36-50.

[49]See: Ashley, *Critique*, 126-127; Ashley and O'Rourke, **Healthcare Ethics** (1989), 211-213; May, **Human Existence**, 99-103, McCarthy and Moraczewski, *Fetal experimentation*, 30-33.

[50]A summary is provided by: Weaver and Hedrick, **Genetics**, 374-406.

[51]See: Ashley, *Critique*, 128; Ashley and O'Rourke, **Healthcare Ethics**, 211-213; May, **Human Existence**, 101-102; McCarthy and Moraczewski, *Fetal experimentation*, 30-33.

[52]See: O'Donnell, *Genetic counseling*, 24. See also: Caspar Ph, "Animation de l'âme et unicité de la forme chez Saint Thomas d'Aquin" *Anthr* 5 (1989) 109-118; "La problématique de l'animation de l'embryon" *NRT* 113 (1991) 239-255, 400-413. An argument in favor of the foundation of the dignity of the human person in being immediately created by God, is found in: Schönborn C, "L'homme créé par Dieu: le fondement de la dignité de l'homme" *Greg* 65 (1984) 337-363.

[53]Classified in: Copeland, *Trophoblastic disease*, 415-421.

[54]See: May, *Zygotes I*, 2-4.

[55]An analysis in: Suarez A, "Hydatidiform moles and teratomas confirm the human identity of the preimplantation embryo" *JMedPhil* 15 (1990) 627-635.

[56]Reporting that: 50-60% of all spontaneous abortions in the first trimester are associated with changes in number or structures of chromosomes; congenital malformations incompatible with human life are found in 80-97% of early spontaneous abortions, and 30% of late one; and only less than 60% of all human zygotes are estimated to ever develop into liveborn babies, are: Campos *et al*, *Spontaneous abortion and fetal wastage*, 125-146.

[57]Described in: Tolmie, *Chromosomal disorders*, 33-45.

[58]See: Ashley, *Critique*, 126; Ashley and O'Rourke, **Healthcare Ethics** (1989), 211-213. See also: Lopez-García G, "La realidad del aborto espontaneo" in: CITM, **Persona**, 333-339.

[59]Photographic laminae of human fetal brain development may be found in: England, **Life Before Birth**, 51-64.

[60]See: England, **Life Before Birth**, 14-19.

[61]Shannon and Wolter, *Pre-embryo*, 620.

[62]See: Ashley and O'Rourke, **Health Care Ethics** (1978), 221-226; May, **Becoming**, 44; Moore, **Developing Human**, 9.

[63]See: Moraczewski, *No brain*, 1-2.

[64]See: Johnson, **Human Developmental Anatomy**, 47-50. See also: Leone S, "L'embrione: soggetto di diritti" *RTMor* 98 (1993) 229-238; Manno AG, "Essere umano dal concepimento" *RTMor* 97 (1993) 89-95.

[65]An appraisal of human phylogeny is given by: Boné, *Paléontologie*, 39-57.

[66]For a review of the ontogenetic and phylogenetic processural development of prenatal human life, see: Serra A, "La realtà biologica del neo-concepito" *CivCat* 126,3 (1975) 9-23.

[67]See: Ashley, *Critique*, 127; McCarthy and Moraczewski, *Fetal experimentation*, 30. A contrasting view distinguishing three differentially-arising dimensions of human beings (organic, psychic and symbolic) in: Malherbe J-F, "The personal status of the human embryo: a philosophical essay on eugenic abortion" in: Malherbe J-F, ed, **Human Life: Its Beginnings and Development**. Paris: L'Harmattan 1988, 101-116, and a strong critique in: Guzzetti GB, "Quando l'embrione è persona? A proposito del pensiero di Jean-François Malherbe" *RTMor* 73 (1987) 67-79.

[68]See: McCormick, *Preembryo*, 1-2; Shannon and Wolter, *Pre-embryo*, 603-613.

[69]See: Ashley, *Constructing*, 507-508; McCarthy and Bayer, **Critical Life Issues**, 80-81; Moraczewski, *Human beings*, 2-3.

[70]See: May, **Human Existence**, 93.

[71]See: McCormick, *Experimentation*, 5.1-5.14.

[72]Described in: Moore, **Developing Human**, 213; Weaver and Hedrick, **Genetics**, 290-314.

[73]For a position on the universality and exclusivity of the teleology of living natural systems, see: Engelman, *Aristotelian teleology*, 297-312.

[74]See: Shannon, *Brain integration*, 138.

[75]See: Curran, *In vitro*, 4.1-4.33; **Moral Theology**, 125-126; **New Perspectives**, 188; **Ongoing Revisions**, 156; **Transition**, 212; McCormick, *Abortion: changing morality*, 39; *Abortion: rules*, 28; **Bioethics**, 124; **Health**, 134-135; **Notes**, 499; *Preembryo*, 11-12; Shannon and Wolter, *Pre-Embryo*, 608, 612-613.

[76]An appraisal of the corporeality of the human "I" in: Documento del Centro di Bioetica della Università Cattolica del Sacro Cuore, "Indentità e statuto dell'embrione umano" *MedMor* 39,4 (1989) 663-676.

[77]See: Moraczewski, *Human beings*, 2-3.

[78]See: May, *Zygotes II*, 2; McCarthy and Bayer, **Critical Life Issues**, 88-90; O'Donnell, *Quality control*, 15-16.

[79]Also arguing in favor of an evaluation of the ontological nature of prenatal human life independent of external decisions regarding its subjective worth or lack thereof, is: De Marco D, "The foetus, his humanity and his rights" *LinacreQ* 41 (1974) 281-284; Fagone V, "Il problema dell'inizio della vita dell'uomo" *CivCat* 124,2 (1973) 531-546. Recognizing the personhood of the human embryo, is: Bueche W, "Destroying human embryos - destroying human lives: a moral issue" *StMor* 29 (1991) 85-115. See also: Carrasco de Paula I, "Personalità dell'embrione e aborto"

in: CITM, **Persona**, 277-290; Daly, *Personhood*, 83-88; Lee, *Personhood*, 80-89; Regan A, "The human conceptus and personhood" *StMor* 30 (1992) 97-127.

CHAPTER XV

ANALYSIS OF THE MORAL ACT

Introduction

In addition to the moral object itself, at the core of human actions are also intentionality and motivation. This can be universally said if one seeks to analyze true moral behavior.

Accordingly, the first section of this chapter briefly examines the relation between human intentionality and motivation, and the role which they both play in a proper analysis of the moral act.

Likewise, vital to a correct analysis of the moral act is as accurate a labeling and evaluating as humanly possible. Granted that here obvious grammatical and hermeneutical limitations will inevitably arise, the fact remains that the best attempt must always be made. Hence, the second section addresses the issues of adequately labeling and evaluating a human action which involves both empirical and moral dimensions, to witness: prenatal diagnosis.

Finally, according to Catholic tradition, when conflict situations arise, the principle of double effect may be invoked. This is precisely what each of the ten authors studied do, as expected, with his or her particular nuances of interpretation. Hence, the third section seeks to critique the various ways in which these ten authors make use of this principle when dealing with prenatal life and conflict situations.

A. INTENTIONALITY AND MOTIVATION

There is no question that, alongside the moral object itself, intentionality and motivation are both also at the root of a proper analysis of the moral act.[1] Lest one succumbs to an unrealistic fragmentation and depersonalization of the significance of human actions, it seems reasonable to admit that behind every true human action is an intention, and behind every intention, a motivation.[2] In fact, if the ahistorical single action is practically unthinkable,[3] this means that one human action flows into another in a more-or-less conscious succession as real life unfolds: intentionality provides the "glue" for the possibility of such succession. Because the true human action is fundamentally a free action, intentionality is that privileged hermeneutical place where the experience of human freedom can be interpreted.[4] This having been said, it must also be recognized that, while intentionality is certainly historically conditioned, it does not remain totally open-ended, facing a future of infinite possibilities.[5] Human action may indeed be the expression of human freedom, but it is never absolute freedom. If anything, it is precisely historical conditioning what renders human action communicable and intelligible, for all human knowing must occur within the realm of history. It is this human knowing what renders possible and intelligible the analysis of the moral act.[6] The fact that intentionality is at the core of the moral act does not mean that it relativizes the norm into absolute possibilities: it rather conditions and delimits it.[7]

If the objective correctness of an action is its clear correspondence with its intention--that is, its achieved mediation between its intermediate ends and its last end--,[8] then in this sense intentionality may be charged with the responsibility of providing the correctness of the action. Motivation, on the other hand, remains one step removed from the actual action by providing the *validity* for the action: its goodness or badness (motivation being that which protends the will to pursue this particular good as perceived good[9]). As such, intentionality must always remain at the service of motivation. It behooves motivation to desire and seek the good; it behooves intentionality to order itself according to the motivation of the agent. To create a chasm between these two is to attack the core of moral truth and intelligibility.[10] It is its presumed intelligibility which renders the analysis of the moral act communicable. Even so, might one realistically expect consensus here without a prior clarification of terms?

B. LABELING AND EVALUATING

This prior clarification points to the necessity of correctly labeling the phenomenon under consideration. That certain actions are always and everywhere wrong is not questioned, what is questioned is the accurate identification of such actions.[11] Have all the possible meanings been explained? Have they been adequately exhausted? What are the various levels of alternatives, given the present conditions?[12] It would seem that here the interdisciplinary work of seeking a common language is indispensable.[13] But one must also ask: is such a search realistic? Or, perhaps, the best that can be hoped for, at least as far as prenatal human life and conflict situations are concerned, is for moral theology and medical science to become aware of each other's terminological differences (PARTS ONE and TWO of this text, respectively). But, what happens when the scientific and the theological horizons necessarily intersect in one and the same action?[14] A case in point is again prenatal diagnosis. While its medical definition may vary according to time, place and circumstances of occurrence, intentionality and motivation are circumscribed to its medical indication and proper procedure in view of the desired results.[15] Morally, intentionality and motivation must consider the values at play, which inevitably implies a prior evaluation. Therefore, at the base of the goodness or badness of an action is found a prior evaluation.[16]

In evaluating the morality of prenatal diagnosis, essential to remember is that there are two *simultaneous* subjects recipient of such action: the mother and the child. How is the agent to evaluate such action when the interests of these two subjects appear to be in conflict?[17]

C. THE PRINCIPLE OF DOUBLE EFFECT

Here, the Catholic tradition has pointed to "direct" and "indirect" voluntariety, and what has come to be known as the principle of double effect.[18] All authors examined invoke the principle in their analyses of the moral act, but invariably arrive at differing conclusions when applied to prenatal life and conflict situations. Some critical observations follow.

1. B. Ashley, OP, and K. O'Rourke, OP

Ashley and O'Rourke sharply distinguish between direct and indirect voluntariety in their analysis.[19] Once again, intentionality is the key element, only that here, they pretend it to take on a certain binding quality. They define an indirect abortion as a procedure which purpose is to treat a threatening maternal pathology, "but in which the death of the fetus is an inevitable result that would have been avoided had it been possible."[20] Why the obligation to avoid it if at all possible? Because for them, human life is intrinsically a moral value, not just and ontic one.[21] In other words, in true human situations, the pre-moral interpretation of the act is not sufficient for a proper evaluation. Determining a "pre-moral" value involves a prior moral evaluation, namely: why is this a "pre-moral" value? This leads them to reject "proportionalism"[22] in favor of "prudential personalism" as a valid system of analysis.[23] However, when they say that: "For proportionalists, the object of a human act, apart from its circumstances and the agent's intention, is only a *premoral* object that involves certain human values and disvalues,"[24] they must be taken to task in that the term "proportionalists" is not being used unequivocally, since it still admits of alternative renditions, such as assessing a premoral evaluation at the psycho-volitive level of the action, while a moral one at the meta-level of its concomitant interpretation.[25] This, in fact, would be a situation much more realistic to the human condition, for it appeals to a necessary mediation between the two levels of reality: metaphysical and historical.[26]

2. C.E. Curran

Curran begins his moral analysis involving prenatal life by distinguishing between two issues: when human life begins, and the possible resolution of conflict situations.[27] Focusing on the latter, he aims at interpreting the act in a manner other than exclusively physical, that is, by including other values which he considers commensurate with human life.[28] Examples of these could be "grave but real threats to the psychological health of the woman and could also include other values of a socio-economic nature in extreme situations."[29] Recognizing the multitude of evaluative levels here operative, the critical question becomes: are these truly commensurable?[30] If there is an acknowledged lack of agreement as to psychological theories and pathologies, there is an even greater discrepancy as to what constitutes "extreme socio-economic situations." Then, one is here plunged into a hopeless subjectivism! Coming now to the actual resolution of conflicts, he rejects the principle of double effect in the case of prenatal life, since he finds the third criterion inapplicable in certain situations. "For example, one cannot abort to save the life of the mother which might be endangered because her heart cannot take the pregnancy."[31] Once again, it must be asked: given the present status of pregnancy management and delivery options, has he sufficiently explored and exhausted all other possible alternatives?[32] In view of current treatment available, it seems not. Finally, what remains even less clear is his suggested alternative: "I am not proposing that the fetus is an unjust aggressor but rather that the ethical model employed in solving problems of unjust aggression avoids some of the problems created by the model of direct and indirect effects when the direct effect is determined by the physical structure of the act itself."[33] However, in this model the motivation is always to *deter* the unjustified aggression, not to *kill* the aggressor (for if the aggressor dies, it remains an "indirect" effect). Therefore, he still fails to avoid alluding to direct and indirect effects, which makes his proposed alternative flawed and useless.

3. W.E. May

May holds the distinction between direct and indirect voluntariety to be basic to his moral analysis: the motive of the agent and the intention of the action are directed, "not upon the life of the fetus, but upon countering the injurious effect that the fetus, simply by its presence, is causing its mother."[34] Even so, it must be admitted that this analysis presumes a strict, literal, physical sense of injurious presence, which is partial and not fully realistic.[35] He develops this position from a deontologism of basic human goods,[36] which finds "consequentionalism" invalid because it fails to adequately evaluate one basic human good against another.[37] Consequentionalism is not, however, an unambiguous term, for no true human action is devoid of consequences.[38] To be concerned with achieving a higher good is not necessarily in contraposition to upholding certain basic human goods. Indeed, the very desire (motivation) to obtain the higher good (*i.e.*, human life) points to a concern for that same good, and thus to the meaning of the action as revelatory of that desire.[39] Hence, his accusation that a concern for a higher good is not revelatory of our being remains unfounded in a deeper analysis of true human experience.

4. D. McCarthy and A. Moraczewski, OP

McCarthy and Moraczewski enter the moral analysis by evaluating risks and benefits,[40] which they hold must center on the same individual, and not on benefits to the community at large.[41] This provides for a double application of the principle of due proportion. On the one hand, benefits to the individual must clearly outweigh the risks involved in pursuing such benefits. On the other, justifying exposing the individual to risks without clear benefits to itself would also justify exposing other disadvantaged individuals or groups in society to be likewise manipulated. Once more, implied in this analysis is that the risks and benefits under discussion directly incumb the individual. Yet, one also detects a broadening interpretation to include some possible indirect benefit (*i.e.*, to allay the mother's fears), which is only justified provided the interests of the individual are safeguarded (*i.e.*, the life of the fetus).[42] Their underlying system is again a brand of "prudential personalism"[43] which takes as normative the "natural" event: embryonic development as a constitutive stage of human life.[44] These two authors are inconsistent, however, because they fail to provide sufficient grounding, not for the inclusion of some obvious indirect benefit (*i.e.*, when the physician is statistically confident that the fetus is normal, while the suspicious mother is contemplating an abortion), but for the shift from direct to indirect benefit under certain conditions: why should such a shift be justified for the fetus and not for the mother?[45]

5. R.A. McCormick, SJ

McCormick places great value on proportionality or commensurate reason, which colors his entire analysis.[46] Hence, "[prenatal] life may be taken only if necessary 'to protect life or other values proportionate to life.'"[47] He notes that these values must be consistent with those justifying the taking of extrauterine life: self-defense, just war, capital punishment, indirect killing.[48] And herein lies the first problem: in the case of these extrauterine examples, the validity of the action arises from the purported legitimacy of a prior evaluation wherein the perpetrator of the evil action was found morally guilty of an unjust aggression; in the case of prenatal life, how can the embryo ever be equally evaluated? Unless he is prepared to renounce to the intentional requirement of a moral action, it seems impossible to do so: he is either making the innocent guilty, or he is ignoring the moral difference between the two.[49]

McCormick also introduces the element of the capacity for intersubjectivity or sociality,[50] which allows him to claim that it is a reasonable assumption to expect from an incompetent (*i.e.*, the fetus) what could be expected if he or she were competent, namely, to choose what ought to be chosen could she or he do so.[51] And he or she ought to choose what is best for her or him and for humanity.[52] Therefore, with minimal or negligible risk to the individual fetus, and notable benefit to fetuses in general and humanity at large, but no benefit to the individual fetus, he permits experimentation.[53] Yet, how reasonable is it to assume that the fetus would choose what it ought to? Is the moral freedom of the human agent to be so radically annihilated? Logical consistency would demand that "society" could impose equivalent experimentation on other (born) incompetents under the aegis of "the common good," a situation which history has invariably condemned, at least when viewed retrospectively. To note also is that, in the particular case of the fetus, minimal risk of grave harm may actually translate into grave risk![54]

6. T.J. O'Donnell, SJ

O'Donnell also analyzes the principle of double effect.[55] He presupposes the action to be a moral action, and therefore the good to be a moral good; the distinction between the good effect ("direct voluntariety") and the evil effect ("indirect voluntariety") residing in the will of the agent.[56] Yet, he is not unaware of the two levels of interpretation.[57] Hence, he contends that even if the evil effect chronologically precedes the good effect, the integrity of the act is salvaged by its overall teleology.[58] Yet, the "due proportion between the intended good and permitted evil" allows for too vague and ambivalent interpretations.[59] Himself admits that it "is not something that can be measured exactly. It is rather a matter of prudent human judgment."[60] And herein the ambivalence: if the morality of the action resides in an *a priori* willing of the objectively good effect, how can it be simultaneously subordinated to a subjective judgment? The contradiction seems to lie in wanting to uphold the free election of a good that *must* be chosen (in order not to vitiate the act).[61] Furthermore, prudence is never innate, but arduously acquired, often only after many "trials and errors;" are such errors to be morally justified under the pretense of the "lack of experience" necessary to acquire prudence? What happens when the "prudent judgment" of two agents leads them to opposite conclusions? In other words, as it stands in his published literature, his analysis admits of further clarification.

7. T.A. Shannon

Shannon accepts as valid the distinction between moral and pre-moral evil in his analysis.[62] Hence, he can state that abortion is at least a pre-moral evil.[63] However, a definite problem arises when he concludes from this that "there is no reasonable basis for arguing that the pre-embryo is morally equivalent to a person or is a person as a basis for prohibiting abortion,"[64] since this would mean that *his* interpretation of current embryological data is the only reasonable possibility: realistically, can one ever claim such interpretative certainty?[65] He then begins a process of evaluation to determine whether, and under what conditions, this also becomes a moral evil, which eventually leads to a gradational argument of increasing claims paralleling organic developmental stages.[66] However, a legitimately critical question is: why should the eventual moral claim of prenatal life hinge primarily on the organic proximity to attainment of the capacity for consciousness? Might this not also presume human consciousness to be an "all-or-none" quality, both ontologically and existentially? In doing so, he is indicating that the fourth element of the principle absolutely predisposes and conditions the entire analysis.[67] Still, the challenge is precisely in determining whether or not these different levels of interpretation of the various stages are truly commensurable so that an adequate comparison between goods and values can be obtained. In this sense, his line of reasoning is also flawed and can therefore withstand further refinement.[68]

Notes

[1]An appraisal of ethical discernment seeking moral estimation, incorporating intentional and motivational personal and social perspectives of the moral act, is found in: Vidal, **Discernimiento**, 13-27. See also: De Virgilio G, "L'analisi dell'atto morale" *RTMor* 98 (1993)

171-176.

[2]It is precisely because of the universal validity of intentionality and motivation that Ashley and O'Rourke can hold some human actions to be intrinsically evil; it is humanly impossible to execute them without *intending* to do evil. See: Ashley and O'Rourke, **Healthcare Ethics** (1989), 214. A critical analysis of the epistemological presuppositions underlying the moral theorem of intrinsic evil in light of an objectivist existential metaphysics of the human act, in: Demmer K, "Erwägungen zum 'intrinsece malum'" *Greg* 68 (1987) 613-637.

[3]See: Demmer K, **Interpretare e Agire: Fondamenti della Morale Cristiana**. (trans. Pedrazzoli M) Milano: Paoline 1989, 164.

[4]See: Demmer, **Interpretare**, 165. A deepened analysis of the role of experience in the moral interpretation of human freedom through insight, is also in: Demmer K, "Sittlich Handeln aus Erfahrung" *Greg* 59 (1978) 661-690.

[5]For a brief historical summary on the role of intentionality in the development of fundamental moral theology over the past thirty years, see: Aubert J-M, "Foi et morale: parcours de moral fondamentale" *Suppl* 155 (1985) 75-80.

[6]Offering a model of the individuating process of the moral norm due to its inherent intelligibility, and of the intersection of the deductive and inductive methods in intuition under the "light of the gospel," is: Privitera S, "Sul processo individuativo della norma morale" *RTMor* 23 (1974) 461-475.

[7]A systematic analysis of the concept and foundation of the Christian moral norm in general and of singular norms, and of the duty of all Christians to discern, in: Chiavacci E, "La fondazione della norma morale nella riflessione teologica contemporanea" *RTMor* 37 (1978) 9-38. See also: Composta D, "L'intenzione come momento costitutivo dell'atto morale" in: AA VV, **Attualità della Teologia Morale: Punti Fermi - Problemi Aperti**. Roma: Urbaniana 1987, 87-110; Di Marino A, "Originalità e origine delle norme morali cristiane" *RTMor* 20 (1973) 515-546.

[8]See: Demmer, **Interpretare**, 169.

[9]For an Aristotelian-Thomistic thesis postulating the specificity of the good thing as the foundation for the possibility of good, see: La Croce E, "Good and goods according to Aristotle" *NewSchol* 63 (1989) 1-17. An argument in favor of a certain binding quality of the truth about goodness regarding the normativity of moral action, in: Kaczynski E, "Verità sul bene nei diversi elementi della morale" *RTMor* 51 (1981) 419-431.

[10]A synthesis on the moral obligation to order human freedom according to right reason, with an openness to Revelation, and leading to true happiness, in: Di Giovanni A, "Etica e valore morale" *CivCat* 127,2 (1976) 371-375.

[11]Here again, for a proper interpretation of O'Donnell, it must be kept in mind that his first hermeneutical principle is the magisterium. Hence, his point of departure for the correct labeling and evaluation of the moral action is always the authentic teaching of the Church, a point which comes forward most clearly in his discussion of "freedom of conscience." See: O'Donnell, **Medicine** (1991), 10-11.

[12]An example of the lack of univocity regarding the autonomy of moral norms, and therefore the crucial need of defining levels of interpretation, in: Privitera S, "Per una interpretazione del dibattito su "L'autonomia morale'" *RTMor* 48 (1980) 565-586.

[13]A strong argument against Christian monopoly in bio-medical ethics and in favor of seeking solidarity with humanism, in: Autiero, "Il rapporto tra medicina e teologia per la prassi dell'etica medica" *Rivista di Teologia Morale* 79 (1988) 47-58.

[14]A review of some unique moral issues associated with prenatal life, in: Tettamanzi D, "Problemi morali circa alcuni interventi sui feti/embrioni umani" *Medicina e Morale* 35,1 (1985)

23-43.

[15]"Diagnosis utilizing procedures available for the recognition of diseases and malformations *in utero*, and the conclusion reached." **Stedman's Medical Dictionary**, s.v. *diagnosis, prenatal.*

[16]See: Demmer, **Interpretare**, 168-174.

[17]For a discussion proposing a mediated alternative between extreme opposite medical ethical systems, see: Attard, *Dimensioni etiche*, 367-384. And a contrasting view, especially seeking to clarify the correct labeling of utilitarianism, consequentialism and proportionalism when it comes to their application in conflict situations, in: Finnis J, **Fundamentals of Ethics**. Oxford; Clarendon 1983, 80-108. An analysis of the meaning of "direct" and "indirect" as applied to the moral evaluation of killing in: Schüller B, "Direct killing/indirect killing" in: Curran CE, McCormick RA, eds, **Readings in Moral Theology 1: Moral Norms and Catholic Tradition.** New York: Paulist 1979, 138-157.

[18]A seminal article contending that the overriding element in the principle, and indeed in all moral judgment, is commensurate reason, in: Knauer P, "The hermeneutic function of the principle of double effect" in: Curran CE, McCormick RA, eds, **Readings in Moral Theology 1: Moral Norms and Catholic Tradition.** New York: Paulist 1979, 1-39. For a review of the origin of "direct" and "indirect" terminology in the tradition, with its present limits and validity of the underlying reality which they seek to elucidate, see: Rossi L, "'Diretto' e 'indiretto' in teologia morale" *RTMor* 9 (1971) 37-65. And a similar assessment of the principle, in: Rossi L, "Il limite del principio del duplice effetto" *RTMor* 13 (1972) 11-37. For a plausible explanation of the present shift in moral theology from norm-theory to act-theory when interpreting the classical fonts of morality regarding resolution of conflict situations, see: Demmer K, "Deuten und Wählen. Vorbemerkungen zu einer Moraltheologischen Handlungstheorie" *Greg* 62 (1981) 231-275. See also: Boyle J, "Who is entitled to double effect?" *JMedPhil* 16 (1991) 475-494; Di Ianni A, "The direct/indirect distinction in morals" in: Curran CE, McCormick RA, eds, **Readings in Moral Theology 1: Moral Norms and Catholic Tradition.** New York: Paulist 1979, 215-243.

[19]See: Ashley and O'Rourke, **Healthcare Ethics** (1989), 214-215.

[20]Ashley and O'Rourke, **Healthcare Ethics** (1989), 214-215.

[21]For a discussion on the equivocity of 'ontic evil' and the ultimate inability to claim that good may come of it, see: Quay PM, "The disvalue of ontic evil" *TS* 46 (1985) 262-286. A critical analysis of ontic and moral evil in Aquinas, and its present application, is also in: Janssens L, "Ontic evil and moral evil" in: Curran CE, McCormick RA, eds, **Readings in Moral Theology 1: Moral Norms and Catholic Tradition.** New York: Paulist 1979, 40-93.

[22]For critique of proportionalism based on its practical inability to adequately choose between basically incommensurable values, see: Kiely B, "The impracticality of proportionalism" *Greg* 66 (1985) 655-687. See also: Connery JR, "Catholic ethics: has the norm for rule-making changed?" *TS* 42 (1981) 232-250; "The teleology of proportionate reason" *TS* 44 (1983) 489-496; Crosby JF, "The creaturehood of the human person and the critique of proportionalism" in: CITM, **Persona**, 195-199.

[23]See: Ashley and O'Rourke, **Healthcare Ethics** (1989), 164-171. For a defense of a personalist anthropology as the grounding of human perfection in the free act of loving God and others by virtue of human substance, see: Walgrave JH, "Personalisme et anthropologie chrétienne" *Greg* 65 (1984) 445-472.

[24]Ashley and O'Rourke, **Healthcare Ethics** (1989), 158.

[25]See: Demmer, **Interpretare**, 182. For a discussion on the different possible meanings of proportionate reason in contemporary literature, see also: Johnstone BV, "The meaning of proportionate reason in contemporary moral theology" *Thom* 49 (1985) 223-247.

[26]See: Demmer, **Interpretare**, 182-183.

[27]See: Curran, **Politics**, 114; **Catholic Moral Theology**, 257.

[28]For a contrasting analysis of seven basic human goods, among which is life, that are considered incommensurable precisely because of their irreducibility, see: Finnis J, **Natural Law and Natural Rights**. Oxford: Clarendon 1980, 85-90.

[29]Curran, **Politics**, 131.

[30]See: Demmer, **Interpretare**, 183.

[31]Curran, *Abortion*, 23. See also; Curran, **Ongoing Revisions**, 157.

[32]Further evidence of his rejection of the principle in these cases can be found in his statement that: "In my judgment abortion can be justified for preserving the life of the mother and for other important values commensurate with life even though the action aims at abortion as a means to an end." Curran, *Abortion*, 24.

[33]Curran, **Themes**, 72. See also: Curran, **Directions**, 163-164.

[34]May, *Abortion*, 75.

[35] This is also evident when he says that: "The death may be direct in an observable way, but the death is definitely not directly intended by the doer of the deed nor is the death of the fetus the moral meaning of the act." May, **Human Existence**, 104.

[36]Such as: "Life, health, justice, peace, friendship and whatever else comprises the whole human good." May, *Human identity*, 37.

[37]"And as a consequentialism the ultimate concern is in the 'higher' good to be achieved as a result of our deeds, not the meaning of our deeds as revelatory of our being." May, *Human identity*, 36. See also: May, *Ethical dilemmas*, 248-265. Another critique along the same lines in: Grisez G, Boyle, Jr. JM, **Life and Death with Liberty and Justice: A Contribution to the Euthanasia Debate**. Notre Dame, IN: U of Notre Dame P 1979, 346-355. See also: Ratzinger Card. J, "Panorama de la théologie dans le monde" *DocCath* 82 (5 may 1985) 505-512, and a critique, in: Chiavacci E, "La questione dei principi fondamentali della morale cristiana" *RTMor* 69 (1986) 21-25.

[38]See: Connery JR, "Morality of consequences: a critical appraisal" in: Curran CE, McCormick RA, eds, **Readings in Moral Theology 1: Moral Norms and Catholic Tradition**. New York: Paulist 1979, 244-266; Demmer, **Interpretare**, 187.

[39]A defense of consequentialism on the basis that it remains essentially open to alternative interpretations of what appears to be good in: McKim R, Simpson P, "On the alleged incoherence of consequentialism" *NewSchol* 62 (1988) 349-352, and a rebuttal in: McDermott JM, "Metaphysical conundrums at the root of moral disagreement" *Greg* 71 (1990) 713-742. See also: Theron S, "Consequentionalism and natural law" in: CITM, **Persona**, 177-193.

[40]This is not to be confused with cost/benefit analysis, which they oppose, as illustrated in the next chapter on: **Prenatal Diagnosis Proper**, in Chapter XVI of PART THREE of this text.

[41]"A risk/benefit estimate in medical procedures normally applies to the risk and benefit of the same individual. If, however, the life and well-being of fetuses can be risked for the benefit of the rest of the community, then what is to prevent application of the same procedure to still other groups of individuals within the community at other stages of development: e.g., infants and children, the retarded and handicapped, the senile?" McCarthy and Moraczewski, **Fetal Experimentation**, 16 (also relevant; 75-80). See also; Atkinson and Moraczewski, **Genetic Counseling**, 19; Moraczewski, *Genetic counseling*, 52-53.

[42]See: McCarthy and Bayer, **Critical Sexual Issues**, 145; Atkinson and Moraczewski, **Genetic Counseling**, 127.

[43]See: McCarthy, *Ethical principles*, 88-92.

[44]This also leads McCarthy to oppose viewing the fetus as an "unjust aggressor," for it is only

living in accordance with its proper stage of development. See: McCarthy, **Beginnings**, 69.

[45]Once again, the level of interpretation is crucial here: from the point of view of the fetus, the benefit might be "indirect;" from the point of view of the mother, it might well be considered "direct." See: Demmer, **Interpretare**, 182-183.

[46]See: McCormick, **Notes**, 473-520; *Bioethics*, 303-318. See also: Cahill, *Teleology*, 601-629. Again, a strong critique of the validity of proportionalism as an applicable theory of moral norms due to its inability to adequately compare incommensurable benefits and harms, in: Grisez G, **The Way of the Lord Jesus: Christian Moral Principles**, Vol I. Chicago: Franciscan Herald Press 1983, 141-171. A rebuttal of that, particularly if one is to maintain some validity of the principle of double effect, including a clearer distinction and a more realistic interpretation between the directness or indirectness of the act intended, in: Hoose B, **Proportionalism: The American Debate and its European Roots**. Washington: Georgetown UP 1987, 101-135. See also: Vacek EV, "Proportionalism: one view of the debate" *TS* 46 (1985) 287-314.

[47]McCormick, **Notes**, 499. Also, a critique of his effort to respond to criticism of relativism by attempting a list of basic human tendencies, in: McKinney RH, "The quest for an adequate proportionalist theory of value" *Thom* 53 (1989) 56-73.

[48]See: McCormick, **Notes**, 515.

[49]For instance, he also seems to expand the concept of aggression when he allows for abortion in a pregnancy resulting from rape or incest, an expansion not without its presuppositions and consequences: is the human being conceived by an act either of rape or incest to be held morally accountable for the manner in which it was conceived? See: McCormick, *Abortion: changing morality*, 41.

[50]Cahill also places great emphasis in the social dimension of the moral analysis. See: Cahill, *Abortion*, 85-97; *Abortion pill*, 5-8; *Catholicism*, 38-54; *Fresh approach*, 20-21. A presentation of ethical analysis surpassing individualism and viewing socialization as integral to moral discernment leading to true personalization also in: Rincón Orduña R, "Introducción a la ética teológica especial" in: López Azpitarte E, Elizari Basterra FJ, Rincón Orduña R, eds, **Praxis Cristiana II: Opción por la Vida y el Amor**. 3ra ed. Madrid: Paulinas 1981, 11-47.

[51]See: McCormick, **Ambiguity**, 22-23; *Experimental*, 2197; *Sociality*, 41-46; *To save*, 172-179.

[52]See: McCormick, *Experimentation*, 5.3-5.4; **Health**, 143; *Proxy consent*, 2-20.

[53]See: McCormick, *Experimentation*, 5.3-5.5.

[54]See: May, **Human Existence**, 89.

[55]"An action, good in itself, which has two effects, an intended and otherwise not reasonably attainable good effect, and a foreseen, but merely permitted, [evil] effect, may licitly be placed, provided there is a due proportion between the intended good and the permitted evil." O'Donnell, **Medicine** (1991), 28-29.

[56]See: O'Donnell, **Medicine** (1991), 29. And a contrasting analysis contending that the principle remains at the level of the rightness or wrongness of the human action or omission in: Schüller B, "The double effect in Catholic thought: a reevaluation" in: McCormick RA, Ramsey P, eds, **Doing Evil to Achieve Good: Moral Choice in Conflict Situations**. Chicago: Loyola 1978, 165-192.

[57]"Here we must distinguish carefully between physical and moral evil. We are speaking of an evil effect in the moral order only. The evil effect is that which, if directly willed, would be morally evil." O'Donnell, **Medicine** (1991), 29.

[58]An appraisal of teleology as the underlying method for establishing moral norms in: Schüller B, "Various types of grounding for ethical norms" in: Curran CE, McCormick RA, eds, **Readings**

in Moral Theology 1: Moral Norms and Catholic Tradition. New York: Paulist 1979, 184-198.

[59]Identifying the intended good and permitted evil do not sufficiently define the absoluteness of a given moral norm. An analysis also questioning in what sense is the absoluteness of moral norms of behavior to be understood, is given by: Fuchs J, **Personal Responsibility and Christian Morality.** (trans. Cleves W *et al*) Washington: Georgetown UP 1983, 115-152. See also: Fuchs J, "The absoluteness of moral terms" in: Curran CE, McCormick RA, eds, **Readings in Moral Theology 1: Moral Norms and Catholic Tradition.** New York: Paulist 1979, 94-137.

[60]O'Donnell, **Medicine** (1991), 30.

[61]"Under no condition can the action be even partially prompted by a desire for the evil effect. Otherwise the evil effect becomes a direct voluntary effect." O'Donnell, **Medicine** (1991), 30.

[62]Also distinguishing between moral and premoral evils, especially in view of the purported intelligibility of intrinsic evil when applied to concrete human acts as valid under all possible circumstances, is: Fuchs J, **Christian Ethics in a Secular Arena.** (trans. Hoose B, McNeil B) Washington: Georgetown UP 1984, 71-90.

[63]"We thus affirm that any abortion is a premoral evil. That is, it is the ending of life." Shannon and Wolter, *Pre-embryo*, 625.

[64]Shannon and Wolter, *Pre-embryo*, 625.

[65]See: Demmer, **Interpretare**, 181.

[66]Thus, in conflict situations, a "Brain Life II" (after synapses have begun to form) embryo has priority over a "Brain Life I" (after the appearance of the cortical plate) embryo, which in turn has priority over a "preembryo." See: Shannon, *Brain integration*, 141-142. Cahill advocates a similar solution: "My position on fetal status might be characterized as 'developmentalist' insofar as I view its values as incremental throughout gestation." Cahill, *Abortion*, 86. See also: Cahill, *Webster*, U:1525-U:1529; Fletcher JC, "Prenatal diagnosis, selective abortion, and the ethics of withholding treatment from the defective newborn" in: Capron AM *et al*, eds, **Genetic Counseling: Facts, Values, and Norms.** New York: Alan R. Liss 1979, 239-254.

[67]"Whereas none of these entities is entitled to the same degree of respect or protection accorded to actual persons because of the absence of biological preconditions necessary (but not sufficient) for personal activity, their own levels of development ground a degree of respect and protection in proportion to their establishing the biological presupposition for morally relevant personal capacities." Shannon, *Brain integration*, 141.

[68]In fact, by grounding the possibility of being human on the capacity for the development of a human brain, Shannon falls prey to the very "naturalistic" system which he seeks to critique. Alternatively, on the need to protect human life at every stage of development, founded on a global vision of the person seeking to overcome partial or unilateral solutions--such as naturalistic or technicistic ones--, see: Lorenzetti L, "Trasmissione della vita umana da un'etica della natura ad un'etica della persona" *Rivista di Teologia Morale* 71 (1986) 117-129.

CHAPTER XVI

PRENATAL DIAGNOSIS PROPER

Introduction

This chapter provides a critical analysis of human prenatal diagnosis proper. It is divided into five sections: indications, benefits, risks, consent, and the particular case of pre-implantation diagnosis.

The first section, on indications, points to the reasons for the observed unanimity of the moral evaluation of prenatal diagnosis among the ten authors examined. Even so, the question of intentionality is not neglected.

The second section, on benefits, is subdivided into four aspects: a true negative diagnosis, a true positive diagnosis, *in utero* therapy and pregnancy management, and early delivery. A true negative diagnosis may contribute both directly and indirectly to the well-being of both mother and child. Likewise, a true positive diagnosis may provide certain benefits, so long as the proper priorities are in place. To this end, as will be seen, a true positive diagnosis can greatly contribute toward exploring the possibilities of *in utero* surgery, or of a more successful pregnancy management. Finally, the prospect of an early delivery may also be a definite benefit of prenatal diagnosis.

The third section, on risks, is also subdivided into four issues: procedures, false positives and false negatives, "therapeutic" abortion, and sex selection. Regarding procedures, a necessary distinction is made between various techniques which afford different degrees of risk. Also, the disadvantages of false positives and false negatives are explored, both to mother and child. Then comes the question of the validity of the concept of "therapeutic" abortion, given the present historical context. Lastly, the controversial issue of sex selection--together with its various implications--is critically analyzed.

The fourth section, on consent, deals with two general areas: informed and proxy consent, and therapeutic and non-therapeutic consent. The first area points to the distinction between these two types of consent, and looks at who has the moral right and responsibility to give consent for the human fetus. The second area addresses the question of the conditions under which consent to undergo prenatal diagnosis is or is not justified.

The fifth section, on pre-implantation diagnosis, seeks to investigate and evaluate the underlying reasons for approving or disapproving this technique as it is becoming available today.

A. INDICATIONS

Addressing the indications for prenatal diagnosis which were previously described,[1] the fundamental question of intentionality retains its full force: why test?[2] In the present state of the art, it is known that: first, not all prenatal defects are lethal.[3] Second, a number of these are becoming treatable during gestation.[4] Accordingly, a moral analysis of benefits and risks afforded by the application of these techniques when indicated is proper.[5] In spite of the philosophical, anthropological and even methodological differences that have been previously exposed, the ten authors examined display a remarkable unanimity of opinion regarding the overall moral evaluation of standard prenatal diagnosis. This is mostly due to the fact that, by the time these tests are done, the pregnancy is well under way,[6] and thus, there is generally no longer any doubt as to the moral status of the human fetus.[7]

B. BENEFITS

1. A True Negative Diagnosis

Over 95% of all prenatal diagnosis is negative, that is, that it detects no fetal deformity or anomaly.[8] However, it is important to mention from the onset that different techniques yield varying degrees of confidence and margins of error, none of them being absolutely predictive or specific.[9] Thus, a false negative result leaves an anomaly undetected, while a false positive "sees" one where none may exist, at least for the defect being tested. Assuming, then, that the result is a true negative, a mother suspecting her pre-born to carry some abnormality may be reassured of a normal fetus. This can be considered a form of indirect therapy in the sense that, if the mother was contemplating an abortion, the threat to the life of the pre-born is now dispelled.[10] Furthermore, a true negative diagnosis may have the benefit of contributing to a less anxious pregnancy altogether, which may actually directly contribute to the welfare of the fetus during months of development.[11]

2. A True Positive Diagnosis

Conversely, if the diagnosis is a true positive one, it may also be instrumental in providing for a better pregnancy management in several ways.[12] First, depending on the type and degree of severity of the anomaly,[13] it helps the physician to enter into dialogue with the parents (the mother)[14] if an adequate cure is presently available, either to eliminate the defect entirely, or to diminish it significantly. Second, it allows the physician to determine whether or not an early delivery is advantageous in the particular case at hand. Third, especially if there is no present *in utero* cure available, it can help the parents in planning for the eventual delivery of a child with some birth defect. Fourth, if the fetus seems non-viable, it may allow the couple to accept the eventuality of a miscarriage or stillbirth.[15] Again, depending on the type and degree of severity of the anomaly, there exist today a host of associations, institutions and support groups that can be very instrumental in providing at least partial relief to the possible suffering and hardships which the parents and the child will have to endure when the pregnancy is carried to term.[16]

3. *In Utero* Therapy and Pregnancy Management

A number of human embryonic and fetal anomalies and deficiencies are very slowly becoming treatable prenatally. First, it might be a question of the pregnant mother managing a restrictive diet, such as in the case of Phenylketonuria.[17] Second, it could involve administering medication to the mother, which is then passed on to the fetus, such as to inhibit preterm labor, or in seeking to prevent IUGR, fetal tachycardia, vitamin deficiencies, and congenital adrenal hyperplasia.[18] Third, it may provide the fetus with medicine through direct injection into his or her umbilical cord, such as in Rh incompatibility. Fourth, some forms of fetal surgery are now also available: shunts to attempt correcting hydrocephaly and aqueductal stenosis, clearing obstructed urinary passages to drain fetal bladder and kidneys, and a variety of other surgical interventions to correct more-or-less serious defects.[19] Time, experience, and collaboration of procedures and results are gradually augmenting the possibilities; indispensably at the core of these possibilities is an accurate prenatal diagnosis.[20]

4. Early Delivery

Another benefit of prenatal diagnosis is the possibility of assessing fetal gestational age and developmental stage so as to plan for an eventual early delivery. Considering an early delivery may be to prevent some (further) damage, such as in special cases of multifetal gestation,[21] or if there is some hope of instituting a concomitant early treatment, such as in particular instances of very low birth weight.[22] In addition, prenatal diagnosis during the third trimester may be instrumental in determining the best route of delivery regarding fetal cranial size related to maternal pelvic size.[23]

In view of all these benefits, it can be sustained that prenatal diagnosis today may present definite medical advantages when properly indicated, both to the fetus and to his or her mother.[24] This, however, is not without its risks.[25]

C. RISKS

1. Procedures

Each invasive prenatal diagnosis technique carries with it a certain percentage of risk of injury and spontaneous abortion or miscarriage.[26] While in general the medical risks are considered to be presently negligible to the mother, it may not be necessarily so for the fetus. For instance, whereas amniocentesis is reported to carry an overall risk of spontaneous abortion of less than 1-2% (and thus compatible with certain of the indications mentioned above), this says nothing about the risk of direct or indirect damage to the fetus itself *without* causing an abortion.[27] It must be recalled here that a "minor" risk to the fetus (*i.e.*, a minuscule needle puncture) may actually represent a major damage, given his or her delicate state of development.[28] Similarly, because CVS is normally performed earlier in pregnancy,[29] it carries with it a somewhat higher risk rate of spontaneous abortion. In addition, since it involves the actual removal of a minute quantity of placental tissue, the long-range effects of this removal on the development of the fetus are as yet unknown.[30] Fetal tissue sampling and fetoscopy carry a higher degree of risk of spontaneous abortion or injury to the fetus, and are therefore more rarely done.[31]

2. False Positives and False Negatives

Currently, the vast majority of pregnant women in the United States who receive a positive prenatal diagnosis choose to abort.[32] Hence, a false positive result is now tantamount to endangering the life of a normal fetus.[33] It could be argued here, however, that since from the Catholic perspective the direct procured abortion of a human fetus, whether normal or carrying some birth defect, is not a licit option,[34] then the moral evaluation of a false positive result should not differ from that of a true positive one. Nonetheless, a false positive diagnosis unnecessarily burdens the parents (the mother) with the erroneous notion that their child is carrying some defect. This misinformation could thus lead them to ponder about an alternative which they would normally not have considered had they known the truth. Conversely, a false negative result may mislead them into thinking that their child is normal, while in fact he or she carries some anomaly. The possible consequences here are again manifold: first, there might have been a cure available for the undetected anomaly. Second, when the anomaly is finally discovered, either at birth or later in life, the physician and the medical facility where the testing took place risk being held liable of negligence. Third, it may lead the parents (the mother) to physically or psychologically neglect or even reject their child due to the false expectation of a totally healthy baby. In sum, false positive and false negative results add a degree of complexity to the moral evaluation of risks in prenatal diagnosis which cannot be ignored in each particular case.[35]

3. "Therapeutic" Abortion

Given the rapid advancements of contemporary medical technology, the uterine gestational development of even a grossly anomalous embryo or fetus today poses no direct threat to the physical life of his or her mother.[36] Hence, when the term "therapeutic" is used to describe the abortion of a fetus carrying some defect, it must be understood that such procedure is never therapeutic for the fetus:[37] it may eliminate the defect in question, but it certainly does not cure the patient; unless, of course, one is willing to recognize as "patient" only the mother.[38] And herein lies a crucial issue: if there are now certain embryonic and fetal anomalies that can be medically treated, does this not make the embryo or the fetus a medical patient too?[39] And, if so, is one willing to accept that the best "treatment" for certain patients is death?[40] This in no way denies the reality that a number of birth defects are extremely serious, that at times they signify a lifetime of severe physical and psychological pain and suffering,[41] not only for the now-born child, but also for his or her parents and other family members, for the medical establishment, and for society at large with its burden of taxes and institutions seeking to care in some measure for many of these individuals. It must be admitted, however, that underneath the concept of "therapeutic" abortion is the erroneous notion that a fetus or embryo is guilty of death simply because he or she is carrying some birth defect.[42] If one is willing to morally justify such rationale, what prevents one from justifying the direct killing of those born individuals who are also carrying the particular defect in question?[43] As can be seen from this brief analysis, the notion of "therapeutic" abortion is a distortion of the legitimate concept of therapy, a distortion which stands in violation of logical consistency and ontological coherence.[44]

4. Sex Selection

One of the "side effects" of prenatal diagnosis is to become aware of the gender of the embryo or fetus being tested. But obtaining this information is not without its moral dilemma either. First, there are a number of defects which are associated with the sex chromosomes: hence, determining the gender of the fetus of a carrier parent may advert the physician to the possibility of he or she carrying a sex-linked anomaly.[45] However, there are instances when strict Mendelian ratios in progeny do not follow, requiring further testing. Even so, aborting a fetus simply on the probability that he or she carries a sex-linked defect is tantamount to risking to abort also a normal fetus.[46] Here again, it must be said that from the Catholic perspective, whether the fetus carries the sex-linked anomaly or not, direct procured abortion is not a licit option.[47] Second, and here lies the greater danger of knowing the gender of the embryo or fetus, from the literature examined, there seems to be a reported bias of the general population in favor of male firstborn children:[48] if true, identified female embryos and fetuses run the risk of being aborted only on the basis of their gender.[49] In fact, given the present legal standing of abortion in the United States, the reality is that either gender may be aborted simply for being of the "wrong" sex.[50]

D. CONSENT

In view of the examined benefits and risks involved in prenatal diagnosis, it must now be asked: who has the moral right to consent to prenatal diagnosis, and under what circumstances?

1. Informed and Proxy Consent

Proxy consent is not a type of informed consent, though it presumes the latter.[51] There is no question that informed consent must be obtained in order to morally justify subjecting a pregnant woman to prenatal diagnosis.[52] This consent normally hinges on the indications mentioned above, once they have been reasonably explained to the expectant mother. Even so, it must be asked: how is one to interpret "reasonably explained"? Again, given the sophisticated level of information and knowledge which is obtained with these techniques regarding the health or ill-health of the fetus (a level that far surpasses any ordinary knowledge of human embryology or pathology which can be expected from the "average" mother or couple), how can one be assured that her consent is correctly informed?[53] A case in point may be when there is a suspicion of some birth defect which is most definitely not life-threatening (*i.e.*, amelia), but that the expectant mother may interpret as sufficiently serious to warrant an abortion.[54] Here enters the second element, namely, proxy consent. Since the ultimate scope of prenatal diagnosis is to appraise the medical condition of the fetus, with a view toward the eventual correction or amelioration of a detected disease or abnormality, and given the fact that it is absolutely impossible for the fetus to provide for his or her own informed consent, then the question arises: can someone morally qualify to give a proxy consent in his or her name?[55] The answer seems in the affirmative, as long as the procedure is ultimately in the best interest of the individual fetus.[56] If found to carry some defect, the best interest of the fetus cannot be considered to be to abort it, for even in the worst case scenario of a fetus carrying the most wretched and painful of diseases: can one ever be absolutely certain that this particular individual would have unquestionably chosen not to live under such conditions? Again, to claim such certainty seems pretentious. If not, then an expectant mother may only give proxy consent, licitly, for her fetus to undergo prenatal diagnosis if she does not consider abortion an option.

2. Therapeutic and Non-therapeutic Consent

Granted that the expectant mother may be morally qualified to give proxy consent on behalf of her pre-born,[57] the question now becomes: under what conditions? In other words, must she have in mind only the best interest of the individual fetus, or of fetuses in general, or even of society at large? If an action posited on a human fetus is morally a particular case of the general category of actions posited on incompetents, then the same rules must apply.[58] Here it is not hard to see that, while it may be medically advantageous for society at large to submit certain individual incompetents against their will to research and experimentation of no particular benefit to them, but of some benefit to society, this procedure would stand in violation of the fundamental values of human dignity and equality elaborated earlier.[59] Furthermore, research and experimentation on an incompetent individual of no therapeutic value to the individual, but of possible value to the particular group of incompetents to which she or he belongs, stands in violation of the dignity of that same individual, and ultimately, of every individual of that group. The moral alternative, then, is for the expectant mother to grant proxy consent only for those therapeutic procedures which benefit her individual pre-born.[60] But it must also be noted here that, often in medicine: first, today's experimental procedure may well be tomorrow's standard procedure. Second, especially in procedures that are similar or closely related, what is still considered experimental in one place may already be considered standard in another. This, moreover, must be further qualified by recognizing that such accepted procedures have in fact evolved and have been sufficiently refined so as to represent some true, albeit tenuous, benefit to the individual patient involved.[61]

E. PRE-IMPLANTATION DIAGNOSIS

Interpretative and evaluative differences become most notable here, though at times they are implicit.[62] As previously described,[63] pre-implantation diagnosis essentially involves analyzing the DNA of a few or even a single blastomere(s) before implantation occurs.[64] At this point, the question must be asked: what is the intention of such analysis? Whereas the eventual goal might certainly be to correct genetic defects at the individual gene level, the present state of the art is far from allowing for this possibility (at least in human systems) without a significantly high risk of damage or destruction. Conversely, if the aim is to detect and destroy those morulae which are found to carry some genetic anomaly, then the moral analysis takes on a different tack altogether, and cannot therefore be accepted.[65] Thus, the issue of hominization once again becomes relevant: those authors maintaining delayed hominization[66] might morally justify this latter course of action simply because they doubt the morula to be a human individual. Conversely, those authors holding for immediate hominization[67] would consider such action the direct killing of an innocent human being.[68] The question then becomes: is such doubt sufficiently grounded so as to morally justify pre-implantation diagnosis? Given the fact that a plausible model has been provided to dispel at least those doubts which have been raised by the delayed hominization authors,[69] it would seem that, presently, to proceed with pre-implantation diagnosis for this purpose is equivalent to be willing to risk the killing of innocent human life *even if* he or she is a human individual.[70]

Notes

[1]See: *Indications*, under **Prenatal Diagnosis**, in Chapter I of PART ONE of this text. An evaluation of indications also in Moraczewski, *Genetic medicine*, 15-25. The vital importance of justified indications may be appreciated in an unwillingness to use prenatal diagnosis solely to target for abortion healthy but incompatible fetuses conceived to serve as organ donors. See: Clark RD, Fletcher J, Petersen G, "Conceiving a fetus for bone marrow donation: an ethical problem in prenatal diagnosis" *PrenatDiag* 9,5 (1989) 329-334; and a follow-up in: Fost N, "Guiding principles for prenatal diagnosis" *PrenatalDiag* 9,5 (1989) 335-337. Questioning the present validity of prenatal diagnosis for psychiatric indications, is: Mattei J-F, "The use of prenatal diagnosis for psychiatric diseases" in: Srám RJ, Bulyzhenkov V, Prilipko L, Christen Y, eds, **Ethical Issues of Molecular Genetics in Psychiatry**. New York: Springer-Verlag 1991, 87-93.

[2]Retaining that the moral liceity of prenatal diagnosis lies in the intention for which it is done, is: Spinsanti S, "La diagnostica prenatale" in: Goffi T, Piana G, eds, **Corso di Morale II: Diakonia (Etica della Persona)**. Brescia: Queriniana 1983, 212-216.

[3]See: **Human Embryonic Disorders**, in Chapter III of PART ONE of this text.

[4]See: *Fetal therapy*, under **Prenatal Interventions**, in Chapter IV of PART ONE of this text.

[5]The increasing popularity of prenatal diagnosis in family planning among both the general population and carrier subgroups calls for ongoing re-evaluation in view of new medical discoveries and perfection of techniques. See: Evers-Kiebooms G, *et al*, "Family planning decisions after the birth of a cystic fibrosis child: the impact of prenatal diagnosis" *ScandJGastroenter* 23,143 (1988) 38-46; "Psychological aspects of amniocentesis: anxiety feelings

in three different risk groups" *ClinGen* 33,3 (1988) 196-206. Pointing to new ethical questions posed by the rapid availability of these techniques, is: Tormey JF, "Ethical considerations of prenatal genetic diagnosis" *ClinObGyn* 19,4 (1976) 957-963, and: MacDonald D, "Prenatal diagnosis: situating the ethical questions" in: Reidy M, ed, **Ethical Issues in Reproductive Medicine.** Dublin: Gill and MacMillan 1982, 4-11. See also: Caffarra C, "Aspetti etici della diagnostica prenatale" *MedMor* 34,4 (1984) 449-457; Delcroix M, Lesage-Desrousseaux E, Lefèvre Ch, "L'anomalie anténatale, croix des moralistes" *MelScRel* 42,3 (1985) 149-167; Leuzzi L, "Indicazioni etiche per la diagnostica prenatale" *MedMor* 34,4 (1984) 458-463; Serra A, "La diagnosi prenatale di malattie genetiche" *MedMor* 34,4 (1984) 433-448; Sgreccia E, **Manuale di Bioetica I: Fondamenti ed Etica Biomedica.** Milano: Vita e Pensiero 1988, 181-197.

[6]See: **Human Embryology** and **Prenatal Interventions**, in Chapters II and IV, respectively, of PART ONE of this text.

[7]See: Ashley and O'Rourke, **Healthcare Ethics** (1989), 320-327; Atkinson and Moraczewski, **Genetic Counseling**, 19-24; Cahill, *Abortion*, 261-276; Curran, *In vitro*, 4.18; **Moral Theology**, 127; May, **Human Existence**, 39-61; McCarthy *et al*, **Critical Sexual Issues** (1989), 144-147; McCormick, **Health**, 140-144; O'Donnell, *Prenatal screening*, 13-14; Shannon, *A survey*, 27-28.

[8]See: Shannon, *A survey*, 27. See also: Rice N, Doherty R, "Reflections on prenatal diagnosis: the consumers' views" *SocWHealthCare* 8,1 (1982) 47-57, especially 47.

[9]See: **Prenatal Interventions**, in Chapter IV of PART ONE of this text.

[10]See: Shannon and DiGiacomo, **Introduction** (1987), 79-92.

[11]See: Ashley and O'Rourke, **Healthcare Ethics** (1989), 320-321; May, **Human Existence**, 116-128; McCarthy *et al*, **Critical Sexual Issues** (1989), 145; Moraczewski, *Moral dimensions*, 52-55; McCormick, **Health**, 141; *Bioethical issues*, 42-45; O'Donnell, *Amniocentesis*, 19; Shannon, *A survey*, 27-28.

[12]See: Ashley and O'Rourke, **Healthcare Ethics** (1989), 320-327. A listing of advantages of prenatal diagnosis to couples who decide not to abort an abnormal gestation, also found in: Clark SL, DeVore GR, "Prenatal diagnosis for couples who would not consider abortion" *ObGyn* 73,6 (1989) 1035-1037.

[13]Note the wide range of anomalies; see **Human Embryonic Disorders**, in Chapter III of PART ONE of this text.

[14]The reason for giving priority to the parents is because of the anthropological and theological priority of favoring decisions concerning progeny done by both spouses. Given the contemporary socio-cultural situation in the United States, one must also be aware of the many unwed mothers and other pregnant women who are constrained by a multitude of reasons to affront their pregnancy, and the decisions taken therein, alone. To this end, a study pointing to some of the marital conflicts which prenatal diagnosis may trigger, is found in: Rice and Doherty, *Reflections*, 47-57.

[15]Sustaining that deliberately aborting a non-viable fetus may actually be more traumatic than allowing "nature to take its course," is: Watkins D, "An alternative to termination of pregnancy" *Pract* 233 (1989) 990-992.

[16]See: McCarthy, *Ethical principles*, 97; Moraczewski, *Trisomy 13*, 1-2; O'Donnell, *Amniocentesis*, 19.

[17]Nevertheless, this continues to be a controversial treatment. A critique of ethical issues in prenatal diagnosis of phenylketonuria, is given by: Holtzman NA, "Ethical issues in the prenatal diagnosis of Phenylketonuria" *Ped* 74,3 (1984) 424-427.

[18]See: *Medical Therapy*, under **Prenatal Interventions**, in Chapter IV of PART ONE of this

text.
[19]See: *Fetal Surgery*, under **Prenatal Interventions**, in Chapter IV of PART ONE of this text.
[20]See: McCarthy *et al*, **Critical Sexual Issues**, 156-159; McCormick, **Health**, 142-143. See also: Calisti A, "diagnosi prenatale e possibilità terapeutiche chirurgiche" *MedMor* 34,4 (1984) 493-497; Spagnolo AG, Di Pietro ML. "Feto a rischio per iperplasia surrenalica congenita: Quali i limiti etici della diagnosi e della terapia fetali?" *MedMor* 4 (1990) 759-778; Tettamanzi D, "Problemi morali circa alcuni interventi sui feti/embrioni umani" *MedMor* 35,1 (1985) 23-43.
[21]See: *Multifetal Gestation*, under **Human Embryology**, in Chapter II of PART ONE of this text.
[22]See: *Very Low Birth Weight*, under **Human Embryology**, in Chapter III of PART ONE of this text.
[23]See: Atkinson and Moraczewski, **Genetic Counseling**, 19, 127-128.
[24]A summary list of medical and ethical recommendations to be implemented by physicians when considering prenatal diagnosis, is provided by: Royal College of Physicians, "Prenatal diagnosis and genetic screening: community and service implications" *JRCPhysLondon* 23,4 (1989) 215-220.
[25]A review of some unique genetic and ethical issues arising from prenatal diagnosis, is also found in: Berg K, "Ethical problems arising from research progress in medical genetics" in: Berg K, Tranoy KE, eds, **Research Ethics**. New York: Alan R. Liss 1983, 261-275; Johnson SR, Elkins TE, "Ethical issues in prenatal diagnosis" *ClinObGyn* 31,2 (1988) 408-417.
[26]See: *Prenatal Diagnosis*, under **Prenatal Interventions**, in Chapter IV of PART ONE of this text.
[27]An early report of fetal distress cases following prenatal diagnosis--some even without evident trauma present--, is reported by: Ron M, Anteby S, Diamant YZ, Polishuk WZ, "Fetal distress following amniocentesis" *IntJGynOb* 12,5 (1974) 172-175.
[28]It is understood that these techniques are done with the concomitant use of ultrasound, a sterile procedure, etc. Nonetheless, they are still heavily dependent on the particular skill and expertise of all the medical personnel involved. See: May, **Human Existence**, 89; O'Donnell, *Amniocentesis*, 9-11.
[29]Evidence that this earlier diagnosis seems to lead to a greater number of abortions due to a lesser capacity of parents to distinguish between different types of abnormalities, is provided by: Verp MS *et al*, "Parental decision following prenatal daignosis of fetal chromosome abnormality" *AJMedGen* 29,3 (1988) 613-622.
[30]See: *Chorionic Villus Sampling*, under **Prenatal Interventions**, in Chapter IV of PART ONE of this text. Appealing for randomized clinical trials of CVS to determine overall risk statistics, is: Fletcher JC, "Ethical aspects of a controlled clinical trial of chorion biopsy approach to prenatal diagnosis" in: Berg K, ed, **Medical Genetics: Past, Present, Future**. New York: Alan R. Liss 1985, 213-248.
[31]A review of some indications and risks of fetal tissue sampling, can be seen in: Rodeck CH, Nicolaides KH, "Fetal tissue biopsy: techniques and indications" *FetalTher* 1,1 (1986) 46-58.
[32]See: McCarthy, *Ethical principles*, 97. See also: Wertz DC, Fletcher JC, "Ethics and medical genetics in the United States: a national survey" *AJMedGen* 29 (1988) 815-827; Rice and Doherty, *Reflections*, 47-57.
[33]See: McCarthy *et al*, **Critical Sexual Issues** (1989), 147.
[34]See: O'Donnell, *Wrongful pregnancy*, 37-40. Confessional differences are most evident here. A review of the influence of religion in prenatal diagnosis decisions, is provided by: Holtam NR,

"Antenatal diagnosis and the termination of pregnancy: what the churches have to say" *JInhMetabDis* 11,suppl 1 (1988) 111-119.

[35]An appeal for guidelines in view of the increasing moral complexity of these techniques, in: Sarto GE, "Ethical and legal considerations of antenatal diagnosis" *ClinObGyn* 7,1 (1980) 135-141. A critique holding that, in view of the present lack of treatment available for the vast majority of anomalies detected, prenatal diagnosis may actually be causing more trauma and overall harm than calm--including increased intolerance of the handicapped--, is found in: Green JM, **Calming Or Harming? A Critical Review of Psychological Effects of Fetal Diagnosis on Pregnant Women.** London: Galton Institute 1990, 4-50.

[36]See: May, **Human Existence**, 104-106; McCarthy and Bayer, **Critical Life Issues**, 101-104.

[37]An example as to what extent this line of reasoning is pervasive--to the point of seeking to "avoid disaster" by killing the fetus carrying some anomaly--, can be blatantly detected in: Fletcher JC, "Prenatal diagnosis of the hemoglobinopathies: ethical issues" *AJObGyn* 135,1 (1979) 53-56. Likewise, an extremely restrictive acceptance of "genetic" abortion, but ultimately under the pretext of the best "interest" for the fetus, is in: Santurri EN, "Prenatal diagnosis: some moral considerations" in: Schneider ED, ed, **Questions about the Beginning of Life: Christian Appraisals of Seven Bioethical Issues.** Minneapolis, MN: Augsburg 1985, 120-150.

[38]See: Atkinson and Moraczewski, **Genetic Counseling**, 19-20; McCarthy, *Ethical principles*, 93-95. Holding that selective termination of pregnancy is also a disregard for the mother, merely offering a "technological solution," is: Overall C, "Selective termination of pregnancy and women's reproductive autonomy" *HastingsCRep* 20,3 (1990) 6-11.

[39]An analysis raising the issue of the fetus as patient, is found in: [no author], "Ethical problems as prenatal diagnosis improves" *ObGynNews* 19,12 (1984) 16. See also: Noia *et al*, "La cordocentesi: indicazioni, utilità e rischi" *MedMor* 4 (1991) 625-640.

[40]Arguing that widespread use of prenatal diagnosis for detecting and destroying "defective" fetuses unduly pressures mothers carrying such "defectives" to do the same, in effect discriminating against certain anomalies (Down's syndrome in this case), is: Smith DJ, "Down's syndrome, amniocentesis, and abortion: prevention or elimination?" *MentalRet* 19,1 (1981) 8-11.

[41]Some ethicists are so adverse to attributing any significance to human suffering, that they condone "therapeutic" abortion of a diseased fetus on the basis that the anomaly might deprive the fetus from obtaining a "human future," even if these ethicists themselves candidly admit to a lack of consensus as to what constitutes a "human future." Fletcher J, "Moral and ethical problems of pre-natal diagnosis" *ClinGen* 8,4 (1975) 251-257.

[42]See: Shannon, *A survey*, 27. Refuting the notion that a "therapeutic" abortion is simply mimicking a missed spontaneous abortion--due to the fact that the fetus carries some anomaly--, since once a natural process passes onto human hands, an essentially different criteriology becomes operative, is: Demmer K, "Genotechnologie e uomo" *VitPens* 67,12 (1984) 46-56. See also: Serra A, "Aborto eugenico: diritto-dovere o delitto?" *CivCat* 124,4 (1973) 110-124.

[43]Pointing to the need for upholding and protecting every human life, regardless of any anomalies it may exhibit, is: Verspieren P, "Prenatal diagnosis and selective abortion: an ethical issue" in: Malherbe J-F, ed, **Human Life: Its Beginnings and Development.** Paris: L'Harmattan 1988, 197-216. See also: Boné E, "A society more intolerant of handicap" in: **Human Life**, 227-237; Doucet H, "Le diagnostic prénatal: interprétation culturelle et réflexions éthiques" *LavalPhilT* 40,1 (1984) 31-48.

[44]See: May, **Human Existence**, 87-90. Also, an early argument on the lack of convincing power of genetic abortion, in: Kass LR, "Implications of prenatal diagnosis for the human right to life" in: Hilton B *et al*, eds, **Ethical Issues in Human Genetics.** New York: Plenum 1973,

185-199. Perhaps the height of absurd reasoning may be seen in the appeal for abortion in order to "protect the defective child from itself," in: Fletcher JC, "Moral problems and ethical guidance in prenatal diagnosis: past, present, and future" in: Milunsky A, ed, **Genetic Disorders and the Fetus: Diagnosis, Prevention, and Treatment**, 2nd ed. New York: Plenum 1986, 819-859, especially 827 ff.

[45]Surveys show that many parents with family histories of hereditary defects are willing to risk even aborting normal fetuses to prevent the possible birth of carriers. See: Costakos D *et al*, "Attitudes toward presymptomatic testing and prenatal diagnosis for Adrenoleukodystrophy among affected families" *AJMedGen* 41 (1991) 295-300.

[46]See: McCarthy *et al*, **Critical Sexual Issues** (1989), 145-146.

[47]Another evaluation of prenatal diagnosis from a Catholic perspective, is found in: Sgreccia E, "Ethical issues in prenatal diagnosis and fetal therapy" *FetalTher* 4,suppl 1 (1989) 16-27.

[48]See: Callahan S, "X versus Y: should parents decide?" *HealthProgr*, 20-21; Russe M, "Genetics and the quality of life" *SocIndRes* 7,1-4 (1980) 419-441, especially 438.

[49]Also reporting a cultural bias for aborting females--yet, surprisingly, upholding its possible licitness under the guise of "not imposing the ethical values of one culture over another"--, is: Dickens BM, "Prenatal diagnosis and female abortion: a case study in medical law and ethics" *JMedEthics* 12 (1986) 143-144, 150.

[50]See: Shannon, *A survey*, 27-28; **Genetic Engineering**, 58. See also: Henifin MS, "Selective termination of pregnancy: commentary" *HastingsCRep* 18,1 (1988) 22; Wertz DC, Fletcher JC, "Fatal knowledge? Prenatal diagnosis and sexual selection" *HastingsCRep* 19,3 (1989) 21-27.

[51]See: May, *Proxy consent*, 73-84. Emphasizing the link between the perceived moral integrity of the attending physician, and the willingness of the patient to grant informed consent, is: Gillett GR, "Informed consent and moral integrity" *JMedEthics* 15 (1989) 117-123. See also: O'Neil R, "Determining proxy consent" *JMedPhil* 8 (1983) 389-403.

[52]A strong position endorsing informed consent considering, however, the mother as the only patient, hence being a partial position, in: Crawfurd MA, "Ethical guidelines in fetal medicine" *FetalTher* 2,3 (1987) 175-180. Similarly, see: Annas GJ, Elias S, "Legal and ethical implications of fetal diagnosis and gene therapy" *AJMedGen* 35,2 (1990) 215-218.

[53]A case study pointing to the pervasive lack of knowledge among the general population regarding genetic diseases and prenatal diagnosis, particularly in reference to inheritance patterns, in: Decruyenaere M *et al*, "Cystic fibrosis: community knowledge and attitudes towards carrier screening and prenatal diagnosis" *ClinGen* 41,4 (1992) 189-196.

[54]Contending that, since the current availability of PND pressures women into acquiring the information it provides, and subsequently into having to act on such information, then only informed consent gives them full control of such decisions, is: Katz Rothman B, "The decision to have or not to have amniocentesis for prenatal diagnosis" in: Michaelson KL, ed, **Childbirth in America: Anthropological Perspectives**. South Hadley, MA: Bergin and Garvey 1988, 90-102.

[55]Also insisting on informed consent by the mother as absolutely necessary to safeguard her just autonomy regarding PND, but again failing to distinguish between it and proxy consent, thus in fact neglecting to realize that precisely in such a case the fetus is the one whose autonomy is unjustly disrespected, is: Faden R, "Autonomy, choice, and the new reproductive technologies: the role of informed consent in prenatal genetic diagnosis" in: Rodin J, Collins A, eds, **Women and New Reproductive Technologies: Medical, Psychosocial, Legal, and Ethical Dilemmas**. Hillsdale, NJ: Lawrence Erlbaum 1991, 37-47.

[56]See: Shannon and DiGiacomo, **Introduction** (1987), 79-92.

---

[57]A parallel case in Shannon and DiGiacomo, **Introduction** (1979), 85-89.

[58]An analysis of limiting access to prenatal diagnosis only to those who can truly benefit from it, in: Juengst ET, "Prenatal diagnosis and the ethics of uncertainty" in: Monagle JF, Thomasma DC, eds, **Medical Ethics: A Guide for Health Professionals**. Rockville, MD: Aspen 1988, 12-25.

[59]See *Human Dignity*, under **Basic Value Systems**, in Chapter XII of PART THREE of this work.

[60]See: O'Donnell, **Medicine** (1991), 112-113, 242. For a contrasting view, see: McCormick, **Health**, 143-144.

[61]Asserting that, in the general case of incompetent patients, there might come a time when the parents may not be capable of upholding the incompetent's best interest--hence the need to resort to a "hierarchical sequence" of surrogates--, are: Pellegrino ED, Thomasma DC, "The role of physicians, families, and other surrogates in decisions concerning incompetent patients" in: their **For the Patient's Good: The Restoration of Beneficence in Health Care**. New York: Oxford UP 1988, 162-171.

[62]Not all authors examined directly address the issue of moral dilemmas in pre-implantation diagnosis. However, since their views regarding the status of pre-implantation human life are known, their possible opinions on the subject may also be tentatively inferred. See: Curran, **Politics**, 171; McCormick, **Health**, 134; Moraczewski, *Test tube*, 3-4.

[63]See: *Pre-Implantation Diagnosis*, under **Prenatal Interventions**, in Chapter IV of PART ONE of this text.

[64]A brief recount of techniques, risks and possibilities, in: Simpson JL, Carson SA, "Preimplantation genetic diagnosis" *NEJM* 327,13 (1992) 951-953.

[65]Contending that preimplantation diagnosis can be considered as no more threatening to human embryos than the presently acceptable practice of selective abortion is: Robertson JA, "Ethical and legal issues in preimplantation genetic screening" *FertSter* 51,1 (1992) 1-11.

[66]Namely: Lisa Cahill, Charles Curran, Richard McCormick, and Thomas Shannon.

[67]Namely: Benedict Ashley, William May, Donald McCarthy, Albert Moraczewski, and Thomas O'Donnell.

[68]See: *Hominization and Personhood*, in Chapter XIV of PART THREE of this text.

[69]See: *Immediate Hominization*, under **Hominization and Personhood**, in Chapter XIV of PART THREE of this text.

[70]Proposing that "contragestation" as the expulsion of a pre-implanted embryo is really a type of procured abortion, is: Di Pietro M-L, Sgreccia E, "La contragestazione ovvero l'aborto nascosto" *MedMor* 38,1 (1988) 5-34.

CHAPTER XVII

SHIFT IN THE SELF-UNDERSTANDING OF MEDICINE

Introduction

Prenatal diagnosis today undoubtedly provides one of the best examples where the current shift in the self-understanding of medicine may be observed. Accordingly, this chapter delves into four aspects which presently typify such shift: what are the first medical principles involved, what are the legitimate rights and responsibilities flowing from such principles, what are the limits of cooperation in prenatal diagnosis, and the particular case of genetic counseling and screening.

Regarding the first medical principles, the will of the patient to be healed must be considered at least on equal footing as the duty of the medical professional to heal. This is because one recognizes that today the patient seeks a greater control of the healing process. This control, however, can never be absolute, lest the physician and indeed the entire health-care profession, be reduced to a mere "fee-for-service" industry. Hence, a fiduciary model of doctor-patient relationship is proposed as the most realistic and effective one.

This model, however, presumes a relation of adults where mutual ligitimate rights and responsibilities may be allocated. In the particular case of prenatal diagnosis, at the forefront are the right to privacy, to information, to procreation, and to be born. However, since to every right there are always corresponding responsibilities, it is also necessary to analyze the range of accountability of the expectant mother, of the father, and of the medical doctor and other healthcare professionals associated with the pregnancy.

This sets the stage for the third section of this chapter, which is a discussion on the possibility of cooperation in prenatal diagnosis, and its limits thereof. Of particular importance are two interrelated issues: when might an attending physician or healthcare facility be guilty of complicity, and when might be the danger of giving scandal.

Finally, the fourth section addresses some contemporary cocerns in prenatal diagnosis regarding the shift toward genetic counseling and screening. Counseling proper may occur: at pre-conception; at post-conception, but pre-testing; and at post-testing. Whereas it can be said that each one of the three stages faces specific moral dilemmas, all stages nontheless touch upon the issue of confidentiality. As regards screening, two possibilities presently arise: negative eugenics and, less likely, positive eugenics.

A. THE FIRST MEDICAL PRINCIPLES

1. The Will of the Patient

In addition to health, one of the first medical principles is also the will of the patient. This is so because it is the patient who first wishes to be healed. In offering his or her expertise, then, the attending physician seeks to accomplish the will of the patient. In this sense, physician and patient always work together; they have a common goal, which brings them to a union of wills. The physician's expertise comes into play precisely in tempering the wishes of the patient as to what is medically possible here and now, all things considered.[1] The physician's role, therefore, continues to be irreplaceable as expert.[2] This notwithstanding, the patient today seeks to be in greater control of the entire healing process, in no small amount, thanks to a greater awareness of social and individual rights springing from a pluralistic society in a democratic system. This is not without its challenges in the prenatal diagnosis situation,[3] some of which are here explored.

2. Control of the Healing Process

If the patient seeks full control of the healing process, to the exclusion of any "doctor's advice," only frustration can ensue.[4] Not that past models in which absolute trust was posited on the physician's competence, indeed at times, beyond the particular area of competence, were not in need of review, but to conclude from this that the attending physician is but a mere "technological expert" who is expected to provide a service for a fee, is to miss the point of medicine altogether.[5] Rather, control of the healing process calls for a system whereby the patient's values can more easily become manifest, so as to truly enter into the decision-making process.[6] This would also have to include those instances when the patient himself or herself may not even be thematically aware of his or her underlying values relevant to the situation at hand. This is particularly true of prenatal diagnosis, where at play are fundamental human values which perhaps have never before been challenged or even summoned in the patient's lifetime to the present.[7] Cognizant of this, one can never say that the patient alone, nor that the physician alone, is in full control of the healing process. Instead, various levels of interaction are inevitably required, which must have a trusting basis to them if any degree of healing is to be expected.[8]

3. A Fiduciary Model

Not that such trust must be uncritically absolute, for it would be absurd to hold that after the current medical "shift" (a shift, in fact, promoted by both, patients *and* doctors), and finding no alternative other than total alienation between the parties concerned, one is to return to some previous situation of unquestionably accepting all "doctor's advice."[9] Nor that this is an option either, given that the medical profession as a whole is no longer accepting this role.[10] At the very minimum, the patient must have some degree of assurance that the attending physician is indeed competent in his or her particular field of medicine. In view of the very intimate nature, relatively long duration, and far-reaching personal consequences of human pregnancy, it would seem that the relationship between an expectant mother and her attending obstetrician/gynecologist is one which likely requires a high level of confidence, trust and respect afforded, not only to her and her physician, but also to her pre-born and his or her father.[11]

B. LEGITIMATE RIGHTS AND RESPONSIBILITIES IN PRENATAL DIAGNOSIS

Every legitimate right entails a corresponding duty, at least to protect such right. Accordingly, when applied to the variety of moral dilemmas present in prenatal diagnosis, certain rights and responsibilities immediately come to the fore. While an exhaustive treatment of the subject is beyond the scope of this work, one cannot escape addressing at least those which appear most frequently in the examined literature.

1. The Rights of Some Persons to Some Services[12]

To privacy

The expectant mother has a right to have her privacy respected. This also includes those personal, marital and family situations which are considered to be intimate by society at large. Now, if one seeks to avoid impinging on another's privacy while in the process of defining one's own, one must have to be content with only a broad and general principle of privacy. In addition, such right, although legitimately recognized by society, cannot be expected realistically to dominate the entire prenatal situation, lest a most basic and universal of human events (*i.e.*, gestation) might fall prey of possession in a negative sense, that is, for a woman to say: "this is *my* pregnancy, and I do with it what I want."[13] Hence, in a true conflict situation, it is not unforeseeable that the expectant mother's right to her privacy might have to be tempered with a more fundamental right (*i.e.*, the right to life, whether her own or her pre-born's).[14] The right to privacy is not an absolute right to the total exclusion of any other claim.[15]

To information

There is no question that the expectant mother, and indeed the couple, also has a right to pertinent information regarding her pregnancy. The word pertinent is key here because it could be maintained that whereas not all information that can be obtained about the fetus by means of prenatal diagnosis is pertinent toward the possible cure or amelioration of an eventual detected anomaly, it could actually be used to his or her detriment, such as in the case of prenatal sex selection.[16] An extremely prudential judgment is then required of the physician. Morally, it is not sufficient to say: "the mother has a right to information."[17] Rather, the physician cannot escape asking: is it not more in line with the healing process to refrain from giving certain information, if it is *not* medically relevant to either patient (the mother or the fetus), but definitely harmful to one of them (the fetus)?[18] Different is the case of the discovery of some prenatal malformation or disease, for now medicine enters into the picture, and a mother cannot be expected to responsibly care for her child if she does not know the medical condition of her child. She also has a right to know of possible treatments and services available concerning the discovered defect. In sum, the mother has a right to pertinent information, and the competent physician never avoids pondering what is medically pertinent to his or her patient.[19]

Always in this light, the physician must also have a right to pertinent information, if she or he is expected to render a professional service. Here the fiduciary model is again crucial, for it incumbs on the physician to seek that information from her or his patient which is relevant to the healing process; it incumbs on the expectant mother to provide it, again, not necessarily being acritical, but certainly underlined by a basic trust in her doctor.[20]

To procreate

Even couples who have tested positive for some genetic anomaly have a right to procreate.[21] But this right must also be tempered by the responsibility and the capacity to properly raise the children originating from that union.[22] There are several concerns at play here. First, there is the evaluation of the severity of the defect in question: is it a minor or correctable one (*i.e.*, polydactyly), or is it indeed serious or life-threatening (*i.e.*, cystic fibrosis)? Second, there is the question of the real physiological capacity of the couple to procreate: Are both partners affected? Are they both carriers, or only one, and how so? What is the actual probability of transmitting the defect? Third, there is an entire cluster of issues of adequate financial, psychological, professional, social and personal resources of the couple: are we talking about a young couple, who is struggling to barely make ends meet, and who might still be very insecure in their new marital relationship; or are they a rather well-established couple, both professionals (perhaps even in the medical fields), with years of marital experience, and quite solid spiritually, financially and otherwise?[23] Finally, to consider is the potential impact on their children's children: assuming that the couple's children will be only carriers, when they become adults, will they also have to contend with the possibility of not marrying or not having children? The right to procreate is not morally unconditional.[24]

To be born

Whereas the right to be born may be a fundamental right,[25] it does not necessarily include a right to be born without defects or anomalies.[26] It could well be that, given contemporary advances in prenatal medicine, a child today might have the right to be born without those illnesses or defects which medicine can reasonably prevent. However, it is not justified to conclude from this that "it is better not to be born than to be born defective."[27] First, because it unrealistically assumes that medicine can now cure prenatally all anomalies. Second, because it considers all anomalies to be equally serious or devastating. Third, even in the worst of cases, because it presumes that the child being born would desire to have been killed rather than to live with such condition.[28] In the final analysis, the incorrectness of the judgment lies precisely in the fact that no one has the right to morally judge the "worthiness" or "unworthiness" of another's life.[29] While it may be said that any number of moral actions are unworthy of the human person, no human life can be said to be unworthy in and of itself, regardless of how "anomalous" it may seem to be.[30] Prenatal diagnosis now allows for the detection of literally thousands of birth defects:[31] the right to be born does not include the right to be born perfect, physiologically or otherwise.[32]

2. Accountability

If to every right did not correspond a duty, no right could be claimed, protected, or promoted. Hence, every subject of rights is accountable in his or her responsibility to uphold the same rights in others. Again, applied to the prenatal situation, specific responsibilities immediately emerge.

Of the expectant mother

Even from a very human perspective, no one normally has greater responsibility over a human fetus than the one at the other end of his or her umbilical cord. This responsibility can indeed be grave or even overwhelming at times, especially if the fetus is diagnosed to carry severe physical and/or mental abnormalities. Once more, the issue at hand is the intrinsic worthiness of human life. The expectant mother is then obliged to care for her pre-born to the best of her ability.[33] This might include prenatal diagnosis if the fetus can benefit from it (directly or indirectly, as seen above[34]), but not to his or her detriment. It must be kept in mind at all times that, as natural as the pregnant condition is, it is nonetheless a supreme act of self-giving; one that extends, not for nine months, but indeed for a lifetime. Thus, an antagonistic model which purports to vie the fetus against his or her mother (and father) is in contraposition to the entire teleology of human pregnancy.[35] At least from a Christian perspective, an antagonistic model of pregnancy seems to serve only do to violence to the human dignity which Christianity seeks to promote: to the expectant mother and her state, to the fetus and his or her predicament, and to a most natural and necessary condition of every humans' life: gestation.

Of the father

Though admittedly they could be quite obvious, seldom does one encounter specific references to the responsibilities of a father regarding prenatal diagnosis of the fetus which he has helped to create. Moreover, at times the entire procedure is done, not only without his knowledge or consent, but actually against his consent. Again, from a Christian perspective, not to include the father in the prenatal diagnosis decision is in principle an antagonistic model which does violence to himself as father, and to the marital relationship as a whole. This having been said, situations can definitely be envisioned whereby a father's handling of prenatal diagnosis information could result in real damage to the fetus, to his or her mother, or to both. Hence, the father's supportive role throughout the entire pregnancy, including the possibility of undergoing prenatal diagnosis if indicated, is unquestionably his utmost responsibility. To fulfill this responsibility is to fulfill his own human condition precisely as father; to neglect it is to neglect himself ultimately into failure.[36] And, by supportive is intended a very realistic provision of such essentials as spiritual, emotional, financial, and time-energy involvement and encouragement. The goal must be clear: the expectant mother should not feel alone or constrained to hiding feelings, doubts, or information from him.[37] Thus, to participate in the creation of a new human life must necessarily include the grave responsibility to participate in the creation of such a conducive and supportive environment to the best of his ability.

Of the medical doctor and other healthcare professionals

Their responsibility of respect and concern is foremost.[38] In the particular setting of medicine and pregnancy, it necessarily extends to the fetus. And, unless one considers medicine to be merely one more fee-for-service industry of a consumer economy,[39] then it must also extend to the value system of his or her mother and father, for at stake is a most human and humane rapport.[40] Hence, it means that the value system of the physician and other medical personnel associated with the pregnancy must also be respected.[41] Since these professionals are responsible for being willing to do what is medically possible for this pregnancy here and now, this might include prenatal diagnosis if indicated. Of the many responsibilities that precede (*i.e.*, to obtain free and informed consent) and follow (*i.e.*, the correct interpretation and communication of pertinent data), intentionality remains central: why test?[42] While the physician cannot realistically be held accountable of his or her patient's intentions (or even fabricated pretenses, as in the case of a mother who claims falsely to have been exposed to teratogens so as to indicate for prenatal diagnosis and thus learn the gender of her fetus), the physician is certainly responsible for his or her own intentions.[43] Hence, knowing that the fetus can now be in fact a medical patient in some cases,[44] if the expectant mother has made it abundantly known that she will abort any "defective" fetus, would not her attending physician be responsible of making it equally clear that killing a patient is not a true medical "cure"?[45]

C. COOPERATION AND ITS LIMITS

The decision whether or not to undergo prenatal diagnosis can never be carried out in isolation. Rather, it involves a host of persons and institutions in cooperation with the expectant mother. From the perspective of the faith,[46] two elements must then be taken into consideration: complicity and scandal.

1. Complicity

An expectant mother indicates for prenatal diagnosis according to any one of the indications mentioned above.[47] If she has also expressed her intention to abort any "defective" fetus discovered, what are the moral possibilities of cooperating in procuring such diagnosis, and the limits thereof?[48] Some preliminary comments apply.

First, the analysis is seen from a Catholic perspective, that is, that direct, procured abortion of a fetus carrying some anomaly is not morally acceptable.[49] Second, despite its moral unacceptability, procured abortion is presently a legal right in the United States of America.[50] Third, over the past twenty years, it has also become accepted by the medical establishment in general,[51] and endured by society at large.[52] Finally, as pointed out earlier, the vast majority of prenatal diagnosis yields a negative result (that is, that the pre-born appears to be healthy, at least regarding the anomaly for which it is being tested).[53]

Given these "facts," a critical analysis of prenatal diagnosis reveals that it can be sufficiently removed from the abortion decision so as to warrant possible moral justification because:[54] first, the procedure itself is not abortifacient to the corresponding observed rate of spontaneous abortion in the general population; second, the attending physician does not have to participate in the mother's intention to abort in order for him or her to have sufficient medical reason for the procedure; third, there still exists the possibility that the mother may be dissuaded from her intention by a careful explanation of the testing results; fourth, the doctor can also make it clear to her that he or she does not partake of her decision, but respects it as coming from a competent adult; fifth, the expectant mother could otherwise have the procedure done by the unscrupulous doctor who sees nothing wrong with "therapeutic" abortion, thus missing an opportunity to attempt to save the life of the fetus in question.[55]

Nevertheless, because prenatal diagnosis provides the specific information that might be used in deciding to abort, the attending physician and associated personnel may be guilty of complicity if a necessary direct relation is established between the information and the abortion. Once again, the prudential judgment of the physician is crucial and unavoidable: first, there must be a medical reason (hence, testing only to find out the fetus' gender, without the suspicion of a sex-linked anomaly, is *not* a medical reason[56]); second, even with a medical reason, the physician must still explore the usefulness of the information for the patient, that is, the fetus: if absolutely no healing benefit is foreseen, while definite harm is (*i.e.*, when his or her mother is completely resolute on aborting any "defective"), then the link might be direct. However, if in the judgment of the physician there is both a medical indication, and the possibility of some direct or indirect benefit, the procedure may be justified. Some could object that this makes the physician responsible for the moral actions of his or her patients, whereas the physician in fact has no control over what the patient does with the information. A counterargument might be that: first, there are *two* patients involved here, and the doctor has a responsibility toward both; second, given the wide-spread acceptance of "therapeutic" abortion, the doctor also has a responsibility to clarify misconceptions and to oppose any manipulation of his or her profession for non-medical reasons, especially those incumbent to his or her specialty.[57] Thus, the attending physician of an expectant mother today cannot avoid discerning whether or not he or she may become involved in complicity due to prenatal diagnosis.[58]

2. Scandal

Whether or not complicity actually occurs, a second necessary consideration of the medical profession in a Catholic facility providing prenatal diagnosis is the possibility of imparting scandal.[59] Again, given the fact that the vast majority of fetuses that test positive are aborted, a physician or medical facility which is routinely involved in prenatal diagnosis may be perceived by the local community as the "antechamber" to the abortion clinic where the "sentence" was declared. Hence, in order to prevent this, these Catholic physicians and medical facilities should at least let it be clearly known that they are not associated with, or referring to, any abortion clinic.[60] Further, if the intention is truly to dissuade the expectant mother from aborting, proper pre-testing and post-testing counseling must be provided in order to correctly address the complexity of issues which inevitably arise from prenatal diagnosis.[61] Once more, some could object to being attributed the task of "dissuading the mother from aborting," yet the alternative may in fact involve falling prey to a discriminatory gradation argument in the negative sense. For example, if the fetus tests positive for unilateral renal agenesis (a condition which is compatible with life), should not the attending physician discourage his or her abortion in order to remain true to the principles of medicine? Or, if a fetus tests positive for Down's, what makes this fetus more deserving of death than the arenal one? The possibility of causing scandal, whether purposely or not, obliges the medical community involved in prenatal diagnosis to do everything in its power to dissociate itself from direct, procured abortion as a form of "healing" in the case of a positive diagnosis.[62]

D. GENETIC COUNSELING AND SCREENING

One very positive way of dissociating from abortion is through genetic counseling.[63] This provides the counselor with an opportunity, not only to properly explain the medical aspects of prenatal diagnosis, but also to explore the different values at play.[64]

1. Pre-Conception Counseling

Briefly, this might involve a woman, a man (or a couple) affected by, or suspecting being carriers of, some genetic or congenital abnormality.[65] Before conception, the counselor has the opportunity to ascertain, to the present extent possible, what, if any, birth defects could be foreseen. Because of the many different degrees of severity, expression and probability of occurrence, each case must be individually evaluated. Some questions to ask would be: is one or both future parents affected? Is the disease sex-linked? What is the extent of its severity? Are there any cures known? What are the overall resources of the couple? Depending on the answer to these and other questions, the conscientious counselor might consider recommending to the married couple not to have any (more) children of their own.[66] If sufficiently before marriage, she or he could counsel the client to seek a partner who is genetically compatible.[67] Needless to say, such delicate discussions deserve the utmost of tact, respect and faith. To insinuate that a person is somehow "less" because she or he is affected by, or is a carrier of, a genetic disease is morally unconscionable.[68]

2. Post-Conception, Pre-Testing Counseling

No expectant mother should undergo prenatal diagnosis without prior counseling.[69] Not that this is realistically possible either, in view of her necessary free and informed consent. However, rather than being a mere formality, *why* and *how* such consent is obtained remains crucial.

Assuming she qualifies due to one of the indications mentioned above,[70] from a Catholic perspective, it seems prudent at this point to advise her that it is not morally licit to consider abortion as "cure" of an eventual fetal anomaly. This allows for a proper respect of all consciences involved, thus minimizing the possibility of misunderstandings later on.[71] If the mother accepts this "precondition," the counselor can then proceed to explain the most appropriate sort of tests, given the particulars of her case, the risks involved, and the possible benefits wihch might be pursued. If the expectant mother does not agree to this precondition, she remains free to seek a different medical professional. Regardless of the outcome, it must be recognized that a proper pre-testing counseling has the potential to set the stage for a truly beneficial diagnosis and prognosis in a fuller sense of "health."

3. Post-Testing Counseling

Perhaps the most delicate of all is the first session after the test results are known. Understandable is a high level of anxiety on the part of the mother, the father, and perhaps even of the counselor and/or attending physician: it is the moment of truth. Again, *how* and *how well* this truth is conveyed remains crucial, for it might actually make the difference between despair and hope (for the parents), between life and death (for the fetus).[72] Now is also when the fruits of pre-testing counseling may be reaped, since the mother (or couple) would have been adequately appraised of at least the foreseeable possibilities. Once more, the cases will vary greatly, ranging from minor deformities, to life-threatening situations. Hence, it could mean counseling the expectant mother to explore *in utero* therapy, if applicable, or to "let nature take its course," that is, to prepare for the eventuality of a miscarriage.

No post-testing counseling would be complete without researching the existence of agencies, foundations, institutions, and support groups available in society for a wide variety of existing handicaps and disabilities.[73] Here again the very human dimension of bearing and caring for a child with birth defects comes to the fore. Though the primary responsibility is theirs, parents ought never to feel alone or abandoned by society in this task. Real, tangible support and encouragement is integral to post-testing counseling.[74] Of particular importance to this author is the spiritual sustenance which can be provided to parents at this critical time in their lives, and the life of their familial and marital relationship.[75]

4. Confidentiality

Unquestionably, confidentiality is at the heart of any successful doctor-patient relationship. This becomes even more evident with prenatal diagnosis, given the intimately personal nature of the information obtained, not only of the fetus, but also of his or her mother, father, and even other ancestors.[76] Thus, the case may arise when, while in the course of testing for some specific sex-linked characteristic, the attending physician or counselor becomes aware that the father of the fetus is not the husband of his or her mother. If this is unbeknownst to her husband, the professional would be bound to confidentiality.[77] Contrary, however, might be the case of discovering a carrier condition in an individual engaged to marry: if this individual does not wish his or her engaged partner to know of such condition, may the counselor break confidentiality? While confidentiality must in principle be scrupulously upheld if one is not to undermine the entire doctor-patient relationship,[78] a foreseeable situation may arise whereby the carrier condition might be severely damaging or even lethal to future offspring if the other partner is also a carrier. It seems that, in the name of justice, a claim could be made where confidentiality might be broken in a true life-threatening predicament.[79] At the very minimum, the counselor who becomes aware of such information is bound to do everything in her or his power to persuade his or her client to mention the condition to his or her engaged partner.[80]

5. Genetic Screening

Negative eugenics

If negative eugenics is the attempt to remove deleterious genes from the human gene pool, then at least ideally, it is a noble goal.[81] Realistically, it might be somewhat less splendid.[82] First, true screening programs which seek to detect genetic abnormalities would have to be totally specific, and thus extremely expensive and intricate.[83] Second, because they have to target certain subgroups within the general population, they could be construed as discriminatory.[84] Third, heterozygotes would go undetected, unless every individual underwent elaborate testing. Fourth, even if heterozygotes were all detected, spontaneous mutations are continuously occurring within the overall gene pool of the population, for evolution by definition is never static.[85] Even so, while negative eugenics may not be a realistic goal for the entire population,[86] it could well serve affected or carrier individuals if practiced voluntarily, that is, if they undergo screening on their own will when suspecting, or being made aware of, some genetic abnormality.[87] A case of true negative eugenics would then be if the affected individual subsequently avoided marriage with a genetically incompatible partner.[88] There is no question that this might involve definite sacrifices. In so doing, the couple would have indeed contributed to a greater humanization in their free exercise of discrete and prudent judgment. Conversely, "eugenic" abortion,[89] while effectively eliminating the patient, still fails to cure the disease.[90]

Positive eugenics

Beyond negative eugenics, trying to actually ameliorate the gene pool is an instance of positive eugenics. Possibilities which were considered science fiction a short time ago are a reality today.[91] In human systems,[92] however, positive eugenics needs to undergo the added and severe scrutiny of its moral licitness, given the potential for enormous genetic damage, both to the individuals involved, and to the population at large. Seeking to genetically better the human race also runs into some formidable questions, such as: What characteristics are to be most valued? How should such research be funded? Who should benefit from it, or have access to it? Who should control it? The magnitude of these issues seems arduous indeed.[93] Nonetheless, it is not inconceivable that individuals and societies could eventually seek to answer such questions.[94] Crucial will then be an anthropology that does not neglect the theological dimension, lest it remain hopelessly defective or wanting.[95] At any rate, it is necessary to note the present exorbitant costs of such programs which, in a system of limited funds, may in effect re-direct resources from other areas of medicine where a much greater number of people would be served in their more immediate needs.[96]

Notes

[1]Entreating medical professionals to resist the temptation of routinely recommending prenatal genetic screening for non-medical, or even medically-invalidated, reasons, are: Elias S, Annas GJ, "Routine prenatal genetic screening" *NEJM* 317,22 (1987) 1407-1409.

[2]A survey showing that, in the United States of America, most medical geneticists are willing to recommend prenatal diagnosis *without* medical indications for patients who refuse abortion, in: Wertz DC, Fletcher JC, "Ethics and medical genetics in the United States: a national survey" *AJMedGen* 29,4 (1988) 815-827, especially 821.

[3]Contending that the present shift towards uncritically complying more and more with patients' rights and wishes may at times actually hurt both, the patients and the practice of medicine, is: O'Donnell, *Abuses*, 15-16.

[4]Surveying a wide range of complex psychological, ethical, legal and social issues raised by the current availability of prenatal diagnosis, hence pointing to the need of a collaborative interaction in the decision making process, are: Beeson D, Douglas R, Lunsford TF, "Prenatal diagnosis of fetal disorders. Part II: issues and implications" *Birth* 10,4 (1983) 233-241.

[5]Warning of the dehumanizing tendency of a rapidly advancing medical technology as one of its current shifts, is: Curran, **Issues**, 75. See also: Godfraind Th, "Les défis posés au chrétien par la technique médicale" *RTLv* 17 (1986) 5-21.

[6]See: Shannon, **Twelve Problems**, 99-112.

[7]An example of a "value-less" description of prenatal diagnostic techniques, combined with a variety of assisted reproductive manipulations and selective abortion, to achieve the product of non-defective human embryos, which in fact betrays an underlying specific set of merely utilitarian values, in: Austin CR, **Human Embryos: The Debate on Assisted Reproduction**. New York: Oxford 1989, 71-81.

[8]Stating that in a rather "unregulated" medical setting such as the one presently operative in the United States, the patient relies mostly on the personal and professional integrity of her or his physician, are: Chervenak FA, McCullough LB, "Ethics in obstetric ultrasound" *JUltrasMed* 8,9 (1989) 493-497.

[9]A summary of guidelines regarding the doctor-patient relationship involving prenatal diagnosis, including that: prenatal diagnosis should be done on a voluntary basis; the expectant mother be left free to choose to abort or not; information be provided when fetal therapy is available; other findings also be disclosed (i.e., XYY genotypes); and, no prenatal diagnosis be done only for sex

selection, is found in: Fletcher JC, "The prenatal state: screening and treating neural tube defects" in: Reiser SJ, Anbar M, eds, **The Machine at the Bedside: Strategies for Using Technology in Patient Care**. New York: Cambridge 1984, 255-260. See also: Fletcher JC, "Ethical issues in genetic screening, prenatal diagnosis, and counseling" in: Weil WB, Benjamin M, eds, **Ethical issues at the Outset of Life**. Boston: Blackwell Scientific 1987, 63-99.

[10]This present "shift" may also be evident in the growing tendency of physicians to fully disclose prenatal diagnosis results for their patients' interpretation, even when the results might be conflicting, controversial, ambiguous or artifactual. See: Wertz and Fletcher, *National survey*, 815-827.

[11]This might again betray a socio-cultural bias, but the fact is that today more than one American expectant mother has to face the prospect of bearing and raising her children without the benefit of their father as her husband; the challenge of raising a *handicapped* child under these conditions, then, becomes that much more onerous. Proposing a medical model wherein both, the patient and the physician, are partners in suffering and hope, is: Brera GR, "La sofferenza nel rapporto medico-paziente: la medicina come scienza della sofferenza" *MedMor* 37,1-2 (1987) 46-57. See also: Coste R, "Passion et compassion: brèves esquisses" *Suppl* 152 (1985) 21-30; Thévenot X, "La compassion: une réponse au mal?" *Suppl* 172 (1990) 79-96.

[12]An early analysis of some of the rights mentioned below, is given by: Shannon and DiGiacomo, **Introduction** (1979), 145-153.

[13]Claiming that due to the exponential rise of prenatal diagnosis information, coupled with an ever greater medicalization of pregnancy, and with the desire to avert any predictable calamity, the "tentative pregnancy" is becoming more and more a standard option, is: Tymstra T, "Prenatal diagnosis, prenatal screening, and the rise of the tentative pregnancy" *IntJTechAssHealthCare* 7,4 (1991) 509-516.

[14]Also advancing that the right to privacy must at times yield to the more basic right to life, including the present tendency of greater privatization of procured abortion, is: Rice CE, "Amniocentesis, coercion, and privacy" in: Nelson LJ, ed, **The Death Decision**. Ann Arbor, MI: Servant 1984, 57-68.

[15]Insisting that society has some saying in the medical technologies affecting prenatal life, particularly against an excessively privatized decision to procure abortion, is: Cahill, *Abortion pill*, 5-8.

[16]See: Atkinson and Moraczewski, **Genetic Counseling**, 23-24.

[17]Pointing to the current exponential growth of information in genetics, with multiple ethical implications, is: Shannon, **Twelve Problems**, 50-72. Acknowledging certain fundamental rights of patients, including the right to know the truth in general--but also recognizing that under certain circumstances discrete silence regarding some specific information is in the best interest of the patient--, is: Perico G, **Problemi di Etica Sanitaria**. Milano: Ancora 1985, 43-51.

[18]Arguing in favor of full disclosure of results, in view of the perceived sense of injustice done to parents who bear children with some genetic defect (in this case, thalassemia) by not having been appraised of their carrier status, is: Modell B, "The ethics of prenatal diagnosis and genetic counselling" *WHealthF* 11,2 (1990) 179-186.

[19]Reporting research demonstrating that some couples actually have *more* difficulty making subsequent reproductive decisions *with* the availability of prenatal diagnosis information and counseling, than without, are: Frets PG, Duivenvoorden HJ, Verhage F, Peters-Romeyn BMT, Neirmeijer MF, "Analysis of problems in making the reproductive decision after genetic counselling" *JMedGen* 28,3 (1991) 194-200. Sustaining that, without adequate information, a person cannot be expected to make mature moral decisions--and that, therefore, there is no "right" to remain uninformed about a given medical condition--, is: Ost DE, "The 'right' not to know"

JMedPhil 9 (1984) 301-312. A contrasting view, maintaining that, at times, a person also has a right not to be told about a certain pathological condition, is found in: Strasser M, "Mill and the right to remain uninformed" *JMedPhil* 11 (1986) 265-278.

[20]The basic right of science to access that genetic information which is relevant to the eventual amelioration of the human condition, especially when seeking to alleviate genetic defects, but always upholding the right to privacy and confidentiality of individuals involved, is attested by: Healy B, "Hearing on the possible uses and misuses of genetic information" *HGeneTher* 3 (1992) 51-56.

[21]See: Shannon and DiGiacomo, **Introduction** (1979), 139-140.

[22]See: Ashley and O'Rouke, **Healthcare Ethics** (1989), 327.

[23]Alluding to the intimidation factor of a "positive" diagnosis, and sustaining that perhaps some women abort children who are carrying defects because they feel incapable of coping with the prospects under the present socio-cultural environment, is: Rapp R, "The power of 'positive' diagnosis: medical and maternal discourses on amniocentesis" in: Michaelson KL, ed, **Childbirth in America: Anthropological Perspectives.** South Hadley, MA: Bergin and Garvey 1988, 103-116.

[24]See: Ashley and O'Rourke, **Healthcare Ethics** (1989), 322. See also: Häring B, "It's wrong to knowingly beget defective children" *USCath* 41,2 (1976) 12-14; Lebel RR, "Genetic decision-making; parental responsibility" *LinacreQ* 43 (1976) 280-291; Verspieren P, "Un droit à l'enfant?" *Ét* 362,5 (1985) 623-628; Vidal M, "¿Existe el 'derecho a procrear'?" *Mor* 9 (1987) 39-50.

[25]Discussing some fundamental rights of the fetus, is: Caffarra C, "The rights of the embryo and the fetus" *FetalTher* 4,suppl 1 (1989) 12-15.

[26]See: Curran, *In vitro*, 4.24; McCormick, *Value impacts*, 38-41. See also: Sgreccia E, "La diagnosi prenatale" in: Congresso Internazionale di Teologia Morale (Roma, 7-12 aprile 1986), **Persona, Verità e Morale.** Roma: Città Nuova 1987, 315-331.

[27]Certainly, no conception is ever totally free of the risk of defect. See: Ashley and O'Rourke, **Healthcare Ethics** (1989), 325-327.

[28]So traumatized by the prospect of a child born with deformities causing its parents and other family members great expense and suffering, and seemingly intimidated by the rise of "wrongful life" or "wrongful birth" legal suits, as to summon prenatal diagnosis followed by selective abortion a "high priority in preventive medicine," which in fact betrays a lack of regard for the possible wishes and interests of the child itself, is: Holder AR, "Amniocentesis, genetic counseling, and genetic screening" in: Holder AR, **Legal Issues in Pediatrics and Adolescent Medicine**, 2nd ed. New Haven, CT: Yale 1985, 25-49.

[29]See: May, *Proxy consent*, 78-82.

[30]Pointing to a social pragmatic bias, which tends to see "eugenic" abortion as "treatment," and therefore to the dangers of prenatal diagnosis as becoming a tool to such "treatment," is: McCarthy, *Pragmatic bias*, 2-3.

[31]See: Shannon, *A survey*, 27. See also **Human Embryonic Disorders**, in Chapter III of PART ONE of this text.

[32]Distinguishing between the right to be born, and the right to be born healthy, is also: Robertson JA, Schulman JD, "Pregnancy and prenatal harm to offspring: the case of mothers with PKU" *HastingsCRep* 17,4 (1987) 23-33.

[33]See: O'Rourke, *Parents and children*, 14-15.

[34]See: *Benefits*, under **Prenatal Diagnosis Proper**, in Chapter XVI of PART THREE of this text.

[35]So, seeking to re-define abortion before implantation as "antigestation" or a type of

"contraception," in order to favor the interests of the mother against those of her pre-born, is deceiving to expectant mothers and also counter to the teleology of pregnancy; such distortion can only serve to further the unjustified antagonism of one innocent life against another. See: Cahill, *Abortion pill*, 5-8.

[36]When parents patently neglect their responsibilities, it is not inappropriate for society to intervene on behalf of their children. See: O'Rourke, *Parents and children*, 14-15.

[37]Research evidence that the success of prenatal screening and counseling depends, at least in part, on the collaboration and participation of the child's father (most certainly if he is either genetically affected, or a carrier), in: Loader S *et al*, "Prenatal screening for hemoglobinopathies. II. Evaluation and counseling" *AJHumGen* 48,3 (1991) 447-451.

[38]For a model of the supportive role of medical personnel, especially in the prenatal diagnosis situation, see: Fibison WJ, Davies BL, "Dilemmas in prenatal diagnosis: a case study" *IssHealth CareW* 4,1 (1983) 57-67.

[39]To that end, the economic tie between prenatal diagnosis and selective abortion must be recognized. Suggesting that professional hesitation and under-referral are contributing to not meeting consumer demands for more, and more accessible, prenatal diagnosis and selective abortion, are: Lippman-Hand A, Piper M, "Prenatal diagnosis for the detection of Down syndrome: why are so few eligible women tested?" *PrenatDiag* 1,4 (1981) 249-257.

[40]A summary statement of ethical principles and concepts for American obstetricians and gynecologists, including the recognition of the fetus as patient, is found in: ACOG, "Ethical decision-making in obstetrics and gynecology" *ACOGTechB* 136 (1989) 1-7. Presenting the validity of a case study where the parents of a possibly affected fetus declined further testing due to "subjective," but very human reasons--not normally falling under any particular ethical system--, are: Smurl JF *et al*, "Ethical considerations in medical genetics: the prenatal diagnosis of Hemophilia B" *AJMedGen* 17,4 (1984) 773-781.

[41]See: Atkinson and Moraczewski, **Genetic Counseling**, 25-29; Moraczewski, *Genetic Counseling*, 52. Arguing that a true Christian medical profession may not be exercised without taking into consideration the personal value system of the professional, including an absolute respect for conscientious objection, is: Spinsanti S, "La normatività etica nel campo bio-medico" in: Goffi T, Piana G, eds, **Corso di Morale II: Diakonia (Etica della Persona)**. Brescia: Queriniana 1983, 127-175.

[42]*I.e.*, 95% of all prenatal diagnosis of women age 35 and older are done only to detect Down's syndrome. Yet, since there is presently no (prenatal) cure for it, prenatal testing may actually endanger the life of the affected fetus by targeting it for selective abortion. See: Atkinson and Moraczewski, **Genetic Counseling**, 22-23. See also: Shannon and DiGiacomo, **Introduction** (1979), 81-82.

[43]Claiming that merely wanting to satisfy the curiosity of the parents regarding the gender of the fetus is not sufficient reason for subjecting it to even minimal risk, are: Ashley and O'Rourke, **Healthcare Ethics** (1989), 324.

[44]See: **Benefits**, in Chapter XVI of PART THREE of this text.

[45]See: McCarthy, *Ethical principles*, 93-95. Holding that, in view of the vast bio-medical advances in the field, the perinatologist today is called to tutor also the legitimate interests of the pre-born human, is: Pascali VL *et al*, "Problemi bioetici, deontologici e medico-legali della medicina perinatale" *MedMor* 42,1 (1992) 43-57.

[46]An in-depth analysis on the topic is found in: Fabbro R, **Cooperation in Evil: A Consideration of the Traditional Doctrine from the Point of View of the Contemporary Discussion about the Moral Act** (Doctoral Dissertation; December 16, 1987). Rome: Gregorian 1989.

---

[47]See: *Indications*, under **Prenatal Diagnosis**, in Chapter I of PART ONE of this text.

[48]From a non-Catholic perspective, moral complicity might be a non-issue for some, since the direct destruction of "defectives" is already seen as a "normal" option, even if this also represents a real danger for the expectant mother (*i.e.*, in selective intrauterine reduction of discordant twins). See: Redwine FO, Hays PM, "Selective birth" *SemPer* 10,1 (1986) 73-81. In fact, some even propose selective abortion of "defectives" to be a mere "extension" of natural selection. See: Ferguson-Smith MA, Ferguson-Smith ME, "Relationships between patient, clinician, and scientist in prenatal diagnosis" in: Dunstan GR, Shinebourne EA, eds, **Doctors' Decisions: Ethical Conflicts in Medical Practice.** New York: Oxford 1989, 18-34.

[49]See: *Dv*, I,2.

[50]See: *Roe v. Wade*, 22 January, 1973.

[51]Procured abortion is presently not opposed by the American Medical Association as a whole.

[52]Though the range of opinions is obviously vast, a majority of the population accepts at least some form of direct abortion.

[53]See: *Indications*, under **Prenatal Diagnosis**, in Chapter I of PART ONE of this text.

[54]See: Atkinson and Morakzewski, **Genetic Counseling**, 22-24; McCormick, **Health**, 140-141; O'Donnell, *Prenatal screening*, 13-14.

[55]See: Ashley and O'Rourke, **Healthcare Ethics** (1982), 316-321; McCarthy, *Ethical principles*, 98; O'Donnell, *Wrongful pregnancy*, 37-40.

[56]See: O'Donnell, *Abuses*, 15-16. A survey claiming lack of consensus among medical geneticists to perform prenatal diagnosis for sex selection in the absence of a sex-linked indication, in: Wertz and Fletcher, *National survey*, 821.

[57]See: Curran, **Politics**, 172.

[58]Also maintaining the possibility of distinguishing between prenatal diagnosis and an eventual subsequent procured abortion, is: Dougherty CJ, "Prenatal diagnosis: a reappraisal" *LinacreQ* 51 (1984) 128-138.

[59]See: O'Donnell, *Wrongful pregnancy*, 38.

[60]Acknowledging that for the medical doctor this might represent loss of income and/or "prestige" among his or her peers, is: O'Donnell, *Abuses*, 16.

[61]See: McCarthy, *Ethical principles*, 97-98.

[62]See: Moraczewski, *Genetic counseling*, 53-55.

[63]Research demonstrating that even genetic counseling does not eliminate all reproductive uncertainty due to variables outside of its scope, in: Wertz DC *et al*, "Genetic counseling and reproductive uncertainty" *AJMedGen* 18,1 (1984) 79-88.

[64]Sustaining that non-directive counseling need not be value-less, are: Atkinson and Moraczewski, **Genetic Counseling**, 25-29; Moraczewski, *Genetic counseling*, 52; **Genetic Medicine**, 101-119. Statistical support for the hypothesis that thorough counseling does not supplant the client's personal values, in: Wertz DC, Sorenson JR, "Client reactions to genetic counseling: self-report of influence" *ClinGen* 30,6 (1986) 494-502. Offering an overview of responsibilities in the counselling situation, including the respect of the conscience of the counselor, is: West R, "Ethical aspects of genetic disease and genetic counselling" *JMedEthics* 14 (1988) 194-197. See also: Seller MJ, "Ethical aspects of genetic counselling" *JMedEthics* 8 (1982) 185-188.

[65]For genetic counseling to be truly effective in helping prospective parents make informed reproductive decisions, merely conveying numeric risk is not sufficient; rather, an in-depth discussion of foreseeable effects must be included, so: Wertz DC *et al*, "Clients' interpretation of risks provided in genetic counseling" *AJHumGen* 39,2 (1986) 253-264.

[66]"In relation to physical, economic, psychological and social conditions, responsible parenthood

is exrecised, either by the deliberate and generous decision to raise a numerous family, or by the decision, made for grave motives and with due respect for the moral law, to avoid for the time being, or even for an indeterminate period, a new birth." *Hv*,10 (USCC transl.). The question of *how* such new birth is avoided is beyond the scope of this work.

[67]See: Ashley and O'Rourke, **Healthcare Ethics** (1989), 325-326.

[68]See: O'Rourke and Brodeur, **Medical Ethics II**, 84-85.

[69]Demonstrating a statistically significant decrease in undergoing prenatal diagnosis due to prior counseling, are: Lorenz RP *et al*, "Encouraging patients to undergo prenatal genetic counseling before the day of amniocentesis: its effect on the use of amniocentesis" *JReprMed* 30,12 (1985) 933-935.

[70]See: *Indications*, under **Prenatal Diagnosis**, in Chapter I of PART ONE of this text.

[71]If a doctor disapproves of abortion on moral grounds, then forcing him or her under penalty of law to reveal information directly leading to abortion might be an infringement on his or her conscience. See: O'Donnell, *Amniocentesis*, 20.

[72] Also against counseling abortion of fetuses carrying defects, are: Ashley and O'Rourke, **Healthcare Ethics** (1989), 324.

[73]See: McCormick, **Health**, 141-142; O'Rourke and Brodeur, **Medical Ethics II**, 84-85.

[74]Asserting that condemning abortion of unwanted pregnancies is not sufficient, rather also providing social and economic alternatives, is: Cahill, *Fresh approach*, 20-21.

[75]See: Baumiller RC, "Clergy involvement: a dimension of real need" *HospPract* 18,4 (1983) 38A,D,E,F; "Genetic decision making and pastoral care" *HospPract* 17,12 (1982) 96A; "Genetic counseling" *NatApostMentRet* Winter (1975) 4-5.

[76]A summary of ethical principles seeking to guide the counselor-patient relationship, in: National Society of Genetic Counselors, "Code of Ethics" *JGenCounsel* 1,1 (1992) 41-43.

[77]Confirming that most medical geneticists would uphold the mother's confidentiality in cases of false paternity, are: Wertz and Fletcher, *National survey*, 815-827.

[78]See: *A fiduciary model*, under **The First Medical Principles**, in Section One of this Chapter.

[79]See: O'Rourke and Brodeur, **Medical Ethics II**, 80-82. See also: Adams J, "Confidentiality and Huntington's chorea" *JMedEthics* 16 (1990) 196-199; Gillon R, "Genetic counselling, confidentiality, and the medical interests of relatives" *JMedEthics* 14 (1988) 171-172.

[80]See: McCarthy and Bayer, **Critical Sexual Issues**, 159.

[81]Advancing the prospect of negative eugenics through human gene therapy (exploring both, somatic and gametic possibilities), is: Fletcher JC, "Moral problems and ethical issues in prospective human gene therapy" *VirgLawR* 69 (1983) 515-546. See also: Lacadena J-R, "Terapia génica: consideraciones éticas" *RazFe* 225 (1992) 510-520. A summary protocol for alpha-fetoprotein screening as one example of negative eugenics, in: American Academy of Pediatrics, "Alpha-fetoprotein screening" *Ped* 80,3 (1987) 444-445.

[82]See: Shannon, **Twelve Problems**, 39-55; *Ethical implications*, 78-98. Pointing to the reality that, since the average entire prenatal diagnosis procedure is more expensive than abortion (and in view of the overall rising cost of maintaining persons with congenital deformities, diseases, or disabilities), even a strictly pragmatical cost-benefit analysis favors abortion *instead* of prenatal diagnosis for health screening, are: Swint JM, Kaback MM, "Intervention against genetic disease: economic and ethical considerations" in: Agich GJ, Begley CE, eds, **The Price of Health.** Boston: D. Reidel 1986, 135-156.

[83]A somber cost/benefit analysis pointing out that even highly specific testing leads to aborting many normal fetuses, so: Garber AM, Fenerty JP, "Costs and benefits of prenatal screening for

cystic fibrosis" *MedCare* 29,5 (1991) 473-489.

[84]Pointing to potential damages to minorities and the poor done by genetic screening programs, is: Russe, *Genetics*, 419-441. See also: Steinbrook R, "In California, voluntary mass prenatal screening" *HastingsCRep* 16,5 (1986) 5-7; Marmion P, "The California alpha-fetoprotein screening program: an advocacy program for handicapped children" *LinacreQ* 54,1 (1987) 77-87.

[85]Retaining that the relatively low rate of increase of defective genes in the human gene pool will remain substantially unaffected, even by significant therapeutic interventions, is: Millard CE, "The effects of modern therapeutics on the human gene pool" *RIMJ* 63,11 (1980) 443-450.

[86]Holding for compulsory screening programs in emergency situations or in cases of contagious diseases, is: Curran, **Politics**, 172-173.

[87]Voluntary screening programs also respect the freedom of those individuals who might not (yet) want to know that they are affected by a future debilitating or fatal disease. See: O'Rourke and Brodeur, **Medical Ethics II**, 83-84.

[88]See: Curran, **Issues**, 106.

[89]Sustaining that often prenatal screening is done only for the purpose of identifying and subsequently aborting "anomalous" fetuses, is: O'Donnell, *Prenatal screening*, 13-14.

[90]Opposing the current trend of eugenic abortion as "medical treatment," is: McCarthy, *Either/or*, 1-2. Holding that the present practice of selective abortion of "defective" fetuses might actually *increase* the amount of deleterious genes, is: Boss JA, "How voluntary prenatal diagnosis and selective abortion increase the abnormal human gene pool" *Birth* 17,2 (1990) 75-79.

[91]This is especially evident in the fields of agriculture, horticulture, and farm animal husbandry.

[92]Exploring main clusters of ethical issues arising from the present international effort to de-code the entire human genome, especially regarding increased genetic information about individuals and populations, and how to effectively manage such data, is: Murray TH, "Ethical issues in human genome research" *FASEBJ* 5,1 (1991) 55-60.

[93]See: Shannon, **Genetic Engineering**, 67-94.

[94]A realistic summary of the present status and future prospects of somatic gene therapy, indicating a slower rate of progress than previously believed, is given by: Orkin SH, Williams DA, "Gene therapy of somatic cells: status and prospects" in: Childs B *et al*, eds, **Molecular Genetics in Medicine (Progress in Medical Genetics**, vol 7). New York: Elserier 1988, 130-142. Offering some hope of future preimplantation therapy based on present recombinant research, are: Ropers H-H, Wieringa B, "The recombinant DNA revolution: implications for diagnosis and prevention of inherited disease" *EurJObGynReprBiol* 32 (1989) 15-27.

[95]See: Shannon, **Twelve Problems**, 50-72. See also: *A Theological System*, under **Basic Value Systems**, in Chapter XII of PART THREE of this text.

[96]Also raising ethical questions of funding and control of human gene therapy research, is: Lappé M, "Ethical Aspects of therapy for genetic diseases" in: Dietz AA, ed, **Genetic Disease: Diagnosis and Treatment: Arnold O. Beckman Conference in Clinical Chemistry** ([*sic*]5th: 1981: Monterey, CA). Washington: American Association for Clinical Chemistry 1983, 282-296. See also: Vidal M, "La 'razón eugenésica': exposición y valoración" *Mor* 9 (1987) 327-340; Cuyás M, "Problematica etica della manipolazione genetica" *RasT* 28 (1987) 471-497.

CHAPTER XVIII

DIALOGUE WITH THE MAGISTERIUM

Introduction

This final chapter contains seven sections which together seek to frame the moral analysis of prenatal diagnosis as seen in the writings of the ten selected American authors regarding a dialogue with the magisterium.

Accordingly, the first section briefly explicates the various levels of magisterial discourse operative in those documents and pronouncements which directly or indirectly touch upon moral dilemmas in prenatal diagnosis.

The second section expresses the need, in any fruitful dialogue, of seeking a common meaning underlying the technical language of both the medical sciences and the theological sciences.

The third section discusses the manner in which both the medical profession and the magisterium exercise moral competence over issues related to prenatal human life and conflict situations, and whether or not probabilism allows for a sufficient distinction between doubts of fact and doubts of law.

The fourth section examines the possibility of consensus within pluralism in an area so controversial that there is lack of agreement among theologians even as to the number and types of different schools of thought evaluating prenatal life and conflict situations in society today. The crucial need for a clearer theological anthropology is thus affirmed once more.

The fifth section acknowledges the reality of theological dissent and its limits in any pluralistic society which seeks to deal with such complex interdisciplinary issues as prenatal diagnosis. Specifically, the validity of a perceived difference in magisterial methodological approach when analyzing sexual or social issues is discussed.

The sixth section explores two underlying attitudes present in any human dialogue: tolerance and intolerance. Whereas it may be maintained that at the root of tolerance is the desire of all parties in the dialogue to arrive at a mutual understanding of the fundamental values involved, it must likewise be recognized that at least from a Catholic perspective, certain situations of intolerance precisely cannot be tolerated. Therefore, two specifically intolerable situations which commonly arise in prenatal diagnosis are critiqued.

Finally, the seventh section touches upon the task of advocacy and witnessing on behalf of the weaker amongst us. Since prenatal diagnosis directly affects two very significant members of society (the preborn human and his or her expectant mother), the charge of advocacy and witnessing on their behalf incumbs, not only the magisterium, but indeed all believers and people of good will.

A. LEVELS OF MAGISTERIAL DISCOURSE

It must at once be recognized that, when the magisterium speaks, it does so at various levels of penetration in the same moral truth. These may be such as: universal principles, general norms, contingent categorial discourse, or informed speculative opinion.[1] The vehicle of communication employed also serves as a hermeneutical key regarding both, the character of the moral truth discussed, and its binding force.[2] A conciliar constitution, conciliar decree or papal encyclical, for instance, may elicit one degree of assent; an apostolic exhortation or declaration another; a Motu Proprio or congregational instruction another; an allocution, pastoral letter or response yet another. In addition, within each one of these vehicles may also be simultaneously contained affirmations of different theological intensity, such as infallible revealed pronouncements, definitive truths intimately connected with revelation, non-definitive doctrine, or conjectural and provisional interventions on debated questions. It must be realized, then, that not all magisterial pronouncements intend to elicit the same level of assent.[3]

Regarding moral dilemmas in prenatal diagnosis facing potentially conflictive situations, some universal values are already to be found at the highest level of moral discourse, such as: the intrinsic dignity of the human person, the obligation to do good and avoid evil, and the fundamental equality of all peoples. These are usually affirmed in conciliar decrees and papal encyclicals.[4] Further along a magisterial discourse may be concrete norms seeking to apply these general principles to a variety of contemporary bio-medical issues.[5] Under this light, specific moral dilemmas related to prenatal diagnosis proper have, so far, been most directly addressed at the level of a congregational instruction.[6] They have been addressed less directly in a number of papal allocutions,[7] and more indirectly in a congregational declaration.[8] Even so, the fundamental principles invoked in their moral evaluation allude to the ordinary magisterial teaching of: no direct killing of innocent human life, and tutelage of the weakest in society.[9] Hence, the specific moral licitness of prenatal diagnosis is always ultimately subordinated to an appraisal of the greater values involved. In this sense, whereas instructions, allocutions or declarations may not be considered in themselves to belong to the highest level of magisterial discourse, the principles appealed to therein in the evaluation of prenatal diagnosis do transcend their specific vehicular mode, thus making them morally binding in character.[10]

B. SEEKING A COMMON MEANING

Basic to a fruitful interdisciplinary dialogue is, if not a common language, at least a common meaning behind the technical language used by each party.[11] In the present historical context, American secular society seeks to employ a language as free as possible of any value judgment or moral connotation. This is done in the interest of creating spaces of freedom for those human actions that tend to be more complex and multifaceted or that lend themselves to a variety of interpretations. It must be understood, however, that even this enterprise reflects a prior value judgment, namely, that of trying not to make a value judgment, particularly when speaking about potentially value-laden topics. Hence, when our contemporary pluralistic society speaks of "termination of pregnancy" as the preferred expression, within the realm of human actions associated with prenatal diagnosis, it implies certain specific value priorities.[12] Clearly stated, the natural termination of a pregnancy is either a spontaneous abortion, a miscarriage, a stillbirth, or a live birth. In the present medical context, it rather implies that a pregnancy has been terminated, not in the involuntary natural course of events, but by a scheduled and premeditated action of all consenting parties involved. Thus, if society is going to prefer this terminology, it must also acknowledge the meaning behind it: the terms describing the action may change, but its meaning remains. In this vein, intellectual and volitive honesty about the meaning of human actions, regarding prenatal human life and conflict situations, is paramount to a profitable dialogue between medicine and the magisterium. Hence, "termination of pregnancy" is not a value-less description of a human action.

Correspondingly, the magisterium must admit that terms such as "natural moral law," "dignity of the human person" and "gravely illicit act" are also not without ambivalent connotation in contemporary pluralistic society.[13] An accurate and articulate explanation of the meaning of these terms is then required if true dialogue is desired.[14] Lest such explanation fall on deaf ears and unimpressed minds, their underlying philosophical and anthropological presuppositions are to be included.[15] This is so, even if it is understood that the magisterium's is a strictly theological proposition which is not subject to any particular philosophical or anthropological system at any given historical time, place and circumstance.[16]

C. MORAL COMPETENCE

Speaking about the meaning of human actions also presupposes moral evaluation. The medical profession may then say that its field of action is restricted to physical healing, and that therefore moral evaluation is beyond its scope, but the fact is that even the desire to fulfill the patient's wishes of being healed is already a value judgment, which requires moral evaluation, namely, health as a good to be sought. The shared subject of science and religion, then, is the human person. Since the Church has a vested interest in defending and upholding the good of the human person, then the magisterium exercises a moral competence when speaking about the human person.[17] It is not questioned here that this competence stems from the authority given to the magisterium by the teaching charism of Christ, but when O'Donnell states that "the credibility of the conclusion rests on the teaching charism with which Christ has endowed His Church, not in the ideas proposed to illustrate the reasonableness of the conclusion,"[18] a problem arises, namely, that such teaching may be considered simply irrelevant in the scientific community. In other words, whereas the authoritative origin of magisterial pronouncement may well be the teaching authority of Christ, its pastoral end is always the salvation of the human person. Since this teaching cannot realistically be expected to attain its end in spite of its very object, it will do so in the manner that it is reasonable. This is why Cahill appeals for reasonable and intelligible arguments from the magisterium when discussing prenatal life and conflict situations.[19] This reasonableness, however, must not be confused with some brand of rationalism. Whereas rationalism seeks to validate all teaching ultimately on a mere human cognitive argumentation, authentic reasonableness aspires at moving the subject to an inner conviction about the truth being conveyed. The truth itself remains always open to a greater reality. Herein lies the present challenge to magisterial moral competence: although in former times an appeal to its teaching authority seemed to suffice for the validity of its argument, today's society, including the medical and healthcare community, demand reasons.[20] However, if the truth is genuinely a human truth, this demand is not inordinate. Rather, it is in some sense already reflecting that very truth: God would not expect us to live and act unreasonably.[21]

Secondly, reasonableness also demands that one make appropriate moral distinctions. Hence, in Tauer's proposal that probabilism can be applied to the abortion debate because the doubt involved is one of law and not of fact, it is necessary to note that at the root of the "probable" argument is precisely a doubt of fact.[22] That is, that those moral theologians who propose the possible validity of an early abortion, do so on the basis of an insufficient acknowledgement of the present biological data; a doubt of fact, not of law.[23] Therefore, when Cahill asks for a revision of magisterial teaching on abortion based on the previous analysis, she is grounding it on an argument which itself needs further revision and clarification if it pretends to address the truth of the issue. Cahill also fails to make appropriate distinctions when stating that, "diverging from the recent magisterium: the fetus, whether a 'person' or not, may be destroyed directly in dire circumstances and/or before a certain stage of development, e.g., threat to maternal life, or evacuation of uterine contents immediately after rape."[24] First, because if the fetus is a "person," then the prohibition of his or her direct destruction is not only part of the recent magisterium, but also of the ongoing magisterium. Second, because if the pathology threatens maternal life (*i.e.*, ectopic pregnancy) the destruction is not direct as she claims, but indirect. Third, because the evacuation of uterine contents immediately after rape is justified precisely only when reasonably presuming that there is as yet no fertilization and therefore no fetus. One who strongly argues against deceptive language elsewhere,[25] should beware of falling prey to it.

D. CONSENSUS WITHIN PLURALISM

It can be unambiguously stated that presently there is no consensus in the United States regarding key decisions of moral agents involving prenatal life and conflict situations.[26] Wishing to achieve such consensus already involves certain value judgments: it presupposes that consensus is both desirable and achievable.[27] Acknowledging this, all ten authors examined seem to agree that a pre-requisite to the eventual approximation of a national consensus leading to due protection of prenatal life is the question of when the human fetus can be considered to be a human person.[28] Toward this end, several of these authors speak of differing schools of thought.[29]

McCormick discerns two general schools: those who assert that the fetus is a nonperson and those who recognize he or she as "protectable humanity."[30] Those belonging to the first school hold that "experimentation on the fetus is legitimate and desirable. If there are to be restrictions, they are rooted in values other than the fetus itself in its present state."[31] The presupposition here is that just because the fetus is not considered a person, he or she has no rights or claims as a subject of research and experimentation, a presupposition that is presently debatable.[32] Regarding the second school, wherein he distinguishes three possible alternatives, he would allow for experimentation "where no discernible risk or discomfort is involved,"[33] which he maintains is based on what is allowable in experimentation in children. Still, it cannot be denied that the overall condition of the fetus is in a much more tender and delicate state than that of a child, even if one considers the most developed fetus and the least developed child. Accordingly, what might be considered risk of minimal damage to a child, might actually mean risk of grave damage to a fetus (*i.e.*, obtaining a tissue sample). Therefore, he is assuming that the extent of risk in experimentation on a fetus is discernible to the same degree of accuracy as it is in experimentation on a child. Finally, the overall comparison between the two general schools is also called into question because, whereas the first school bases its moral decisions on whether the fetus is a person or not, the second school never explicitly maintains that the fetus is in fact a person, but only "protectable humanity." Therefore, he is using two different sets of criteria which are not necessarily comparable.[34]

Moraczewski perceives three schools: social, developmental, and genetic.[35] When evaluating the first school, he notes that there doesn't seem to be an objective standard for establishing who has a right to belong in society, which presupposes an individual's right to belong in society. Given this assumption, he rejects the criteria of this school because "contained within the social school of thought is an implicit feature tending to justify an arbitrary community decision about the unborn's right to life."[36] But in doing so, he is presuming that if society is not able to recognize the unborn as a person, it is also unable to recognize it as a human life. Then, when evaluating the second school, he rejects it for similar reasons, maintaining that "one of the most serious difficulties facing any developmentalist is that of convincing fellow developmentalists that the proposed criterion is *the* unique characteristic or set of characteristics that makes human beings valued by others."[37] As difficult as this task might be, it does not necessarily mean that it is impossible to achieve. In fact, in accepting the criteria of the third school, he is presupposing that an equally difficult consensus is indeed achievable when he states that "only the genetic approach to the human being or person which identifies the beginning of human personhood with the time of fertilization can provide a stable and principled basis for protecting the unborn child afflicted with a genetic disease."[38]

Curran advances four different schools: individual-biological, relational, multiple, and conferred rights.[39] Rejecting the last three as not sufficiently accurate, he endorses the first school, which he further subdivides into five chronological possibilities: at birth, at viability, at the formation of brain-morphism, at fertilization, or at implantation. Discarding the first four, he espouses the latter, for he maintains that only at implantation is there the possibility of the beginning of the development of an individual human life. The flaw in this argument is not so much in making individuality a necessary, if not sufficient, condition for the existence of human personhood, but rather the reason which he cites as confirmatory of this condition. He holds that "before this time [implantation] there is no organizer that directs the differentiation of the pluripotential cells so that without this organizer hominization cannot occur."[40] The error here is two-fold: first, that the blastocyst has not undergone any differentiation before implantation; second, that no organizer is needed before implantation for hominization to occur. Unless he intends "organizer," "differentiation" and "hominization" in very peculiar ways, his hypothesis cannot be considered to be substantiated by current biological evidence.[41]

From the brief analysis above, it can be seen that lack of consensus exists among theologians even in perceiving the number and types of schools of thought operative today. At a deeper level, consensus within a pluralistic society means that absolute unanimity regarding the public regulation of specific moral dilemmas involving prenatal life and conflict situations is not realistic (a limit factor inherent to any contemporary pluralistic society).[42] The believer then has to make some choices: for the sake of peaceful and respectful coexistence, what is negotiable and what is not? Of the non-compromisable, what is the proper means of upholding its integrity?[43] To note is the fact that the various national committees evaluating what may and may not be done to prenatal human life are all using as a basis a utilitarian, pragmatical analysis of both content and methods, which leads them to settle for the minimal common denominator among differing social interest groups.[44] While the minimal common denominator may well be the dignity of the human person, at the level of application this principle collapses into the perception that, since there is no consensus on whether or when the fetus is a human person, then a partial and gradual protection is sufficient. In an issue such as prenatal diagnosis, partial and gradual protection may actually be more damaging than none, since it erroneously conveys the notion that the issue is settled morally and is in no further need of review.[45]

E. THEOLOGICAL DISSENT AND ITS LIMITS

To be safeguarded are the legitimate spaces of freedom of conscience created by a truly pluralistic society and by the magisterium itself.[46] These spaces are best utilized in the research of truth.[47] The ensemble of truths associated with prenatal diagnosis, because they deal ultimately with the human person, cut across boundaries of biology, medicine, technology, psychology, sociology and theology. Therefore the same intellectual space can be said to be simultaneously inhabited by the scientist, the technician, the parent, and the theologian. All having an interest in the truth, communication of their findings is crucial, each in their particular area of expertise and peculiar mode of expression.[48] Of these, the theologian finds herself or himself at once in the privileged and risky position of interlocutor.[49] Integrity in theological research demands that he or she first ponder, then seek to articulate the truth learnt to the best of her or his ability.[50] Because of the various disciplines and strata which make up the truth about prenatal diagnosis, one major task of the moral theologian is to constantly evaluate new evidence and trends.[51]

It seems that these ten American theologians are seeking to incorporate into their analyses the apparent crisis of traditional moral values gripping contemporary U.S. marriages and families,[52] combined with another apparent expansion of freedom of choice and action afforded by an exponential rise in recourse to biomedical technology.[53] The danger is that, in doing so, a number of the revisionists may also become habitually over-critical of magisterial documents: for them, any analysis of sexual morality coming from Rome may immediately be seen as suspect of being "out of touch" with the present American reality. In such light, some are claiming a lack of consistency in magisterial methodology. They sustain that while Rome now considers social ethics issues within a historical approach ("particular, contingent, individual realities"), sexual ethics issues are still regulated by the use of a classicist approach ("an eternal, immutable, unchanging reality").[54] This leads Curran to conclude that while the historical approach allows for grey areas, the classicist does not. One needs to question, however, how accurate and profound an assessment this is, since the overall impression is rather a certain degree of compartmentalization of key concepts into merely two mutually exclusive methodological categories which follow some predetermined scheme. In reality, these key concepts afford a richer and more nuanced expression.[55] Hence, he states that "whereas the official social teaching [of the Church] has evolved so that it now employs historical consciousness, personalism, and a relationality-responsibility ethical model, the sexual teaching still emphasizes classicism, human nature and faculties, and a law model of ethics."[56] The difficulty is in perceiving how these two "categories" are indeed mutually exclusive: can personalism ever be understood without delving into human nature and human faculties? Is relationality-responsibility at all meaningful without some code of conduct to regulate it? True revision seeks a much deeper and realistic analysis: moral dilemmas in prenatal diagnosis involve simultaneously sexual *and* social ethical issues.[57]

F. TOLERANCE AND INTOLERANCE

Tolerance in a pluralistic society is a deep respect for the conscience of the other, not the tacit acceptance of given multiple convictions, therefore also calling for ongoing evaluation.[58] True dialogue between the healthcare profession and the magisterium demands tolerance, lest it become rather a monologue (of which either side may be at fault). Tolerance demands that both scientist and theologian seek to engage in earnest self criticism and mutual understanding. Tolerance also implies a former prioritizing, for it means that civil coexistence is valued even above the possibility of differences of moral opinion and action. Tolerance also implies valuing dialogue to the extent of foregoing one's own opinion for the sake of maintaining the dialogue alive.[59] Tolerance, however, cannot be unlimited, for then the dialogue collapses into nothing at all, both parties ceasing to make any significant contribution whatsoever. What are, then, the limits of tolerance?

One limit may be an intolerance toward the intolerance of others. That is, if individuals or groups within society begin to display a definitive and programmatic intolerance toward certain other individuals or groups (*i.e.*, pre-born humans), justice and civility demand that society not tolerate such a degrading state of affairs. Prenatal diagnosis today affords the prospect of a fetus who carries some anomaly to be targeted for selective abortion on the sole basis of being a carrier of that anomaly. When this becomes more and more "standard medical practice," it betrays an underlying intolerant situation.[60]

Another limit may be if it begins to compromise the conscience of any one of the parties involved in the dialogue. If prenatal diagnosis is becoming routine, the physician with legitimate reservations as to its medical indication may nonetheless be expected to prescribe or perform it. Furthermore, pressure may come from fear of adverse legal action. This would represent an invasion of authentic discretionary judgement in medical practice.[61] Similarly, a Catholic healthcare facility providing prenatal counseling and diagnosis may also be erroneously expected to counsel, or even provide for, "therapeutic" abortions. Likewise, an expectant mother undergoing prenatal diagnosis who is informed of carrying a pre-born with some defect, might feel pressured by the medical establishment into aborting rather than "burdening society" with such a child. Finally, the magisterium itself may come under pressure to restrict its teaching to the private sphere under the charge of interfering with the freedom of conscience of others, a freedom misconstrued as encompassing the right not to be exposed to a "religious" message.[62] For tolerance not to be overpowered by intolerance, then, realistic limits respecting freedom of conscience must be set. This requires both, ongoing revision and prophetic announcement.[63]

G. ADVOCACY AND WITNESSING

Tolerance in a truly pluralistic society also means providing the necessary spaces for advocacy and witnessing.[64] It must be understood here that none of the partners of an interdisciplinary dialogue ever come to the negotiating table *tabula rasa*, that is, without a set of interests and proposals to champion. The very fact of wanting to engage in dialogue already speaks of certain values to be sought. To this end, from the point of view of the magisterium is always the desire to defend and promote the intrinsic dignity of the human person at every stage of his or her development.[65] This is why McCarthy and Moraczewski exhort, not only the Church's hierarchy, but all believers, to give witness of their faith by advocating on behalf of those affected by genetic defects, whether born or unborn.[66] This is not to say that only believers are capable of sustaining such vision of the human person. Rather, it means this advocacy and witnessing is integral to the gospel message.

It must be noted that each stage of human development presents itself with its particular needs, challenges, incongruities, and contributions. Furthermore, history has proven that it is totally foreign to the human condition to pretend to require no interaction with other persons, both human and divine. In this sense, O'Rourke rightly comments that an overly autonomous model of the human person, while in itself not contrary to magisterial teaching, when taken to the extreme may actually fail to render sufficient witness to both: the person's natural need for community, and his or her destiny of eternal life in communion with God.[67]

A practical application of this may be seen in the disparate moral evaluations which are arrived at by the Catholic magisterium, on one side, and the various national and international ethical committees,[68] on the other, when studying bio-medical issues involving prenatal life: these committees, failing to agree on a transcendental vision of the human person, are constrained to using an autonomous model, but a partial one at that. Partial because true autonomy does not mean total self-sufficiency. Rather, it seeks to appeal to the conscience of each individual as fundamental when making moral decisions.

Finally, O'Donnell brings out the sobering reality that, in living the gospel today, a physician may well suffer peer isolation and discrimination, and also financial and legal martyrdom.[69] Liberating truth is never free, it always comes at a price.

In sum, due to a deeply rich and penetrating Christocentric theological anthropology,[70] the moral theologian and the magisterium today are in a privileged position to witness on behalf of those who cannot advocate their own dignity due to their utterly hidden life and radical state of dependency: the pre-born.[71] Concurringly, this vision is periodically augmented and refined as they ponder and incorporate the theological meaning of new scientific evidence available. Regarding the moral evaluation of prenatal diagnosis, critical solidarity and vigilance interweave in the ongoing dialogue between science and theology.[72]

Notes

[1]Each one of these four attempts to illustrate a different level of penetration. For an explication of magisterial pronouncement levels from within the magisterium itself, see: CDF, *Istruzione sulla vocazione ecclesiale del teologo* (Bologna: Dehoniane 1990),IV,23-24. See also: *LG*,25.

[2]Pointing to both, the character of the document and the peculiarity of the language therein, as interpretative keys, is: Demmer K, **Introduzione alla Teologia Morale**. Casale Monferrato, AL: PIEMME 1993, 58.

[3]The magisterium has always distinguished various levels of discourse regarding moral truths. Acknowledging different levels of authority and acceptance of official Church teaching, and recognizing the possibility of dialogue within certain levels, is: Pilarczyk D, "Dissent in the Church" in: Curran CE, McCormick RA, eds, **Readings in Moral Theology No. 6: Dissent in the Church**. Mahwah, New Jersey: Paulist 1988, 152-163.

[4]See: *GS*, PART ONE,I,12-22; II,23-32; PART TWO,I,47-52; *FC*, PART TWO,11-16; PART THREE,17-41; PART FOUR,77.

[5]A compendium of magisterial teaching on biological and medical issues (from Pius XII to 1987), is found in: Verspieren P, ed, **Biologie, Médicine et Éthique**, *Les Dossiers de la Documentation Catholique*. Paris: Centurion 1987, especially 13-216.

[6]See: *Dv*,I,2. Highlighting the complexity of themes and discursive levels within *Dv*, is: Rubio M. "El método en el discurso teológico-ético de la Instrucción 'Donum vitae'" *Mor* 9 (1987) 251-263. See also: Albacete LM, **Commentary on Instruction on Respect for Human Life in Its Origin and on the Dignity of Procreation**. Boston, MA: Daughters of St. Paul 1987, 5-22.

[7]See: Pius XII, *Allocution à VII Congrès International d'Hematologie*, Vatican: AAS L (1958) 732-740; John Paul II, *Address to the XV International Congress of Catholic Doctors* (3 October 1982), Vatican: Osservatore Romano (Oct. 25, 1982) 9-10; *Address to I International Congress of Pro-Life Movement on the Theme: "Pre-natal diagnosis and surgical treatment of congenital malformations"* (Dec. 3-5, 1982), Vatican: Osservatore Romano (Jan. 3-10, 1983) 19.

[8]See: CDF, *Declaration on Procured abortion* (Boston, MA: Daughters of St. Paul 1974).

[9]See: O'Donnell, *Catholic honesty*, 33-36.

[10]Pointing to a certain development of the magisterium in moral matters, especially toward a more personalist approach, yet remaining faithful to the ongoing teaching of the church regarding the personal dignity of the human embryo, is: Chapelle A, "Pour lire 'Donum vitae'" *NRT* 109 (1987) 481-508. See also: Elizari FJ, "Valor teológico-moral de la Instrucción vaticana" *Mor* 9 (1987) 239-250.

[11]Pointing to a lack of consistency in the use of key terminology by recent magisterial documents

regarding prenatal human life, is: McCormick, *Preembryo*, 6-8.

[12]See: Crawfurd MA, *Ethical and legal*, 310-314.

[13]See: *Dv*, Introduction,3; I,2. Defending a more common opinion that particular norms of natural law are not object of infallible teaching, is: Sullivan FA, "The authority of the magisterium on questions of natural moral law" in: Curran CE, McCormick RA, eds, **Readings in Moral Theology No. 6: Dissent in the Church.** Mahwah, New Jersey: Paulist 1988, 42-57. And a rebuttal, in: Grisez G, "Infallibility and specific moral norms: a review discussion" in: Curran CE, McCormick RA, eds, **Readings in Moral Theology No. 6: Dissent in the Church.** Mahwah, New Jersey: Paulist 1988, 58-96.

[14]An appeal for dialogue regarding certain open procreative issues and *Dv*, is found in: Rollin R, "L'éthique de la procréation à travers trois documents" *Lum Vie* 37,187 (1988) 67-89.

[15]For an explanation of magisterial use of natural moral law as identified with the concept of human nature, nonetheless, requiring both an anthropological and a philosophical grounding in Covenant theology at the theoretical level, see: Famerée J, "La fonction du magistère ecclésial en morale" *NRT* 107 (1985) 722-739. See also: Rubio M, "El esquema antropológico subyacente en la Instruccción 'Donum vitae'" *Mor* 9 (1987) 283-296.

[16]See: Ashley, *Ethical decisions*, 66.

[17]See: *HV*,4. Maintaining that the magisterium has the right to critique bio-medical technology which may affect the dignity of the human person, is: Kaczynski E, "Rispetto per la vita nascente e dignità della procreazione" *Ang* 64 (1987) 583-591. Holding that the search for truth is what ultimately propels the Church to speak on issues considered fundamental to human life, is: Faivre A, "'Où est la vérité?' Déplacements et enjeux d'une question" *Lum Vie* 35,180 (1986) 5-16. See also: Lawler RD, "The magisterium and Catholic moral teaching" in: CITM, **Persona**, 217-233.

[18]O'Donnell, *Beyond*, 11. See also; O'Donnell, **Medicine** (1991), 7.

[19]See: Cahill, *Catholicism*, 38-54.

[20]Arguing for the present need for reasonableness in magisterial moral pronouncements, is: López Azpitarte E, "El magisterio moral de la Iglesia: tensiones actuales" *SalTer* 75 (1987) 503-514. See also: Vidal M, "Referencias al magisterio eclesiástico en la Instrucción 'Donum vitae'" *Mor* 9 (1987) 265-281.

[21]Also pointing at the use of reasonableness to diffuse some of the present tension and confliction between the magisterium and the theologian in ethical issues, is: López Azpitarte E, "Magisterio de la Iglesia y problemas éticos: discusiones actuales" *RazFe* 213 [215] (1987) 371-381.

[22]See: Tauer, *Probabilism*, 3-33.

[23]See: McCormick, *Therapy*, 396-403. See also: **Immediate Hominization,** in Chapter XIV of PART THREE of this text.

[24]Cahill, *Seamless garment*, 71.

[25]See: Cahill, *Abortion pill*, 5-8.

[26]A survey of U.S. geneticists on issues of prenatal life and conflict situations, in: Wertz DC, Fletcher JC, "Ethics and medical genetics in the United States: a national survey" *AJMedGen* 29 (1988) 815-827.

[27]An analysis of "anthropological constants" mediating moral estimation toward consensus in: Vidal M, **El Discernimiento Ético: Hacia Una Estimativa Moral Cristiana.** Madrid: Cristiandad 1980, 13-27. Appealing for the need of an interdisciplinary dialogue when addressing contemporary bio-medical issues, including those issues incumbent to prenatal life, is: Demmer K, "Gene technologies and man: the ethical implications of a contemporary challenge" in: Malherbe J-F, ed, **Human Life: Its Beginnings and Development.** Paris: L'Harmattan 1988, 315-332. See also: Demmer K, "La sfida teologica del dialogo interdisciplinare" *Laurent* 33 (1992) 403-

420.
[28]See: Shannon and Cahill, **Religion and Artificial Reproduction**, 116.
[29]So also regarding different schools of thought, is: Elizari Basterra FJ, "Moral de la vida y la salud" in: López Azpitarte E, Elizari Basterra FJ, Rincón Orduña R, eds, **Praxis Cristiana II: Opción por la vida y el amor**. 3rd ed. Madrid: Paulinas 1981, 86-93.
[30]See: McCormick, *Experimentation*, 5.4-5.5.
[31]McCormick, *Experimentation*, 5.4.
[32]In fact, even nonhuman subjects of research and experimentation are afforded certain decorous treatment precisely as living beings.
[33]McCormick, *Experimentation*, 5.4.
[34]For a discussion on the possible rights of the human fetus, see: Fagot-Largeault A, Delaisi de Parseval G, "Le droits de l'embryon (foetus) humain, et la notion de personne humaine potentielle" *RMetaphMor* 92 (1987) 361-385.
[35]See: Atkinson and Moraczewski, **Genetic Counseling**, 60-75.
[36]Atkinson and Moraczewski, **Genetic Counseling**, 64.
[37]Atkinson and Moraczewski, **Genetic Counseling**, 66.
[38]Atkinson and Moraczewski, **Genetic Counseling**, 75.
[39]See: Curran, *Abortion*, 18-22.
[40]Curran, *Abortion*, 23.
[41]See: *Immediate Hominization*, under **Hominization and Personhood**, in Chapter XIV of PART THREE of this text.
[42]Pointing to a fundamental methodological dissimilarity between objectivist and subjectivist ethics, is: Ashley, *Ethical decisions*, 50-53, 66. Sustaining that there has always been a certain amount of pluralism in the entire history of theology, is: Marlè R, "La question du pluralisme en theologie" *Greg* 71 (1990) 465-486.
[43]Sustaining that even the availability of magisterial pronouncements does not excuse the believer from engaging in his or her own mature moral discernment, is: Thévenot X, "Magistère et discernement moral" *Et* 362 (1985) 231-244.
[44]See: Shannon and Cahill, **Religion and Artificial Reproduction**, 97-98.
[45]Observing that, in seeking to uphold the dignity of all human life, it must be clarified that this is a fundamental value--and not an absolute one--, is: Gafo J, "El documento Vaticano sobre bioética" *RazFe* 215 (1987) 461-471. Affirming that--from conception--the human embryo is not a potential human being, but an actual human being with potential for further development, is: Lorenzetti L, "Etica e tecniche bio-mediche: criteri di lettura del documento <<Ratzinger>>" *RTMor* 74 (1987) 83-88. Attesting that it is also proper of the church to seek to illumine bio-medical technology regarding what is the real good of society, is: Serra A, "Embrione umano, scienza e medicina: in margine al recente documento" *CivCat* 138,2 (1987) 247-261.
[46]For a brief summary of norms on legitimate theological dissent, see: NCCB, "Norms of licit theological dissent" in: Curran CE, McCormick RA, eds, **Readings in Moral Theology No. 6: Dissent in the Church**. Mahwah, New Jersey: Paulist 1988, 127-128. Warning against three specific dangers for the theologian in today's pluralistic society, is: Novak M, "Dissent in the Church" in: Curran CE, McCormick RA, eds, **Readings in Moral Theology No. 6: Dissent in the Church**. Mahwah, New Jersey: Paulist 1988, 112-126.
[47]A strong case in favor of legitimate freedom of investigation to the theologians by the magisterium, rooted in fidelity to God and his people, without denying the task of the magisterium in guaranteeing the faith, thus pointing to different but complimentary functions of magisterium and theologians, is given by: Sanchíz A, "Magisterio y teologos ante el reto de la nueva cultura"

EscrVedat 17 (1987) 127-142. Distinguishing between the way truth comes about as perceived by secular society--more as welling up from below, through a process of trial and error--, and by the church--more as sought in divine revelation, and authoritatively transmitted over the ages--, is: Mahony R, "The magisterium and theological dissent" in: Curran CE, McCormick RA, eds, **Readings in Moral Theology No. 6: Dissent in the Church**. Mahwah, New Jersey: Paulist 1988, 164-175.

[48]Underscoring the need for interdisciplinary dialogue between moral theology and empirical sciences, precisely because of the different methodologies operant, is: Privitera S, **Temi Etici di Dialogo Ecumenico: Sull'Universalità dell'Esigenza Dialogica dell'Etica**. Palermo: Edi Oftes 1992, 143-158. See also: Thévoz J-M, "Une recherche interdisciplinaire: la bioéthique" *RTPhil* 118 (1986) 67-79.

[49]Distinguishing between private and public dissent--and advancing that frequent, public dissent from the non-infallible, ordinary magisterium may in fact be questioning the authority and not the teaching--, is: Malone R, "Magisterium and dissent" in: AA VV, **Attualità della Teologia Morale: Punti Fermi - Problemi Aperti**. Roma: Urbaniana 1987, 211-229.

[50]Claiming that, throughout the entire history of the church, there is no one paradigm which adequately describes the relationship between the theologian and the magisterium--therefore proposing a list of responsibilities and rights of the theologian applicable to the present historical moment--, is: Nilson J, "The rights and responsibilities of theologians: a theological perspective" in: Curran CE, McCormick RA, eds, **Readings in Moral Theology No. 6: Dissent in the Church**. Mahwah, New Jersey: Paulist 1988, 5-34.

[51]Also appealing for freedom of investigative research by the theologian, underlining the fact that in any living community--such as the Church--tensions will always exist, is: Flecha J-R, "Estatuto eclesial del teólogo moralista" *Mor* 10 (1988) 445-466.

[52]To witness: very high overall divorce rate; many couples intending never to have children; *de facto* wide spread use of contraception, contraceptive sterilization and procured abortion. To this end, Ashley sees in McCormick's position on technologically assisted human reproduction a further weakening of the already precarious family bond. See: Ashley, *Chill factor*, 67-77.

[53]To note, the present availability of: assisted reproduction, therapeutic abortion, selective fetal reduction, surrogacy, gametic banks, prenatal diagnosis and prenatal therapy.

[54]See: Curran, **Tensions**, 88-107.

[55]For a brief description of the classicist and the historical world-views of Catholic theological interpretation--and their limitations--, proposing an alternative contemporary model re-incorporating symbolic consciousness, see: Bohr D, **Catholic Moral Tradition: In Christ, a New Creation**. Huntington, IN: Our Sunday Visitor 1990, 67-74.

[56]Curran, **Tensions**, 87-109; here 107.

[57]A recent critique of Curran's position is found in: Grabowski JS, Naughton MJ, "Catholic social and sexual ethics: inconsistent or organic?" *Thom* 57 (1993) 555-578.

[58]See: Demmer, **Interpretare**, 192.

[59]See: Demmer K, "Der Anspruch der Toleranz" *Greg* 63 (1982) 701-720.

[60]An analysis of secular and sacred philosophical tendencies, having as a consequence the desmystification of traditional and transcendental moral values by questioning the very sense and non-sense of human existence, but sustaining its sense precisely in the intolerant situation--springing the subject to transcendence, since the subject can never be reduced to his or her external conditions --, is found in: Colomber J, "Résistance à l'intolérable" *LumVie* 38,191 (1989) 69-84.

[61]See: O'Donnell, *Basic determinants*, 22-23.

[62]Research demonstrating that religious affiliation and participation level do have some influence

on the eventual decision to undergo prenatal diagnosis, are: Seals BF, Ekwo EE, Williamson RA, Hanson JW, "Moral and religious influences on the amniocentesis decision" *SocBiol* 32,1-2 (1985) 13-30.

[63]Also holding prophecy as the original competence of the magisterium at the theoretical level, is: Demmer K, "La competenza normativa del magistero ecclesiastico in morale" in: Demmer K, Schüller B, eds, **Fede Cristiana e Agire Morale**. (Riva G, trad.) Assisi: Cittadella 1980, 144-170.

[64]Affirming that intrinsic to the freedom of the believer is his or her capacity for witnessing as a particular aspect of moral decision and action, is: Demmer K, "Sittlich handeln als Zeugnis geben" *Greg* 64 (1983) 453-485. Distinguishing two irreducible functions, one of the magisterium and another of the theologian--yet both having the duty of prophecy as a common ground--, is: Goffi T, "Magistero ecclesiale ed etica cristiana" *RTMor* 63 (1984) 431-439. Also addressing the relationship between the magisterium and the theologian, is: Testa B, "La funzione del magistero ordinario nell'elaborazione teologica" *Anthr* 7 (1991) 67-82.

[65]See: *DH*,2; CDF, *Procured abortion*,6; *Dv* Introduction; *GS*, 12; *HV*,7; *RH*,10.

[66]See: McCarthy and Moraczewski, **Genetic Counseling**, 141-161.

[67]See: O'Rourke, *Two ethical approaches*, 49-50.

[68]*I.e.*, Australian Study Group, International Bioethics Summit Conference, U.S. President's Commission for the Study of Ethical Problems in Medicine and Biomedical and Behavioral Research, Warnok Committee. See also: O'Rourke, *Two ethical approaches*, 48-51, 58.

[69]O'Donnell, *Questions*, 3-4.

[70]See: Pinckaers S, "La morale chrétienne et ses sources: ecriture, tradition et magistère" *Anthr* 3 (1987) 25-42.

[71]Summarizing the Church's advocacy on behalf of those who cannot promote their own cause--such as the unborn--, is: May, *Abortion*, 38-44.

[72]See: Cuyás M, "Il progresso biomedico interpella la teologia morale" in: Latourelle, ed, **Vaticano II: Bilancio e Prospettive. Venticinque Anni Dopo (1962-1987)**. Assisi 1987, 1480-1506; Demmer, **Introduzione**, 133-135; Vatican II, *Humanae Personae Dignitatem*, 1002-1014.

CONCLUSIONS

PART ONE of this work (BIO-MEDICAL CONSIDERATIONS OF PRENATAL DIAGNOSIS) has sought to convey a sense of the intricate complexity involved in human embryonic development and in prenatal diagnosis. In former times, the human pre-born appeared for months to be in a rather tranquil and restful state; nourished, bathed and protected within his or her mother's womb. However, we now know otherwise, thanks in no small part to the pronounced achievements of contemporary bio-medical technology. This means that currently the human conceptus can be monitored during its entire gestational development practically from the first time it comes into existence as a single microscopic zygote. Such observation reveals a high level of organization and coordination already present even during the initial stages of embryonic development. In fact, considering all that could "go wrong," from the time of fusion of the two parental gametic pro-nuclei to the moment of birth nine months later, a sheer probabilistic analysis would indicate a much higher rate of children born with congenital defects.

Yet, as has been observed, more than 95% of all PND reveals a normal embryo or fetus. Nonetheless, the grievous fact remains that, of the few expectant mothers who are informed of carrying a child with some birth defect, over 90% procure an abortion. This, however, is a totally recent phenomenon in that, before the advent of PND, birth defects were only confirmed *after* birth. With increased knowledge comes increased power. As usual, this power is ambivalent; it can further humanize, or dehumanize.

Whereas a "negative" PND is always welcomed news, there is no doubt that the expectant parents who receive a "positive" diagnosis will be challenged in ways that were simply unimaginable a few short years ago. Indeed, few incidents in a person's life could match the levels of frustration, anger, sorrow, fear, anxiety and helplessness which conceivably may develop as a consequence of receiving a "positive" PND.

This is where PART TWO (the writings of TEN NORTH AMERICAN CATHOLIC MORAL THEOLOGIANS on the subject at hand) and PART THREE (A CRITICAL EVALUATION thereof) of this work may be most useful: in the sense that the complexity of moral dilemmas associated with prenatal diagnosis defies theological and pastoral minds and hearts of all backgrounds and acumen.

Even so, not all is lost, for if through the proper use of contemporary advancements in bio-medical technology and the concomitant theological reflection which should always accompany them, human life is better understood and appreciated, then it can be argued that a greater humanization has already occurred. This is particularly true when it applies to that realm which has been traditionally considered to be the "sanctuary of the womb."

In their moral evaluation of PND, all ten authors examined seek to contribute to a greater humanization. How this humanization is brought about varies from author to author according to a wide range of nuanced arguments and perspectives. On a number of crucial issues, they arrive at conclusions which are clearly incompatible with one another (as in the case of pre-implantation human life, or of the degree of risk or harm that an embryo or fetus may be exposed to). Yet, in their evaluation of standard PND, the writings of these ten moral theologians display a surprisingly unanimous condemnation of its use for "therapeutic abortion," for "multifetal reduction," or for "fetal sex selection;" while at the same time maintaining the moral validity of its use for any medical treatment that might directly benefit the individual fetus or embryo and its mother. Therefore, the key to interpreting these conclusions lies in the critical evaluation of their particular hermeneutical and epistemological presuppositions--something which was attempted in PART THREE. These presuppositions, in turn, are never immune from the socio-cultural *ethos* in which they occur. Hence, it is at this last level that the moral evaluation of PND is presently at once most challenging and most challenged.

The existing American *ethos* of "abortion on demand" is most challenged by the increasing possibility of treating the pre-born human as a medical patient and, as such, as full recipient of the fundamental right afforded all patients: the right to live. Being fundamental, such right to live is not subordinate to state of dependency or condition of health, for if it were, then logical and ontological consistency would demand that other (born) individuals in similar state or condition be similarly treated. For instance, whereas an adult suffering from severe mental retardation may find him- or herself for all practical purposes in a state of total dependency upon others for her or his survival, his or her health condition and dependent state certainly do not warrant that she or he be killed as a form of treatment. On the other hand, if a particular health condition is such that no degree of dependent state would offer any hope of survival whatsoever (cf. complete acardia or anencephalia), then "allowing nature to follow its course" may indeed be the most human--and Christian--response. Hence, the difference between commission and omission becomes crucial: allowing a patient (born or unborn) with a terminal pathology to die by omitting any heroic intervention is not to be confused with intervening on a patient with a viable pathology in such a way as to directly procure the patient's death as a means of "healing" such pathology. Thus, at the core of the discussion of moral dilemmas in prenatal diagnosis lies the very definition of "medical treatment." It is the belief of this author that history has amply demonstrated that whenever direct killing of the patient has been considered a form of "treatment," society has been invariably dehumanized.

Conversely, this *ethos* of "abortion on demand" is most challenging in its pervasiveness and in its perception of being at the root of respecting the freedom of conscience of every individual that lives in a pluralistic society. And herein lies also the possible contribution of PND as a tool for greater humanization: in that in order for it to render true benefit, one must recognize both, the embryo or fetus *and* its mother as medical patients. As such, they are both subjects of authentic medical treatment, that is, of that cure and care which is possible and available here and now. Hence, genuine respect for freedom of conscience must never rest satisfied with a given socio-cultural *ethos*, especially one in which a whole class of individuals within that society is being systematically discriminated against. Rather, it must seek to raise that consciousness to a higher freedom, namely, a freedom not granted or allotted to any of its members by society itself, but quite the opposite: a freedom of existence of each individual so as to make the very existence of society possible. The key question here is not "which was first: the individual or the community?" Instead, it is the realization that: first, no society can pretend to exist for any length of time without upholding the right of each of its members to exist--particularly if such members have not been lawfully convicted of a punishable criminal action. Second, is the further realization that no member of society exists as a mere "part" of society (as an organ or appendage exists as a part to its body), for whereas it is acceptable that a diseased organ or appendage may be sacrificed in order to promote or safeguard the health of the entire organism, it is never acceptable for an innocent individual to be sacrificed--even for the purported benefit of the entire community. Such willful sacrifice by society of an innocent individual would constitute a direct violation of her or his dignity and integrity, which would result in an overall lessening of freedom of conscience rather than the desired opposite (This does not exclude the possibility, however, of any given member of society to freely and consciously sacrifice his or her life for the perceived benefit of that society--even if such perception may be objectively erroneous. This conscious freedom, then, is always the proper realm of the first person, not of the third).

One definite ramification of these conclusions, then, is the real impact which PND may have on the proper formulation of public policy. Again, recognizing the human pre-born as a medical patient demands certain consequential protection afforded all medical patients. And herein abides the very kernel of the present paradoxical status of the human pre-born in the United States: on one hand, it is a potential medical patient; on the other, no further reason than "psychological or emotional distress to its mother" is needed to warrant its destruction--even if diagnostically "normal." One must then ask: how much longer can a society which prides itself on being at the forefront of championing inalienable individual human rights maintain such flagrant inconsistency?

Needless to say, the answer to this question depends on whether a nation as a whole, and particular professional groups comprising its leadership (legislators, the medical profession, the judiciary, civil rights leaders), are themselves willing to admit a judgment error of such magnitude. This admittance, in turn, is also linked to a very complex system of interrelated factors, not the least of which has been the ongoing anthropological, philosophical and theological speculation on the ontological status of the human embryo at its various stages of development. In the name of the latter, key men and women in positions of national leadership have "abstained" from passing judgment on such ontological status. The tragic consequence of this, however, is that by the very nature of a democratic, pluralistic society, when the leadership fails to give direction on fundamental issues (such as defining who qualifies as a member of society, entitling him or her to due protection under the law), then the issues become decided nonetheless, but skewed by interest groups who at best are ignorant of the deeper realities involving human life, or at worst seek to secure the rights of certain individuals above those of other. The most patent instance of this is when those others are so defenseless, that they are totally dependent upon third party advocacy for their very survival.

And yet, because this situation is not without historical precedent, both in America and in other parts of the world, then one can also look at the reconciling unfolding of previous analogies with a sense of optimism and hope. Indeed, if past generations have had the courage eventually to admit such judgment error, then in principle there is no reason why a similar admission cannot take place presently. The danger, of course, is that typically these previous recognitions have not happened before much blood has been shed; the greater shedding corresponding to the longer sustained time of the particular injustice. Hence, time is of essence: the longer time passes with this sustained paradox, the more the error compounds, the more painful the eventual reconciliation, and the less willing the population may be to forgive such sustained deception.

But the deeper question remains: why *should* society recognize the human unborn as a member of society, given the ongoing anthropological, philosophical and theological speculation? The reason why it should is admittedly at least provisional, yet nonetheless urgent: if the real possibility exists that it is a human individual, then not receiving the benefit of the doubt would be tantamount to condoning its destruction even *if it is* human. Lest we regress to former times of greater human rights abuses, on fundamental issues such as human life, the benefit of the doubt must be in favor of life, especially when empirical data is more and more in its favor.

The measure of a coherent and civilized society--the alleged hallmark of a pluralistic society--is the respect for the dignity and integrity of *all* its members, regardless of state of dependency or condition of health.

I believe that, in the end, the answer to the moral dilemmas which arise in prenatal diagnosis lies precisely in the answer to the question: who is the subject of PND? The subject of PND is both, the human fetus or embryo and his or her mother and, by association, his or her father. Whenever any of these subjects are manipulated, violated or disregarded, prenatal diagnosis has failed to live up to its medical definition, namely: "diagnosis utilized in procedures available for the recognition of diseases and malformations in utero, and the conclusion reached."[1]

[1]Stedman's **Medical Dictionary**: *diagnosis, prenatal..*

BIBLIOGRAPHY

I. MAGISTERIAL LITERATURE

John Paul II, *Address to the I International Congress of Pro-Life Movement on the Theme: "Pre-natal diagnosis and surgical treatment of congenital malformations"* (Dec. 3-5, 1982), Vatican: Osservatore Romano (Jan. 3-10, 1983) 19.

--------, *Address to the XV International Congress of Catholic Doctors* (3 October 1982), Vatican: Osservatore Romano (Oct. 25, 1982) 9-10.

--------, *The Redeemer of Man (Redemptor Hominis)*, (Vatican trans.) Boston, MA: Daughters of St. Paul 1979.

--------, *The Role of the Christian Family in the Modern World (Familiaris Consortio)*, (Vatican trans.) Boston, MA: Daughters of St. Paul 1981.

Paul VI, *On the Regulation of Birth (Humanae Vitae)*, (NCCB trans.) Washington, DC: United States Catholic Conference 1968.

Pius XII, *Allocution à VII Congrès International d'Hematologie*, Vatican: AAS L (1958) 732-740.

Sacred Congregation for the Doctrine of the Faith, *Declaration on Certain Problems of Sexual Ethics*, in: Vatican Council II: More Postconciliar Documents, vol 2, Flannery A, ed. Northport, NY: Costello 1975, 486-499.

--------, *Declaration on Procured Abortion*, (Vatican trans.) Boston, Ma: Daughters of St. Paul 1974.

--------, *Instruction on Respect for Human Life in its Origin and on the Dignity of Procreation: Reply to Certain Questions of the Day (Donum vitae)*, (Vatican trans.) Boston, MA: Daughters of St. Paul 1987.

--------, *Istruzione sulla Vocazione Ecclesiale del Teologo*, Bologna: Dehoniane 1990.

U.S. National Conference of Catholic Bishops, "Norms of licit theological dissent" in: Curran CE, McCormick RA, eds, **Readings in Moral Theology No. 6: Dissent in the Church**. Mahwah, New Jersey: Paulist 1988, 127-128.

Vatican Council II, *Declaration on Religious Liberty (Dignitatis Humanae)*, in: Vatican Council II: The Conciliar and Post Conciliar Documents, Flannery A, ed, Northport, NY: Costello 1979, 799-812.

--------, *Dogmatic Constitution on the Church (Lumen Gentium)*, in: Vatican Council II: The Conciliar and Post Conciliar Documents, Flannery A, ed, Northport, NY: Costello 1979, 350-426.

--------, *On Dialogue with Unbelievers (Humanae Personae Dignitatem)*, in: Vatican Council II: The Conciliar and Post Conciliar Documents, Flannery A, ed, Northport, NY: Costello 1979, 1002-1014.

--------, *Pastoral Constitution on the Church in the Modern World (Gaudium et Spes)*, in: Vatican Council II: The Conciliar and Post Conciliar Documents, Flannery A, ed, Northport, NY: Costello 1979, 903-1001.

II. ETHICAL AND MORAL THEOLOGICAL LITERATURE

1. PRIMARY SOURCES

BOOKS

Ashley BM, **Theologies of the Body: Humanist and Christian**. Braintree, MA: Pope John XXIII Medical-Moral Research and Education Center 1985.

Ashley BM, O'Rourke DK, **Ethics of Health Care**. St. Louis, MO: Catholic Health Association 1986.

--------, **Health Care Ethics: A Theological Analysis**, 2nd ed. St. Louis, MO: The Catholic Hospital Association 1982.

--------, **Health Care Ethics: A Theological Analysis**. St. Louis, MO: The Catholic Hospital Association 1978.

--------, **Healthcare Ethics: A Theological Analysis**, 3rd ed. St. Louis, MO: The Catholic Hospital Association 1989.

Atkinson GM, Moraczewski AS, eds, **Genetic Counseling, The Church, and The Law**. St. Louis, MO: Pope John XXIII Medical-Moral Research and Education Center 1980.

Curran CE, **Catholic Moral Theology in Dialogue**. Notre Dame, IN: Fides 1972.

--------, **Directions in Fundamental Moral Theology**. Notre Dame, IN: U. of Notre Dame 1985.

--------, **Issues in Sexual and Medical Ethics**. Notre Dame, IN: U. of Notre Dame 1978.

--------, **Moral Theology: A Continuing Journey**. Notre Dame, IN: U. of Notre Dame 1982.

--------, **New Perspectives in Moral Theology**. Notre Dame, IN: Fides 1974.

--------, **Ongoing Revision in Moral Theology**. Notre Dame, IN: Fides 1975.

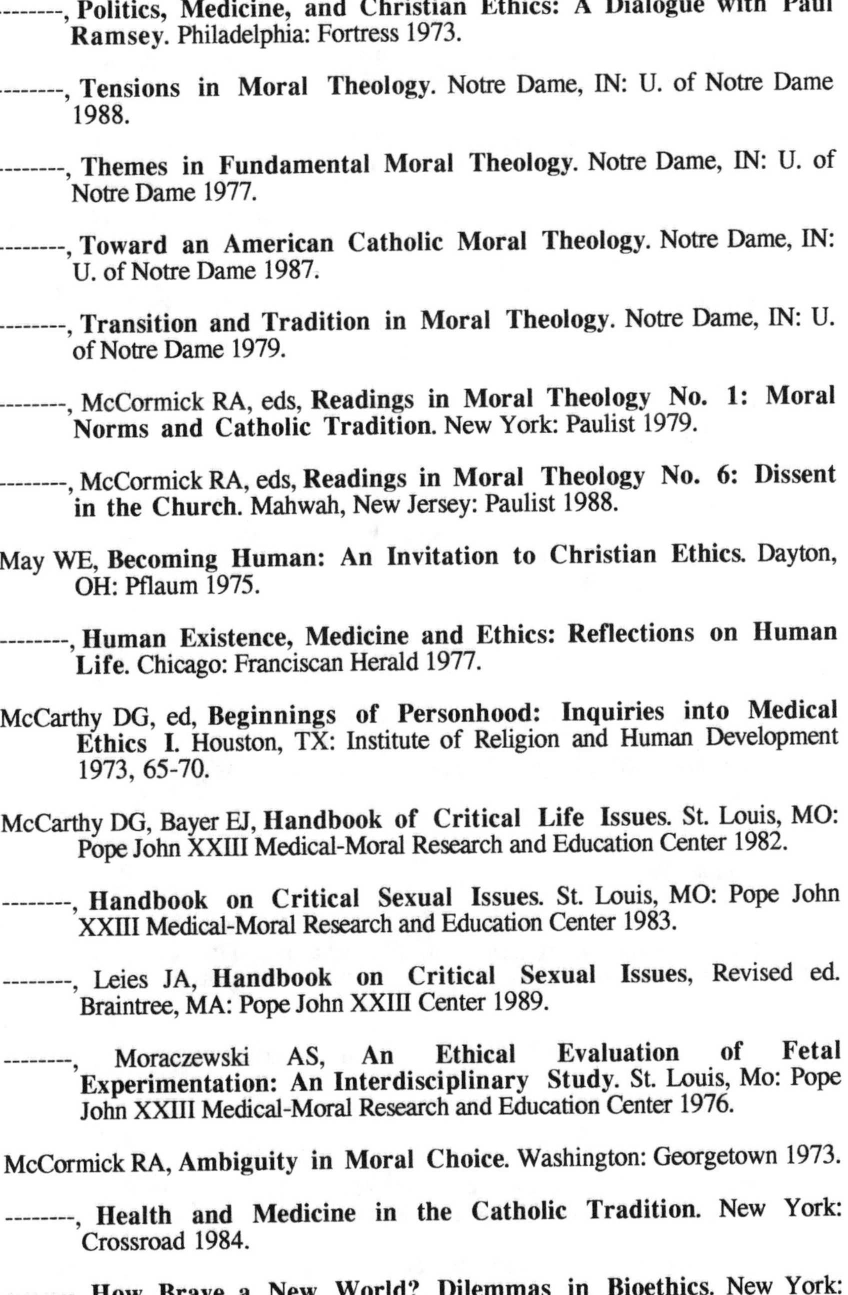

--------, **Politics, Medicine, and Christian Ethics: A Dialogue with Paul Ramsey**. Philadelphia: Fortress 1973.

--------, **Tensions in Moral Theology**. Notre Dame, IN: U. of Notre Dame 1988.

--------, **Themes in Fundamental Moral Theology**. Notre Dame, IN: U. of Notre Dame 1977.

--------, **Toward an American Catholic Moral Theology**. Notre Dame, IN: U. of Notre Dame 1987.

--------, **Transition and Tradition in Moral Theology**. Notre Dame, IN: U. of Notre Dame 1979.

--------, McCormick RA, eds, **Readings in Moral Theology No. 1: Moral Norms and Catholic Tradition**. New York: Paulist 1979.

--------, McCormick RA, eds, **Readings in Moral Theology No. 6: Dissent in the Church**. Mahwah, New Jersey: Paulist 1988.

May WE, **Becoming Human: An Invitation to Christian Ethics**. Dayton, OH: Pflaum 1975.

--------, **Human Existence, Medicine and Ethics: Reflections on Human Life**. Chicago: Franciscan Herald 1977.

McCarthy DG, ed, **Beginnings of Personhood: Inquiries into Medical Ethics I**. Houston, TX: Institute of Religion and Human Development 1973, 65-70.

McCarthy DG, Bayer EJ, **Handbook of Critical Life Issues**. St. Louis, MO: Pope John XXIII Medical-Moral Research and Education Center 1982.

--------, **Handbook on Critical Sexual Issues**. St. Louis, MO: Pope John XXIII Medical-Moral Research and Education Center 1983.

--------, Leies JA, **Handbook on Critical Sexual Issues**, Revised ed. Braintree, MA: Pope John XXIII Center 1989.

--------, Moraczewski AS, **An Ethical Evaluation of Fetal Experimentation: An Interdisciplinary Study**. St. Louis, Mo: Pope John XXIII Medical-Moral Research and Education Center 1976.

McCormick RA, **Ambiguity in Moral Choice**. Washington: Georgetown 1973.

--------, **Health and Medicine in the Catholic Tradition**. New York: Crossroad 1984.

--------, **How Brave a New World? Dilemmas in Bioethics**. New York:

Doubleday 1981.

--------, **Notes on Moral Theology: 1965 through 1980**. Washington: University Press of America 1981.

--------, **The Critical Calling: Reflections on Moral Dilemmas Since Vatican II**. Washington: Georgetown 1989.

--------, Ramsey P, eds, **Doing Evil to Achieve Good: Moral Choice in Conflict Situations**. Chicago: Loyola 1978.

Moraczewski AS, ed, **Genetic Medicine and Engineering: Ethical and Social Dimensions**. St. Louis, MO: Pope John XXIII Medical-Moral Research and Education Center 1983.

O'Donnell TJ, **Medicine and Christian Morality**, 2nd Revised and Updated ed. New York: Alba House 1991.

--------, **Medicine and Christian Morality**. New York: Alba House 1976.

O'Rourke KD, Brodeur D, **Medical Ethics: Common Ground for Understanding**. St. Louis, MO: Catholic Health Association of the United States 1986.

--------, **Medical Ethics: Common Ground for Understanding**, vol. II. St. Louis, MO: Catholic Health Association of the United States 1989.

Shannon TA, **An Introduction to Bioethics**, 2nd ed. New York: Paulist 1987.

--------, **Twelve Problems in Health Care Ethics**. New York: Edwin Mellen 1984.

--------, **What Are They Saying about Genetic Engineering**? New York: Paulist 1985.

--------, Cahill LS, **Religion and Artificial Reproduction: An Inquiry into the Vatican "Instruction on Respect for Human Life in Its Origin and on the Dignity of Human Reproduction"**. New York: Crossroad 1988.

--------, DiGiacomo JJ, **An Introduction to Bioethics**. New York: Paulist 1979.

ARTICLES

Ashley BM, "A child's rights to his own parents: a look at two value systems" *Hospital Progress* 61,8 (1980) 47-49.

--------, "A critique of the theory of delayed hominization" in: McCarthy DG, Moraczewski AS, eds, **An Ethical Evaluation of Fetal**

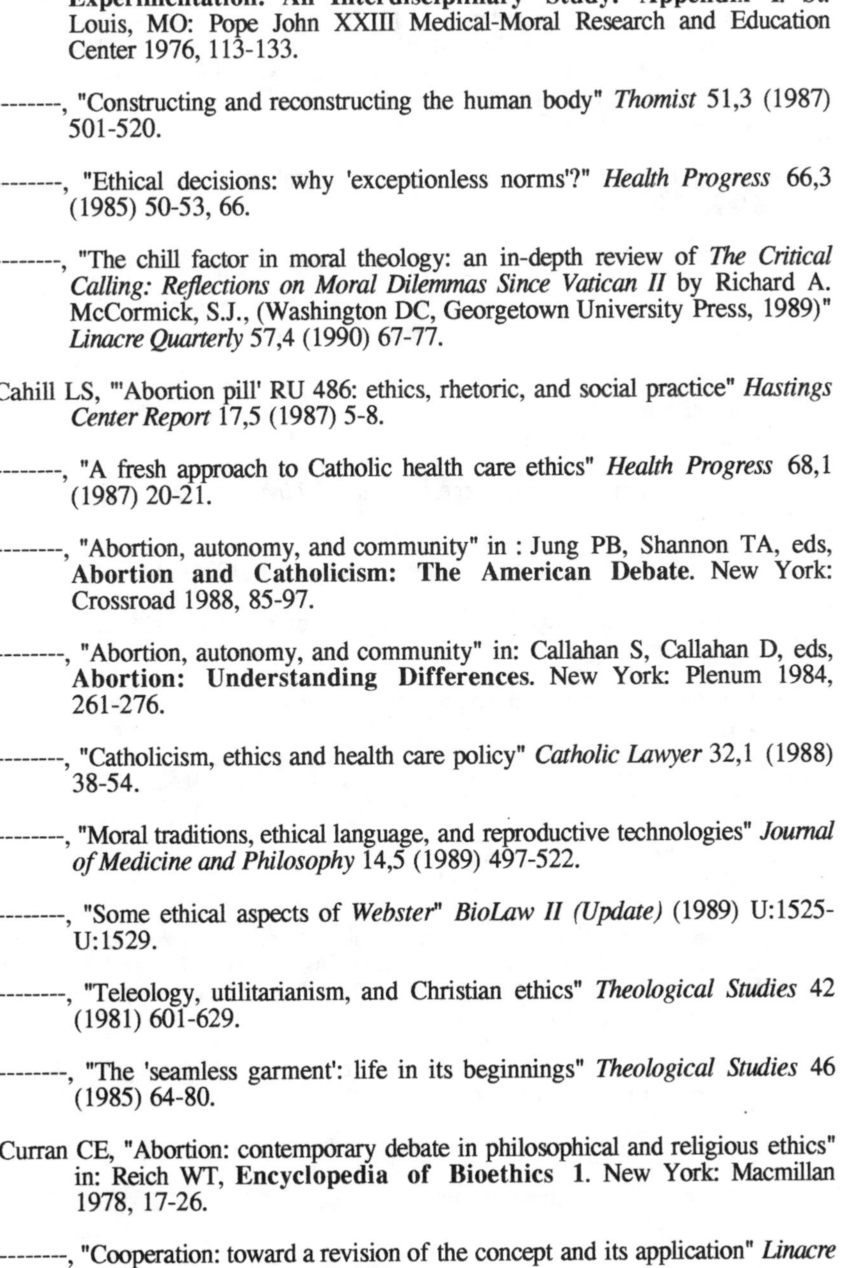

Experimentation: An Interdisciplinary Study. Appendix I. St. Louis, MO: Pope John XXIII Medical-Moral Research and Education Center 1976, 113-133.

--------, "Constructing and reconstructing the human body" *Thomist* 51,3 (1987) 501-520.

--------, "Ethical decisions: why 'exceptionless norms'?" *Health Progress* 66,3 (1985) 50-53, 66.

--------, "The chill factor in moral theology: an in-depth review of *The Critical Calling: Reflections on Moral Dilemmas Since Vatican II* by Richard A. McCormick, S.J., (Washington DC, Georgetown University Press, 1989)" *Linacre Quarterly* 57,4 (1990) 67-77.

Cahill LS, "'Abortion pill' RU 486: ethics, rhetoric, and social practice" *Hastings Center Report* 17,5 (1987) 5-8.

--------, "A fresh approach to Catholic health care ethics" *Health Progress* 68,1 (1987) 20-21.

--------, "Abortion, autonomy, and community" in : Jung PB, Shannon TA, eds, **Abortion and Catholicism: The American Debate**. New York: Crossroad 1988, 85-97.

--------, "Abortion, autonomy, and community" in: Callahan S, Callahan D, eds, **Abortion: Understanding Differences**. New York: Plenum 1984, 261-276.

--------, "Catholicism, ethics and health care policy" *Catholic Lawyer* 32,1 (1988) 38-54.

--------, "Moral traditions, ethical language, and reproductive technologies" *Journal of Medicine and Philosophy* 14,5 (1989) 497-522.

--------, "Some ethical aspects of *Webster*" *BioLaw II (Update)* (1989) U:1525-U:1529.

--------, "Teleology, utilitarianism, and Christian ethics" *Theological Studies* 42 (1981) 601-629.

--------, "The 'seamless garment': life in its beginnings" *Theological Studies* 46 (1985) 64-80.

Curran CE, "Abortion: contemporary debate in philosophical and religious ethics" in: Reich WT, **Encyclopedia of Bioethics 1**. New York: Macmillan 1978, 17-26.

--------, "Cooperation: toward a revision of the concept and its application" *Linacre Quarterly* 41,3 (1974) 152-167.

--------, "*In vitro* fertilization and embryo transfer: from a perspective of moral theology" in: U.S. Department of Health, Education, and Welfare: Ethics Advisory Board, Appendix: **HEW Support of Research Involving Human *In Vitro* Fertilization and Embryo Transfer.** Washington: Department of Health, Education, and Welfare, Ethics Advisory Board, May 4, 1979, 4.1-4.33.

May WE, "Abortion, Catholic teaching, and public policy" *Linacre Quarterly* 52,1 (1985) 38-44.

--------, "Ethics and human indentity: the challenge of the new biology" *Horizons* 3,1 (1976) 17-37.

--------, "Experimenting on human subjects" *Linacre Quarterly* 41,4 (1974) 238-252.

--------, "Meeting ethical dilemmas in health care: some basic criteria" *Linacre Quarterly* 49,3 (1982) 248-265.

--------, "Proxy consent to human experimentation" *Linacre Quarterly* 43,2 (1976) 73-84.

--------, "The morality of abortion" *Linacre Quarterly* 41,1 (1974) 66-77.

--------, "What makes a human being to be a being of moral worth?" *Thomist* 40 (1976) 416-443.

--------, "Zygotes, embryos, and persons: Part I" *Ethics and Medics* 16,10 (1991) 2-4.

--------, "Zygotes, embryos, and persons: Part II" *Ethics and Medics* 17,1 (1992) 1-3.

McCarthy DG, "Amniocentesis and our pragmatic bias" *Ethics and Medics* 4,4 (1979) 2-3.

--------, "Ethical principles and genetic medicine" in: Moraczewski AS, ed, **Genetic Medicine and Engineering: Ethical and Social Dimensions.** St. Louis, MO: Pope John XXIII Medical-Moral Research and Education Center 1983, 87-99.

--------, "Testimony for the Subcommittee on investigations and oversights" *Linacre Quarterly* 51 (1984) 315-321.

--------, "The either/or of genetic defect" *Ethics and Medics* 8,3 (1983) 1-2.

McCormick RA, "1973-1983: value impacts of a decade" *Hospital Progress* 63,12 (1982) 38-41.

--------, "A commentary on the commentaries" in: McCormick RA, Ramsey P, eds,

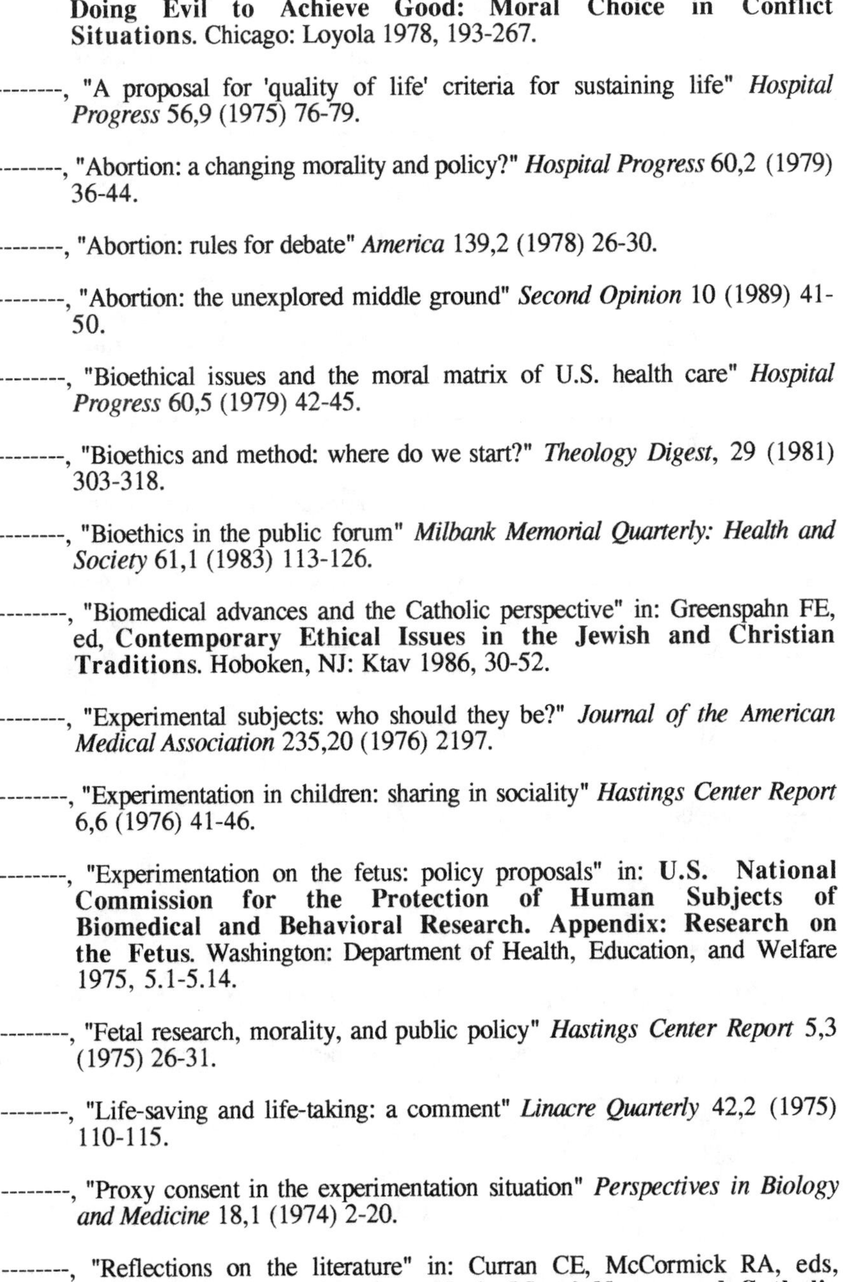

Doing Evil to Achieve Good: Moral Choice in Conflict Situations. Chicago: Loyola 1978, 193-267.

--------, "A proposal for 'quality of life' criteria for sustaining life" *Hospital Progress* 56,9 (1975) 76-79.

--------, "Abortion: a changing morality and policy?" *Hospital Progress* 60,2 (1979) 36-44.

--------, "Abortion: rules for debate" *America* 139,2 (1978) 26-30.

--------, "Abortion: the unexplored middle ground" *Second Opinion* 10 (1989) 41-50.

--------, "Bioethical issues and the moral matrix of U.S. health care" *Hospital Progress* 60,5 (1979) 42-45.

--------, "Bioethics and method: where do we start?" *Theology Digest*, 29 (1981) 303-318.

--------, "Bioethics in the public forum" *Milbank Memorial Quarterly: Health and Society* 61,1 (1983) 113-126.

--------, "Biomedical advances and the Catholic perspective" in: Greenspahn FE, ed, **Contemporary Ethical Issues in the Jewish and Christian Traditions**. Hoboken, NJ: Ktav 1986, 30-52.

--------, "Experimental subjects: who should they be?" *Journal of the American Medical Association* 235,20 (1976) 2197.

--------, "Experimentation in children: sharing in sociality" *Hastings Center Report* 6,6 (1976) 41-46.

--------, "Experimentation on the fetus: policy proposals" in: **U.S. National Commission for the Protection of Human Subjects of Biomedical and Behavioral Research. Appendix: Research on the Fetus**. Washington: Department of Health, Education, and Welfare 1975, 5.1-5.14.

--------, "Fetal research, morality, and public policy" *Hastings Center Report* 5,3 (1975) 26-31.

--------, "Life-saving and life-taking: a comment" *Linacre Quarterly* 42,2 (1975) 110-115.

--------, "Proxy consent in the experimentation situation" *Perspectives in Biology and Medicine* 18,1 (1974) 2-20.

--------, "Reflections on the literature" in: Curran CE, McCormick RA, eds, **Readings in Moral Theology No.1: Moral Norms and Catholic**

Tradition. New York: Paulist 1979, 294-340.

--------, "Saving defective infants: options for life or death" *America* 148,16 (1983) 313-317.

--------, "The moral right to privacy" *Hospital Progress* 57,8 (1976) 38-42.

--------, "The preservation of life" *Linacre Quarterly* 43,3 (1976) 94-100.

--------, "The quality of life, the sanctity of life" *Hastings Center Report* 8,1 (1978) 30-36.

--------, "Theology and bioethics: Christian foundations" in: Shelp EE, ed, **Theology and Bioethics: Exploring the Foundations and Frontiers.** Boston: Reidel 1985, 95-113.

--------, "Therapy or tampering? The ethics of reproductive technology" *America* 153,17 (1985) 396-403.

--------, "To save or let die: the dilemma of modern medicine" *Journal of the American Medical Association* 229,2 (1974) 172-179.

--------, "Who or what is the preembryo?" *Kennedy Institute of Ethics Journal* 1,1 (1991) 1-15.

--------, Walters L, "Fetal research and public policy" *America* 132,24 (1975) 473-476.

Moraczewski AS, "Can science identify human beings?" *Ethics and Medics* 6,7 (1981) 2-3.

--------, "No brain and yet alive" *Ethics and Medics* 16,12 (1991) 1-2.

--------, "Some moral dimensions in genetic counseling" *Hospital Progress* 61,10 (1980) 52-55.

--------, "Test tube embryo testing" *Ethics and Medics* 17,5 (1992) 3-4.

--------, "Trisomy 13 - a dilemma" *Ethics and Medics* 11,2 (1986) 1-2.

Moussa M, Shannon TA, "The search for the new pineal gland: brain life and personhood" *Hastings Center Report* 22,3 (1992) 30-37.

O'Donnell TJ, "'Abortion and Catholic honesty'" *Medical-Moral Newsletter* 20,9 (1983) 33-34.

--------, "Ambivalent current medical attitudes toward abortion" *Medical-Moral Newsletter* 18,9 (1981) 33-35.

--------, "Amniocentesis and abortion - the courts and the moral conscience"

Medical-Moral Newsletter 17,5 (1980) 17-20.

--------, "Amniocentesis and the defective child" *Medical-Moral Newsletter* 16,3 (1979) 9-11.

--------, "Beyond bioethics" *Medical-Moral Newsletter* 27,3 (1990) 9-11.

--------, "Catholic doctors, Catholic hospitals and the prenatal diagnosis of anencephaly" *Medical-Moral Newsletter* 18,10 (1981) 37-39.

--------, "Coherently consistent or morally meaningless?" *Medical-Moral Newsletter* 28,3 (1991) 9-10.

--------, "Early diagnosis of tubal pregnancy: new issues" *Medical-Moral Newsletter* 25,6 (1988) 23-24.

--------, "Ethics and production-line quality control of human life" *Medical-Moral Newsletter* 28,4 (1991) 15-16.

--------, "Genetic counseling, the Church, and the law" *Medical-Moral Newsletter* 17,6 (1980) 21-24.

--------, "Issues or objective truth?" *Medical-Moral Newsletter* 29,5 (1992) 19-20.

--------, "Medical double-talk on abortion" *Medical-Moral Newsletter* 24,1 (1987) 1-2.

--------, "Mifepristone: the new 'abortion pill'" *Medical-Moral Newsletter* 26,2 (1989) 7.

--------, "Morality of using aborted fetal tissue" *Medical-Moral Newsletter* 26,4 (1989) 13-15.

--------, "Prenatal screening: some moral considerations" *Medical-Moral Newsletter* 29,4 (1992) 13-14.

--------, "Questions regarding genetic counseling" *Medical-Moral Newsletter* 25,1 (1988) 3-4.

--------, "Roe vs. Wade: have the abuses helped turn the tide?" *Medical-Moral Newsletter* 26,4 (1989) 15-16.

--------, "Selective abortion in multiple pregnancy" *Medical-Moral Newsletter* 26,2 (1989) 8.

--------, "The basic determinants of the morality of human action" *Medical-Moral Newsletter* 27,6 (1990) 21-23.

--------, "The roots of Catholic moral teaching" *Medical-Moral Newsletter* 25,9 (1988) 33-36.

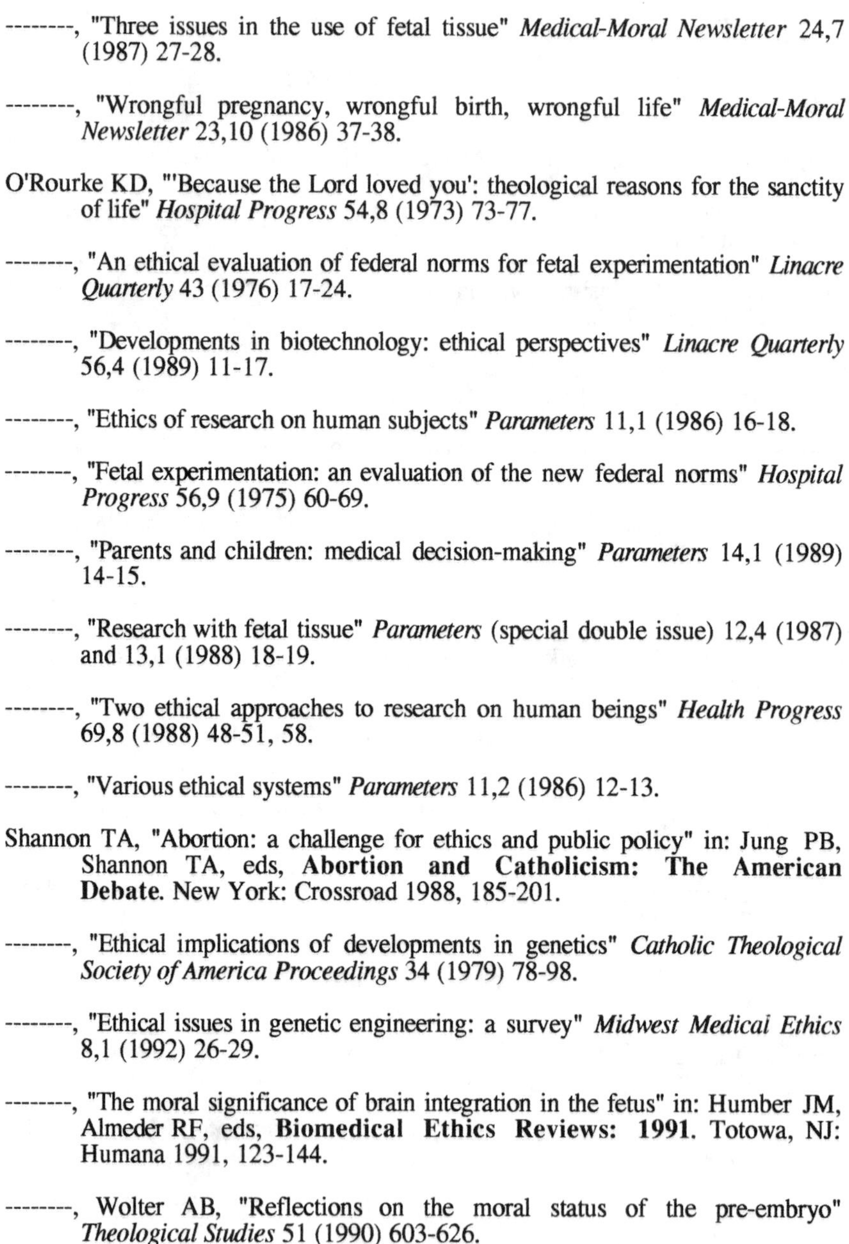

--------, "Three issues in the use of fetal tissue" *Medical-Moral Newsletter* 24,7 (1987) 27-28.

--------, "Wrongful pregnancy, wrongful birth, wrongful life" *Medical-Moral Newsletter* 23,10 (1986) 37-38.

O'Rourke KD, "'Because the Lord loved you': theological reasons for the sanctity of life" *Hospital Progress* 54,8 (1973) 73-77.

--------, "An ethical evaluation of federal norms for fetal experimentation" *Linacre Quarterly* 43 (1976) 17-24.

--------, "Developments in biotechnology: ethical perspectives" *Linacre Quarterly* 56,4 (1989) 11-17.

--------, "Ethics of research on human subjects" *Parameters* 11,1 (1986) 16-18.

--------, "Fetal experimentation: an evaluation of the new federal norms" *Hospital Progress* 56,9 (1975) 60-69.

--------, "Parents and children: medical decision-making" *Parameters* 14,1 (1989) 14-15.

--------, "Research with fetal tissue" *Parameters* (special double issue) 12,4 (1987) and 13,1 (1988) 18-19.

--------, "Two ethical approaches to research on human beings" *Health Progress* 69,8 (1988) 48-51, 58.

--------, "Various ethical systems" *Parameters* 11,2 (1986) 12-13.

Shannon TA, "Abortion: a challenge for ethics and public policy" in: Jung PB, Shannon TA, eds, **Abortion and Catholicism: The American Debate**. New York: Crossroad 1988, 185-201.

--------, "Ethical implications of developments in genetics" *Catholic Theological Society of America Proceedings* 34 (1979) 78-98.

--------, "Ethical issues in genetic engineering: a survey" *Midwest Medical Ethics* 8,1 (1992) 26-29.

--------, "The moral significance of brain integration in the fetus" in: Humber JM, Almeder RF, eds, **Biomedical Ethics Reviews: 1991**. Totowa, NJ: Humana 1991, 123-144.

--------, Wolter AB, "Reflections on the moral status of the pre-embryo" *Theological Studies* 51 (1990) 603-626.

2. SECONDARY SOURCES

BOOKS

AA VV, **Attualità della Teologia Morale: Punti Fermi - Problemi Aperti.** Roma: Urbaniana 1987.

Agich GJ, Begley CE, eds, **The Price of Health.** Boston: D. Reidel 1986.

Albacete LM, **Commentary on Instruction on Respect for Human Life in Its Origin and on the Dignity of Procreation.** Boston, MA: Daughters of St. Paul 1987.

Austin CR, **Human Embryos: The Debate on Assisted Reproduction.** New York: Oxford 1989.

Azpitarte E, Elizari Basterra FJ, Rincón Orduña R, eds, **Praxis Cristiana II: Opción por la Vida y el Amor**, 3ra ed. Madrid: Paulinas 1981.

Biolo S, ed, **Nascita e Morte dell'Uomo.** Atti del 46 Convegno del Centro Studi Filosofici di Gallarate, Genova: Marietti 1993.

Bohr D, **Catholic Moral Tradition: In Christ, a New Creation.** Huntington, IN: Our Sunday Visitor 1990.

Capron AM *et al*, eds, **Genetic Counseling: Facts, Values, and Norms.** New York: Alan R. Liss 1979.

Catholic Health Association of Canada, **Health Care Ethics Guide.** Ottawa, ON: Catholic Health Association of Canada 1991.

Catholic Health Association of the United States, **Human Genetics: Ethical Issues in Genetic Testing, Counseling, and Therapy.** St. Louis, MO: Catholic Health Association 1990.

Center for Disease Control and Prevention (Dec. 18, 1992), **MMWR 1992**, vol. 41,50, Atlanta, GA: Department of Health and Human Services 1992.

Childs B *et al*, eds, **Molecular Genetics in Medicine: Progress in Medical Genetics**, vol. VII. Hew York: Elserier 1988.

Congresso Internazionale di Teologia Morale (Roma, 7-12 aprile 1986), **Persona, Verità e Morale.** Roma: Città Nuova 1987.

Demmer K, **Interpretare e Agire: Fondamenti della Morale Cristiana.** (trans. Pedrazzoli M) Milano: Paoline 1989.

--------, **Introduzione alla Teologia Morale.** Casale Monferrato, AL: PIEMME 1993.

--------, Schüller B, eds, **Fede Cristiana e Agire Morale.** (Riva G, trad.) Assisi: Cittadella 1980.

Dietz AA, ed, **Genetic Diesase: Diagnosis and Treatment: Arnold O. Beckman Conference in Clinical Chemistry** ([*sic*]5th: 1981: Monterey, CA). Washington: American Association for Clinical Chemistry 1983.

Dunstan GR, Shinebourne EA, eds, **Doctors' Decisions: Ethical Conflicts in Medical Practice.** New York: Oxford 1989.

Evans MI, Fletcher JC, Dixler AO, Schulman JD, eds, **Fetal Diagnosis and Therapy: Science, Ethics and the Law.** Philadelphia: Lippincott 1989.

Fabbro R, **Cooperation in Evil: A Consideration of the Traditional Doctrine from the Point of View of the Contemporary Discussion about the Moral Act** (Doctoral Dissertation; Dec. 16, 1987). Rome: Gregorian 1989.

Finnis J, **Fundamentals of Ethics.** Oxford: Clarendon 1983.

Finnis J, **Natural Law and Natural Rights.** Oxford: Clarendon 1980.

Ford NM, **When Did I Begin? Conception of the Human Individual in History, Philosophy, and Science.** Cambridge: Cambridge University 1988.

Fuchs J, **Christian Ethics in a Secular Arena.** (trans. Hoose B, McNeil B) Washington: Georgetown UP 1984.

--------, **Personal Responsibility and Christian Morality.** (trans. Cleves W *et al*) Washington: Georgetown UP 1983.

Goffi T, Piana G, eds, **Corso di Morale II: Diakonia (Etica della Persona).** Brescia: Queriniana 1983.

Green JM, **Calming Or Harming? A Critical Review of Psychological Effects of Fetal Diagnosis on Pregnant Women.** London: Galton Institute 1990.

Grisez G, Boyle, Jr. JM, **Life and Death with Liberty and Justice: A Contribution to the Euthanasia Debate.** Notre Dame, IN: U of Notre Dame P 1979.

--------, **The Way of the Lord Jesus: Christian Moral Principles**, vol. I. Chicago: Franciscan Herald Press 1983.

Holder AR, **Legal Issues in Pediatrics and Adolescent Medicine**, 2nd ed. New Haven, CT: Yale 1985.

Hoose B, **Proportionalism: The American Debate and its European Roots**. Washington: Georgetown UP 1987.

Latourelle R, ed, **Vaticano II: Bilancio e Prospettive. Venticinque Anni Dopo (1962-1987)**. Assisi 1987.

López Azpitarte E, Elizari Basterra FJ, Rincón Orduña R, eds, **Praxis Cristiana II: Opción por la Vida y el Amor**, 3ra ed. Madrid: Paulinas 1981.

Malherbe J-F, ed, **Human Life: Its Beginnings and Development. Bioethical Reflections by Catholic Scholars** (International Federation of Catholic Universities). Paris: L'Harmattan 1988.

Michaelson KL, ed, **Childbirth in America: Anthropological Perspectives**. South Hadley, MA: Bergin and Garvey 1988.

Milunsky A, ed, **Genetic Disorders and the Fetus: Diagnosis, Prevention, and Treatment**, 2nd ed. New York: Plenum 1986.

Monagle JF, Thomasma DC, eds, **Medical Ethics: A Guide for Health Professionals**. Rockville, MD: Aspen 1988.

National Center for Health Statistics, *Advance Report of Final Natality Statistics, 1991*, **Monthly Vital Statistics Report**, vol. 42,3 Supplement. Hyattsville, MD: Public Health Services 1993.

Nelson LJ, ed, **The Death Decision**. Ann Arbor, MI: Servant 1984.

Pellegrino ED, Langan JP, Harvey JC, eds, **Catholic Perspectives on Medical Morals: Foundational Issues**. Netherlands: Kluwer 1989.

--------, Thomasma DC, **For the Patient's Good: The Restoration of Beneficence in Health Care**. New York: Oxford UP 1988.

Perico G, **Problemi di Etica Sanitaria**. Milano: Ancora 1985.

Pinckaers S, **Les Sources de la Morale Chrétienne: sa Méthode, son Contenu, son Histoire**. Fribourg, Suisse: Éditions Universitaires Fribourg 1985.

Privitera S, **Temi Etici di Dialogo Ecumenico: Sull'Universalità dell'Esigenza Dialogica dell'Etica**. Palermo: Edi Oftes 1992.

Reidy M, ed, **Ethical Issues in Reproductive Medicine**. Dublin: Gill and MacMillan 1982.

Reiser SJ, Anbar M, eds, **The Machine at the Bedside: Strategies for Using Technology in Patient Care**. New York: Cambridge 1984.

Rincón Orduña R, Mora Bartrés G, López Azpitarte E, eds, **Praxis Cristiana I:**

Fundamentación, 5ta ed. Madrid: Paulinas 1980.

Rodin J, Collins A, eds, **Women and New Reproductive Technologies: Medical, Psychosocial, Legal, and Ethical Dilemmas**. Hillsdale, NJ: Lawrence Erlbaum Associates 1991.

Schneider ED, ed, **Questions about the Beginning of Life: Christian Appraisals of Seven Bioethical Issues**. Minneapolis, MN: Augsburg 1985.

Serra A, Santosuosso F, Bompiani A, Manni C, Cotta S, eds, **Medicina e Genetica Verso il Futuro**. L'Aquila-Roma: Japadre 1986.

Sgreccia E, **Bioetica: Manuale per Medici e Biologi**. Milano: Vita e Pensiero 1986.

--------, **Manuale di Bioetica I: Fondamenti ed Etica Biomedica**. Milano: Vita e Pensiero 1988.

Spicker SC, Engelhardt, Jr. HT, eds, **Philosophical Medical Ethics**. Boston: Reidel 1977.

Srám RJ, Bulyzhenkov V, Prilipko L, Christen Y, eds, **Ethical Issues of Molecular Genetics in Psychiatry**. New York: Springer-Verlag 1991.

Tettamanzi D, **Bioetica: Nuove Frontiere per l'Uomo**, 2da ed. Casale Monferrato, AL: Piemme 1990.

Vidal M, **El Discernimiento Ético: Hacia una Estimativa Moral Cristiana**. Madrid: Cristiandad 1980.

Wattiaux H, **Génétique et Fécondité Humaines**. Louvain-la-Neuve: Cahiers de la Revue Théologique de Louvain 1986.

Weil WB, Benjamin M, eds, **Ethical Issues at the Outset of Life**. Boston: Blackwell Scientific 1987.

ARTICLES

ACOG, "Ethical decision-making in obstetrics and gynecology" *ACOG Technical Bulletin* 136 (1989) 1-7.

Adams J, "Confidentiality and Huntington's chorea" *Journal of Medical Ethics* 16 (1990) 196-199.

American Academy of Pediatrics, "Alpha-fetoprotein screening" *Pediatrics* 80,3 (1987) 444-445.

Annas GJ, Elias S, "Legal and ethical implications of fetal diagnosis and gene therapy" *American Journal of Medical Genetics* 35,2 (1990) 215-218.

Attard M, "Dimensioni etiche della medicina genetica: la moralità dei bambini in provetta" *Rivista di Teologia Morale* 43 (1979) 367-384.

Aubert J-M, "Foi et morale: parcours de moral fondamentale" *Le Supplement* 155 (1985) 75-80.

Autiero A, "Etica della vita prenatale: fatti, problemi, prospettive" *Rivista di Teologia Morale* 17,68 (1985) 31-44.

--------, "Il rapporto tra medicina e teologia per la prassi dell'etica medica" *Rivista di Teologia Morale* 79 (1988) 47-58.

--------, "Natura e leggi di natura" in: Goffi T, Piana G, eds, **Corso di Morale II: Diakonia (Etica della Persona)**. Brescia: Queriniana 1983, 106-109.

Barry R, "Personhood: the conditions of identification and description" *Linacre Quarterly* 45 (1978) 64-81.

Baumiller RC, "Clergy involvement: a dimension of real need" *Hospital Practice* 18,4 (1983) 38A,D,E,F.

--------, "Genetic counseling" *National Apostolate for the Mentally Retarded* Winter (1975) 4-5.

--------, "Genetic decision making and pastoral care" *Hospital Practice* 17,12 (1982) 96A.

Bausola A, "Riflessione filosofica sulla fondazione della morale" in: Congresso Internazionale di Teologia Morale, **Persona, Verita e Morale**. Roma: Citta Nuova 1987, 37-48.

Bedate CA, "Reflections concerning questions of life and death: towards a new paradigm for understanding the ethical value of the biological human entity" in: Malherbe J-F, ed, **Human Life: Its Beginnings and Development**. Paris: L'Harmattan 1988, 67-97.

--------, Cefalo RC, "The zygote: to be or not to be a person" *Journal of Medicine and Philosophy* 14 (1989) 642.

Beeson D, Douglas R, Lunsford TF, "Prenatal diagnosis of fetal disorders. Part II: issues and implications" *Birth* 10,4 (1983) 233-241.

Berg K, "Ethical problems arising from research progress in medical genetics" in: Berg K, Tranoy KE, eds, **Research Ethics**. New York: Alan R. Liss 1983, 261-275.

Bigger CP, "St. Thomas on essence and participation" *New Scholasticism* 62 (1988) 319-348.

Biggers JD, "Arbitrary partitions of prenatal life" *Human Reproduction* 5,1 (1990) 1-6.

Birch AC, "The dialectic of discovery" *New Scholasticism* 63 (1989) 295-312.

Böckle F, "Le magistère de l'église en matière morale" *Revue Théologique de Louvain* 19 (1988) 3-16.

Bompiani A, "Metodi e problemi della riproduzione umana 'artificiale' o 'assistita'" in: Serra A, Santosuosso F, Bompiani A, Manni C, Cotta S, eds, **Medicina e Genetica Verso il Futuro.** L'Aquila-Roma: Japadre 1986, 41-72.

Bondolfi A, "Statuto dell'embrione. Considerazioni di metodo" *Rivista di Teologia Morale* 90 (1991) 223-241.

Boné E, "A society more intolerant of handicap" in: Malherbe J-F, ed, **Human Life: Its Beginnings and Development.** Paris: L'Hrmattan 1988, 227-237.

--------, "Paléontologie et reconnaissance de l'homme" *Études* 352,1 (1980) 39-57.

--------, "Le génie génétique au prisme de l'éthique" *Revue Théologique de Louvain* 17 (1986) 156-191.

Boss JA, "How voluntary prenatal diagnosis and selective abortion increase the abnormal human gene pool" *Birth* 17,2 (1990) 75-79.

Boyle J, "Who is entitled to double effect?" *Journal of Medicine and Philosophy* 16 (1991) 475-494.

Boyle, Jr, JM, Grisez G, Tollefson O, "Determinism, freedom, and self referential arguments" *Review of Metaphysics* 26,1 (1972) 3-37.

Brera GR, "La sofferenza nel rapporto medico-paziente: la medicina come scienza della sofferenza" *Medicina e Morale* 37,1-2 (1987) 46-57.

Brown M, "St. Thomas Aquinas and the individuation of persons" *American Catholic Philosophical Quarterly* 65 (1991) 29-44.

Bueche W, "Destroying human embryos - destroying human lives: a moral issue" *Studia Moralia* 29 (1991) 85-115.

Caffarra C, "Aspetti etici della diagnostica prenatale" *Medicina e Morale* 34,4 (1984) 449-457.

--------, "The rights of the embryo and the fetus" *Fetal Therapy* 4,suppl 1 (1989) 12-15.

Calisti A, "Diagnosi prenatale e possibilità terapeutiche chirurgiche" *Medicina e*

Morale 34,4 (1984) 493-497.

Callahan S, "X versus Y: should parents decide?" *Health Progress* 70 (1989) 20-21.

Campos L, Tejedo A, Abel F, Cefalo RC, "Genetics and scope of spontaneous abortion and fetal wastage" in: Malherbe J-F, ed, **Human Life: Its Beginnings and Development**. Paris: L'Harmattan 1988, 125-146.

Carrasco de Paula I, "Personalità dell'embrione e aborto" in: Congresso Internazionale di Teologia Morale (Roma, 7-12 aprile 1986), **Persona, Verità e Morale**. Roma: Città Nuova 1987, 277-290.

Caspar Ph, "Animation de l'âme et unicité de la forme chez Saint Thomas d'Aquin" *Anthropotes* 5 (1989) 109-118.

--------, "La problématique de l'animation de l'embryon" *Nouvelle Revue Théologique* 113 (1991) 239-255, 400-413.

Centore FF, "Potency, space, and time: three modern theories" *New Scholasticism* 63 (1989) 435-462.

Chapelle A, "Pour lire 'Donum vitae'" *Nouvelle Revue Théologique* 109 (1987) 481-508.

Chervenak FA, McCullough LB, "Ethics in obstetric ultrasound" *Journal of Ultrasound Medicine* 8,9 (1989) 493-497.

Chiavacci E, "La fondazione della norma morale nella riflessione teologica contemporanea" *Rivista di Teologia Morale* 37 (1978) 9-38.

--------, "La questione dei principi fondamentali della morale cristiana" *Rivista di Teologia Morale* 69 (1986) 21-25.

Cinque B, Pelagalli M, Daini S, Dell'Acqua S, Spagnolo AG, "Aborto ripetuto spontaneo: aspetti scientifici e obbligazioni morali" *Medicina e Morale* 42,5 (1992) 889-908.

Clark RD, Fletcher J, Petersen G, "Conceiving a fetus for bone marrow donation: an ethical problem in prenatal diagnosis" *Prenatal Diagnosis* 9,5 (1989) 329-334.

Clark SL, DeVore GR, "Prenatal diagnosis for couples who would not consider abortion" *Obstetrics and Gynecology* 73,6 (1989) 1035-1037.

Colomber J, "Résistance à l'intolérable" *Lumière et Vie* 38,191 (1989) 69-84.

Composta D, "L'intenzione come momento costitutivo dell'atto morale" in: AA VV, **Attualità della Teologia Morale: Punti Fermi - Problemi Aperti.** Roma: Urbaniana 1987, 87-110.

Connery JR, "Catholic ethics: has the norm for rule-making changed?" *Theological Studies* 42 (1981) 232-250.

--------, "Morality of consequences: a critical appraisal" in: Curran CE, McCormick RA, eds, **Readings in Moral Theology No. 1: Moral Norms and Catholic Tradition.** New York: Paulist 1979, 244-266.

--------, "The teleology of proportionate reason" *Theological Studies* 44 (1983) 489-496.

Costakos D, Abramson RK, Edwards JG, Rizzo WB, Best RG, "Attitudes toward presymptomatic testing and prenatal diagnosis for Adrenoleukodystrophy among affected families" *American Journal of Medical Genetics* 41 (1991) 295-300.

Coste R, "Passion et compassion: brèves esquisses" *Le Supplement* 152 (1985) 21-30.

Crawfurd Md'A, "Ethical guidelines in fetal medicine" *Fetal Therapy* 2,3 (1987) 175-180.

Crescini A, "La natura della vita: una indagine filosofica" **Giornale di Metafisica** 14 (1992) 277-330.

Crosby JF, "The creaturehood of the human person and the critique of proportionalism" in: Congresso Internazionale di Teologia Morale (Roma, 7-12 aprile 1986), **Persona, Verità e Morale.** Roma: Città Nuova 1987, 195-199.

Cuyás M, "Il progresso biomedico interpella la teologia morale" in: Latourelle, ed, **Vaticano II: Bilancio e Prospettive. Venticinque Anni Dopo (1962-1987).** Assisi 1987, 1480-1506.

--------, "Problematica etica della manipolazione genetica" *Rassegna di Teologia* 28 (1987) 471-497.

Daly TV, "The personhood of the human embryo" *Linacre Quarterly* 57,1 (1990) 83-88.

De Marco D, "The foetus, his humanity and his rights" *Linacre Quarterly* 41 (1974) 281-284.

De Virgilio G, "L'analisi dell'atto morale" *Rivista di Teologia Morale* 98 (1993) 171-176.

Decruyenaere M, Evers-Kiebooms G, Denayer L, Van den Berghe H, "Cystic fibrosis: community knowledge and attitudes towards carrier screening and prenatal diagnosis" *Clinical Genetics* 41,4 (1992) 189-196.

Delcroix M, Lesage-Desrousseaux E, Lefèvre Ch, "L'anomalie anténatale, croix des moralistes" *Mélanges de Science Religieuse* 42,3 (1985) 149-167.

Demmer K, "Christliches Ethos und Menschenrechte. Einige moraltheologische Erwägungen" *Gregorianum* 60 (1979) 453-479.

--------, "Der Anspruch der Toleranz" *Gregorianum* 63 (1982) 701-720.

--------, "Deuten und Wählen. Vorbemerkungen zu einer Moraltheologischen Handlungstheorie" *Gregorianum* 62 (1981) 231-275.

--------, "Erwägungen zum 'intrinsece malum'" *Gregorianum* 68 (1987) 613-637.

--------, "Gene technologies and man: the ethical implications of a contemporary challenge" in: Malherbe J-F, ed, **Human Life: Its Beginnings and Development**. Paris: L'Harmattan 1988, 315-332.

--------, "Genotechnologie e uomo" *Vita e Pensiero* 67,12 (1984) 46-56.

--------, "La competenza normativa del magistero ecclesiastico in morale" in: Demmer K, Schüller B, eds, **Fede Cristiana e Agire Morale**. (Riva G, trad.) Assisi: Cittadella 1980, 144-170.

--------, "La sfida teologica del dialogo interdisciplinare" *Laurent* 33 (1992) 403-420.

--------, "Man's appropriate stewardship of his biological nature" in: Malherbe J-F, ed, **Human Life: Its Beginnings and Development.** Paris: L'Harmattan 1988, 259-271.

--------, "Sittlich handeln als Zeugnis geben" *Gregorianum* 64 (1983) 453-485.

--------, "Sittlich Handeln aus Erfahrung" *Gregorianum* 59 (1978) 661-690.

--------, "Theological argument and hermeneutics in bioethics" in: Pellegrino ED, Langan JP, Harvey JC, eds, **Catholic Perspectives on Medical Morals: Foundational Issues**. Netherlands: Kluwer 1989, 103-122.

Di Giovanni A, "Etica e valore morale" *La Civiltà Cattolica* 127,2 (1976) 371-375.

Di Ianni A, "The direct/indirect distinction in morals" in: Curran CE, McCormick RA, eds, **Readings in Moral Theology No. 1: Moral Norms and Catholic Tradition**. New York: Paulist 1979, 215-243.

Di Marino A, "Originalità e origine delle norme morali cristiane" *Rivista di Teologia Morale* 20 (1973) 515-546.

Di Pietro M-L, Sgreccia E, "La contragestazione ovvero l'aborto nascosto" *Medicina e Morale* 38,1 (1988) 5-34.

Dickens BM, "Prenatal diagnosis and female abortion: a case study in medical law and ethics" *Journal of Medical Ethics* 12 (1986) 143-144, 150.

Documento del Centro di Bioetica della Università Cattolica del Sacro Cuore, "Indentità e statuto dell'embrione umano" *Medicina e Morale* 39,4 (1989) 663-676.

Doran K, "Person - a key concept for ethics" *Linacre Quarterly* 56 (1989) 38-49.

Doucet H, "Le diagnostic prénatal: interprétation culturelle et réflexions éthiques" *Laval Philosophique et Théologique* 40,1 (1984) 31-48.

Dougherty CJ, "Prenatal diagnosis: a reappraisal" *Linacre Quarterly* 51 (1984) 128-138.

Elias S, Annas GJ, "Routine prenatal genetic screening" *New England Journal of Medicine* 317,22 (1987) 1407-1409.

Elizari Basterra FJ, "Moral de la vida y la salud" in: López Azpitarte E, Elizari Basterra FJ, Rincón Orduña R, eds, **Praxis Cristiana II: Opción por la Vida y el Amor**. 3rd ed. Madrid: Paulinas 1981, 86-93.

--------, "Valor teológico-moral de la Instrucción vaticana" *Moralia* 9 (1987) 239-250.

--------, "Valoración de la vida humana antes de nacer -- condicionamientos sociales --" *Moralia* 13 (1991) 187-204.

Engelhardt, Jr. HT, "Some persons are humans, some humans are persons, and the world is what we persons make it" in: Spicker SC, Engelhardt, Jr. HT, eds, **Philosophical Medical Ethics.** Boston: Reidel 1977, 183-194.

Engelman E, "Aristotelian teleology, presocratic hylozoism, and 20th century interpretation" *American Catholic Philosophical Quarterly* 64 (1990) 297-312.

Evers-Kiebooms G, Denayer L, Cassiman J-J, Van den Berghe H, "Family planning decisions after the birth of a cystic fibrosis child: the impact of prenatal diagnosis" *Scandinavian Journal of Gastroenterology* 23,143 (1988) 38-46.

--------, Swerts A, Van den Berghe H, "Psychological aspects of amniocentesis: anxiety feelings in three different risk groups" *Clinical Genetics* 33,3 (1988) 196-206.

Faden R, "Autonomy, choice, and the new reproductive technologies: the role of informed consent in prenatal genetic diagnosis" in: Rodin J, Collins A, eds, **Women and New Reproductive Technologies: Medical, Psychosocial, Legal, and Ethical Dilemmas.** Hillsdale, NJ: Lawrence Erlbaum Associates 1991, 37-47.

Fagone V, "Essere umano ed essere umanizzato: Nuove prospettive antropologiche sul problema dell'aborto" *La Civiltà Cattolica* 124,3 (1973) 20-36.

--------, "Il problema dell'inizio della vita dell'uomo" *La Civiltà Cattolica* 124,2 (1973) 531-546.

--------, "Vita prenatale e soggetto umano" *La Civiltà Cattolica* 126,1 (1975) 441-460.

Fagot-Largeault A, Delaisi de Parseval G, "Le droits de l'embryon (foetus) humain, et la notion de personne humaine potentielle" *Revue de Métaphysique et de Morale* 92 (1987) 361-385.

Faivre A, "'Où est la vérité?' Déplacements et enjeux d'u question" *Lumière et Vie* 35,180 (1986) 5-16.

Famerée J, "La fonction du magistère ecclésial en morale" *Neuvelle Revue Théologique* 107 (1985) 722-739.

Ferguson-Smith MA, Ferguson-Smith ME, "Relationships between patient, clinician, and scientist in prenatal diagnosis" in: Dunstan GR, Shinebourne EA, eds, **Doctors' Decisions: Ethical Conflicts in Medical Practice**. New York: Oxford 1989, 18-34.

Fibison WJ, Davies BL, "Dilemmas in prenatal diagnosis: a case study" *Issues in Health Care of Women* 4,1 (1983) 57-67.

Filice FP, "Twinning and recombination: a review of the data" *Linacre Quarterly* 48 (1981) 40-51.

Flecha J-R, "Estatuto eclesial del teólogo moralista" *Moralia* 10 (1988) 445-466.

Fletcher J, "Moral and ethical problems of pre-natal diagnosis" *Clinical Genetics* 8,4 (1975) 251-257.

Fletcher JC, "Ethical aspects of a controlled clinical trial of chorion biopsy approach to prenatal diagnosis" in: Berg K, ed, **Medical Genetics: Past, Present, Future**. New York: Alan R. Liss 1985, 213-248.

--------, "Ethical issues in genetic screening, prenatal diagnosis, and counseling" in: Weil WB, Benjamin M, eds, **Ethical Issues at the Outset of Life**. Boston: Blackwell Scientific 1987, 63-99.

--------, "Ethics in experimental fetal therapy: is there an early consensus?" in: Evans MI *et al*, eds, **Fetal Diagnosis and Therapy: Science, Ethics and the Law**. Philadelphia: Lippincott 1989, 438-446.

--------, "Moral problems and ethical guidance in prenatal diagnosis: past, present, and future" in: Milunsky A, ed, **Genetic Disorders and the Fetus: Diagnosis, Prevention, and Treatment**, 2nd ed. New York: Plenum

1986, 819-859.

--------, "Moral problems and ethical issues in prospective human gene therapy" *Virginia Law Review* 69 (1983) 515-546.

--------, "Prenatal diagnosis of the hemoglobinopathies: ethical issues" *American Journal of Obstetrics and Gynecology* 135,1 (1979) 53-56.

--------, "Prenatal diagnosis, selective abortion, and the ethics of withholding treatment from the defective newborn" in: Capron AM *et al*, eds, **Genetic Counseling: Facts, Values, and Norms.** New York: Alan R. Liss 1979, 239-254.

--------, "The prenatal state: screening and treating neural tube defects" in: Reiser SJ, Anbar M, eds, **The Machine at the Bedside: Strategies for Using Technology in Patient Care.** New York: Cambridge 1984, 255-260.

Ford NM, "**When Did I Begin?** A reply to Nicholas Tonti-Filippini" *Linacre Quarterly* 57 (1990) 59-66.

Fost N, "Guiding principles for prenatal diagnosis" *Prenatal Diagnosis* 9,5 (1989) 335-337.

Frets PG, Duivenvoorden HJ, Verhage F, Peters-Romeyn BMT, Neirmeijer MF, "Analysis of problems in making the reproductive decision after genetic counselling" *Journal of Medical Genetics* 28,3 (1991) 194-200.

Fuchs J, "The absoluteness of moral terms" in: Curran CE, McCormick RA, eds, **Readings in Moral Theology No. 1: Moral Norms and Catholic Tradition.** New York: Paulist 1979, 94-137.

Gafo J, "El documento Vaticano sobre bioética" *Razón y Fe* 215 (1987) 461-471.

Garber AM, Fenerty JP, "Costs and benefits of prenatal screening for cystic fibrosis" *Medical Care* 29,5 (1991) 473-489.

Gesché A, "L'homme créé créateur" *Revue Théologique de Louvain* 22 (1991) 153-184.

Gillett GR, "Informed consent and moral integrity" *Journal of Medical Ethics* 15 (1989) 117-123.

Gillon R, "Ethics and clinical practice" *Journal of Inherited Metabolic Disease* 11,1 (1988) 120-124.

--------, "Genetic counselling, confidentiality, and the medical interests of relatives" *Journal of Medical Ethics* 14 (1988) 171-172.

Godfraind Th, "Les défis posés au chrétien par la technique médicale" *Revue*

Théologique de Louvain 17 (1986) 5-21.

Goffi T, "Magistero ecclesiale ed etica cristiana" *Rivista di Teologia Morale* 63 (1984) 431-439.

--------, Piana G, "La persona all'origine dell'etica" in: Goffi T, Piana G, eds, **Corso di Morale II: Diakonia (Etica della Persona)**. Brescia: Queriniana 1983, 9-15.

Grisez G, "Infallibility and specific moral norms: a review discussion" in: Curran CE, McCormick RA, eds, **Readings in Moral Theology No. 6: Dissent in the Church**. Mahwah, New Jersey: Paulist 1988, 58-96.

Guinchedi F, "Considerazioni sullo statuto embrionario" *Rassegna di Teologia* 34 (1993) 62-76.

Guzzetti GB, "Quando l'embrione è persona? A proposito del pensiero di Jean-François Malherbe" *Rivista di Teologia Morale* 73 (1987) 67-79.

Hamel E, "La morale cristiana e la cultura contemporanea" in: AA VV, **Attualità della Teologia Morale: Punti Fermi - Problemi Aperti**. Roma: Urbaniana 1987, 11-22.

Häring B, "It's wrong to knowingly beget defective children" *U.S. Catholic* 41,2 (1976) 12-14.

--------, "New dimensions of responsible parenthood" *Theological Studies* 37 (1976) 120-132.

Healy B, "Hearing on the possible uses and misuses of genetic information" *Human Gene Therapy* 3 (1992) 51-56.

Henifin MS, "Selective termination of pregnancy: commentary" *Hastings Center Report* 18,1 (1988) 22.

Herranz G, "Scienze biomediche e qualità della vitta" in: Congresso Internazionale di Teologia Morale (Roma, 7-12 aprile 1986), **Persona, Verità e Morale**. Roma: Città Nuova 1987, 79-87.

Holder AR, "Amniocentesis, genetic counseling, and genetic screening" in: Holder AR, **Legal Issues in Pediatrics and Adolescent Medicine**, 2nd ed. New Haven, CT: Yale 1985, 25-49.

Holtam NR, "Antenatal diagnosis and the termination of pregnancy: what the churches have to say" *Journal of Inherited Metabolic Disease* 11,suppl 1 (1988) 111-119.

Holtzman NA, "Ethical issues in the prenatal diagnosis of Phenylketonuria" *Pediatrics* 74,3 (1984) 424-427.

Janssens L, "Ontic evil and moral evil" in: Curran CE, McCormick RA, eds, **Readings in Moral Theology No. 1: Moral Norms and Catholic Tradition.** New York: Paulist 1979, 40-93.

Johnson SR, Elkins TE, "Ethical issues in prenatal diagnosis" *Clinical Obstetrics and Gynecology* 31,2 (1988) 408-417.

Johnstone BV, "The meaning of proportionate reason in contemporary moral theology" *The Thomist* 49 (1985) 223-247.

Jonas H, "Tecnica, libertà e dovere" *Rivista di Teologia Morale* 77 (1988) 25-35.

Juengst ET, "Prenatal diagnosis and the ethics of uncertainty" in: Monagle JF, Thomasma DC, eds, **Medical Ethics: A Guide for Health Professionals.** Rockville, MD: Aspen 1988, 12-25.

Kaczynski E, "Rispetto per la vita nascente e dignità della procreazione" *Angelicum* 64 (1987) 583-591.

--------, "Verità sul bene nei diversi elementi della morale" *Rivista di Teologia Morale* 51 (1981) 419-431.

Kass LR, "Implications of prenatal diagnosis for the human right to life" in: Hilton B *et al*, **Ethical Issues in Human Genetics.** New York: Plenum 1973, 185-199.

Katz Rothman B, "The decision to have or not to have amniocentesis for prenatal diagnosis" in: Michaelson KL, ed, **Childbirth in America: Anthropological Perspectives.** South Hadley, MA: Bergin and Garvey 1988, 90-102.

Kiely B, "The impracticality of proportionalism" *Gregorianum* 66 (1985) 655-687.

Klein E, "Introduction au débat quantique" *Études* 375,6 (1991) 633-645.

Knauer P, "The hermeneutic function of the principle of double effect" in: Curran CE, McCormick RA, eds, **Readings in Moral Theology No. 1: Moral Norms and Catholic Tradition.** New York: Paulist 1979, 1-39.

La Croce E, "Good and goods according to Aristotle" *New Scholasticism* 63 (1989) 1-17.

Lacadena J-R, "Terapia génica: consideraciones éticas" *Razón y Fe* 225 (1992) 510-520.

--------, "Status of the embryo prior to implantation" in: Malherbe J-F, ed, **Human Life: Its Beginnings and Development.** Paris: L'Harmattan 1988, 39-45.

Lachièze-Rey M, "Big bang et formation de l'universe" *Études* 366,5 (1987) 627-648.

Lappé M, "Ethical aspects of therapy for genetic diseases" in: Dietz AA, ed, **Genetic Disease: Diagnosis and Treatment: Arnold O. Beckman Conference in Clinical Chemistry** ([*sic*]5th: 1981: Monterey, CA). Washington: American Association for Clinical Chemistry 1983, 282-296.

Lawler RD, "The magisterium and Catholic moral teaching" in: Congresso Internazionale di Teologia Morale (Roma, 7-12 aprile 1986), **Persona, Verità e Morale.** Roma: Città Nuova 1987, 217-233.

Lebacqz KA, "Prenatal diagnosis and selective abortion" *Linacre Quarterly* 40 (1973) 109-127.

Lebel RR, "Genetic decision-making; parental responsibility" *Linacre Quarterly* 43 (1976) 280-291

Lee P, "Personhood, the moral standing of the unborn, and abortion" *Linacre Quarterly* 57,2 (1990) 80-89.

Leone S, "L'embrione: soggetto di diritti" *Rivista di Teologia Morale* 98 (1993) 229-238.

Leuzzi L, "Indicazioni etiche per la diagnostica prenatale" *Medicina e Morale* 34,4 (1984) 458-463.

Lippman-Hand A, Piper M, "Prenatal diagnosis for the detection of Down syndrome: why are so few eligible women tested?" *Prenatal Diagnosis* 1,4 (1981) 249-257.

Lizotte A, Reflexions philosophiques sur l'âme et la personne de l'embryon" *Anthropotes* 3 (1987) 155-195.

Loader S, Sutera CJ, Walden M, Kozyra A, Rowley PT, "Prenatal screening for hemoglobinopathies. II. Evaluation and counseling" *American Journal of Human Genetics* 48,3 (1991) 447-451.

Lonchamp J-P, "Le principe anthropique" *Études* 374,4 (1991) 493-502.

López Azpitarte, "Decisiones de conciencia en un mundo tecnificado" *Moralia* 10 (1988) 65-89.

--------, "El magisterio moral de la Iglesia: tensiones actuales" *Sal Terrae* 75 (1987) 503-514.

--------, "El proyecto ético: la realización del hombre como persona" in: Rincón Orduña R, Mora Bartrés G, López Azpitarte E, eds, **Praxis Cristiana I: Fundamentación.** 5ta ed. Madrid: Paulinas 1980, 263-278.

--------, "La génesis de la moral: autonomía y autenticidad del comportamiento" in: Rincón Orduña R, Mora Bartrés G, López Azpitarte E, eds, **Praxis Cristiana I: Fundamentación.** 5th ed. Madrid: Paulinas 1980, 243-261.

--------, "Magisterio de la Iglesia y problemas éticos: discusiones actuales" *Razón y Fe* 213 [215] (1987) 371-381.

Lopez-García G, "La realidad del aborto espontaneo" in: Congresso Internazionale di Teologia Morale (Roma, 7-12 aprile 1986), **Persona, Verità e Morale.** Roma: Città Nuova 1987, 333-339.

Lorenz RP, Botti JJ, Schmidt CM, Ladda RL, "Encouraging patients to undergo prenatal genetic counseling before the day of amniocentesis: its effect on the use of amniocentesis" *Journal of Reproductive Medicine* 30,12 (1985) 933-935.

Lorenzetti L, "Etica e tecniche bio-mediche: criteri di lettura del documento <<Ratzinger>>" *Rivista di Teologia Morale* 74 (1987) 83-88.

--------, "Trasmissione della vita umana da un'etica della natura ad un'etica della persona" *Rivista di Teologia Morale* 71 (1986) 117-129.

Lustiger J-M, "L'homme sans fin: ou le redoutable paradoxe de la culture contemporaine" *Études* 359,4 (1983) 293-301.

MacDonald D, "Prenatal diagnosis: situating the ethical questions" in: Reidy M, ed, **Ethical Issues in Reproductive Medicine.** Dublin: Gill and MacMillan 1982, 4-11.

Maguire DC, "Abortion: a question of Catholic Honesty" *Christian Century* 100,26 (1983) 803-807.

Mahony R, "The magisterium and theological dissent" in: Curran CE, McCormick RA eds, **Readings in Moral Theology No. 6: Dissent in the Church.** Mahwah, New Jersey: Paulist 1988, 164-175.

Makin S, "Aquinas, natural tendencies and natural kinds" *New Scholasticism* 63 (1989) 253-274.

Malherbe J-F, "The personal status of the human embryo: a philosophical essay on eugenic abortion" in: Malherbe J-F, ed, **Human Life: Its Beginnings and Development.** Paris: L'Harmattan 1988, 101-116.

Malone R, "Magisterium and dissent" in: AA VV, **Attualità della Teologia Morale: Punti Fermi - Problemi Aperti.** Roma: Urbaniana 1987, 211-229.

Manno AG, "Essere umano dal concepimento" *Rivista di Teologia Morale* 97 (1993) 89-95.

Marlè R, "La question du pluralisme en theologie" *Gregorianum* 71 (1990) 465-486.

Marmion P, "The California alpha-fetoprotein screening program: an advocacy program for handicapped children" *Linacre Quarterly* 54,1 (1987) 77-87.

Marra B, "L'embrione e la sua natura" *Sapientia* 46 (1993) 87-89.

Mattai G, "Le difficoltà della morale cattolica" *Rivista di Teologia Morale* 84 (1989) 49-53.

Mattei J-F, "The use of prenatal diagnosis for psychiatric diseases" in: Srám RJ, Bulyzhenkov V, Prilipko L, Christen Y, eds, **Ethical Issues of Molecular Genetics in Psychiatry**. New York: Springer-Verlag 1991, 87-93.

Mayaud P-N, "Une histoire de la matière" *Études* 353,1 (1980) 5-21.

McDermott JM, "Metaphysical conundrums at the root of moral disagreement" *Gregorianum* 71 (1990) 713-742.

McKim R, Simpson P, "On the alleged incoherence of consequentialism" *New Scholasticism* 62 (1988) 349-352.

McKinney RH, "The quest for an adequate proportionalist theory of value" *The Thomist* 53 (1989) 56-73.

Millard CE, "The effects of modern therapeutics on the human gene pool" *Rhode Island Medical Journal* 63,11 (1980) 443-450.

Modell B, "The ethics of prenatal diagnosis and genetic counselling" *World Health Forum* 11,2 (1990) 179-186.

Murray TH, "Ethical issues in human genome research" *FASEB Journal* 5,1 (1991) 55-60.

National Society of Genetic Counselors, "Code of Ethics" *Journal of Genetic Counseling* 1,1 (1992) 41-43.

Nilson J, "The rights and responsibilities of theologians: a theological perspective" in: Curran CE, McCormick RA, eds, **Readings in Moral Theology No. 6: Dissent in the Church**. Mahwah, New Jersey: Paulist 1988, 5-34.

Noia G, Masini L, De Santis M, Di Lieto MP, Trivellini C, Bianchi A, Caruso A, Mancuso S, "La cordocentesi: indicazioni, utilità e rischi" *Medicina e Morale* 4 (1991) 625-640.

Novak M, "Dissent in the Church" in: Curran CE, McCormick RA, eds, **Readings in Moral Theology No. 6: Dissent in the Church.**

Mahwah, New Jersey: Paulist 1988, 112-126.

O'Neil R, "Determining proxy consent" *Journal of Medicine and Philosophy* 8 (1983) 389-403.

O'Reilly S, "The ethics of genetic counseling" *Acta Geneticae Medicae Gemellologiae* 23 (1974) 207-210.

Orkin SH, Williams DA, "Gene therapy of somatic cells: status and prospects" in: Childs B *et al*, eds, **Molecular Genetics in Medicine (Progress in Medical Genetics**, vol 7). New York: Elserier 1988, 130-142.

Ost DE, "The 'right' not to know" *Journal of Medicine and Philosophy* 9 (1984) 301-312.

Overall C, "Selective termination of pregnancy and women's reproductive autonomy" *Hastings Center Report* 20,3 (1990) 6-11.

Paoletti RA, "Developmental-genetic and psycho-social positions regarding the ontological status of the fetus" *Linacre Quarterly* 44 (1977) 243-261.

Pascali VL, Bottone E, Fiori A, "Problemi bioetici, deontologici e medico-legali della medicina perinatale" *Medicina e Morale* 42,1 (1992) 43-57.

Pellegrino ED, Thomasma DC, "The role of physicians, families, and other surrogates in decisions concerning incompetent patients" in: their **For the Patient's Good: The Restoration of Beneficence in Health Care.** New York: Oxford UP 1988, 162-171.

Pilarczyk D, "Dissent in the Church" in: Curran CE, McCormick RA, eds, **Readings in Moral Theology No. 6: Dissent in the Church.** Mahwah, New Jersey: Paulist 1988, 152-163.

Possenti V, "La bioetica alla ricerca dei principi: la persona" *Medicina e Morale* 42,6 (1992) 1075-1094.

Privitera S, "Per una interpretazione del dibattito su 'L'autonomia morale'" *Rivista di Teologia Morale* 48 (1980) 565-586.

--------, "Riflessioni sullo status morale e giuridico dell'embrione" *Rivista di Teologia Morale* 89 (1991) 93-100.

--------, "Sul processo individuativo della norma morale" *Rivista di Teologia Morale* 23 (1974) 461-475.

Quay PM, "The disvalue of ontic evil" *Theological Studies* 46 (1985) 262-286.

Rapp R, "The power of 'positive' diagnosis: medical and maternal discourses on amniocentesis" in: Michaelson KL, ed, **Childbirth in America: Anthropological Perspectives.** South Hadley, MA: Bergin and Garvey

1988, 103-116.

Ratzinger Card. J, "Panorama de la théologie dans le monde" *La Documentation Catholique* 82 (May 5, 1985) 505-512.

Redwine FO, Hays PM, "Selective birth" *Seminars in Perinatology* 10,1 (1986) 73-81.

Regan A, "The human conceptus and personhood" *Studia Moralia* 30 (1992) 97-127.

Ricard K, "Une révolution en biologie: a propos du code génétique" *Études* 364,3 (1986) 355-366.

Rice CE, "Amniocentesis, coercion, and privacy" in: Nelson LJ, ed, **The Death Decision**. Ann Arbor, MI: Servant 1984, 57-68.

Rice N, Doherty R, "Reflections on prenatal diagnosis: the consumers' views" *Social Work in Health Care* 8,1 (1982) 47-57.

Richards MPM, "Social and ethical problems of fetal diagnosis and screening" *Journal of Reproductive and Infant Psychology* 7,3 (1989) 171-185.

Rincón Orduña R, "Introducción a la ética teológica especial" in: López Azpitarte E, Elizari Basterra FJ, Rincón Orduña R, eds, **Praxis Cristiana II: Opción por la Vida y el Amor**. 3ra ed. Madrid: Paulinas 1981, 11-47.

Rioja A, "La filosofía de la complementariedad y la descripción objetiva de la naturaleza" *Revista de Filosofía* 5,8 (1992) 257-282.

Riou G, "Les défis de l'environnement: seuils, limites et irréversibilité" *Études* 355,7 (1981) 43-58.

Robertson JA, "Ethical and legal issues in preimplantation genetic screening" *Fertility and Sterility* 51,1 (1992) 1-11.

--------, Schulman JD, "Pregnancy and prenatal harm to offspring: the case of mothers with PKU" *Hastings Center Report* 17,4 (1987) 23-33.

Rodeck CH, Nicolaides KH, "Fetal tissue biopsy: techniques and indications" *Fetal Therapy* 1,1 (1986) 46-58.

Rollin R, "L'éthique de la procréation à travers trois documents" *Lumière et Vie* 37,187 (1988) 67-89.

Ron M, Anteby S, Diamant YZ, Polishuk WZ, "Prenatal distress following amniocentesis" *International Journal of Gynaecology and Obstetrics* 12,5 (1974) 172-175.

Ropers H-H, Wieringa B, "The recombinant DNA revolution: implications for diagnosis and prevention of inherited disease" *European Journal of Obstetrics & Gynecology and Reproductive Biology* 32 (1989) 15-27.

Rossi L, "'Diretto' e 'indiretto' in teologia morale" *Rivista di Teologia Morale* 9 (1971) 37-65.

--------, "Il limite del principio del duplice effetto" *Rivista di Teologia Morale* 13 (1972) 11-37.

Royal College of Physicians, "Prenatal diagnosis and genetic screening: community and service implications" *Journal of the Royal College of Physicians of London* 23,4 (1989) 215-220.

Rubio M, "El esquema antropológico subyacente en la Instrucción 'Donum vitae'" *Moralia* 9 (1987) 283-296.

--------, "El método en el discurso teológico-ético de la Instrucción 'Donum vitae'" *Moralia* 9 (1987) 251-263.

Russe M, "Genetics and the quality of life" *Social Indicators Research* 7,1-4 (1980) 419-441.

Russo F, "L'evolution: une théorie en crise" *Études* 370,3 (1989) 345-350.

Sanchíz A, "Magisterio y teologos ante el reto de la nueva cultura" *Escritos del Vedat* 17 (1987) 127-142.

Santurri EN, "Prenatal diagnosis: some moral considerations" in: Schneider ED, ed, **Questions about the Beginning of Life: Christian Appraisals of Seven Bioethical Issues.** Minneapolis, MN: Augsburg 1985, 120-150.

Sarto GE, "Ethical and legal considerations of antenatal diagnosis" *Clinics in Obstetrics and Gynaecology* 7,1 (1980) 135-141.

Schönborn C, "L'homme créé par Dieu: le fondement de la dignité de l'homme" *Gregorianum* 65 (1984) 337-363.

Schüller B, "Direct killing/indirect killing" in: Curran CE, McCormick RA, eds, **Readings in Moral Theology No. 1: Moral Norms and Catholic Tradition.** New York: Paulist 1979, 138-157.

--------, "The double effect in Catholic thought: a reevaluation" in: McCormick RA, Ramsey P, eds, **Doing Evil to Achieve Good: Moral Choice in Conflict Situations.** Chicago: Loyola 1978, 165-192.

--------, "Various types of grounding for ethical norms" in: Curran CE, McCormick RA, eds, **Readings in Moral Theology No. 1: Moral Norms and Catholic Tradition.** New York: Paulist 1979, 184-198.

Seals BF, Ekwo EE, Williamson RA, Hanson JW, "Moral and religious influences on the amniocentesis decision" *Social Biology* 32,1-2 (1985) 13-30.

Seller MJ, "Ethical aspects of genetic counselling" *Journal of Medical Ethics* 8 (1982) 185-188.

Serra A, "Aborto eugenico: diritto-dovere o delitto?" *La Civiltà Cattolica* 124,4 (1973) 110-124.

--------, "Embrione umano, scienza e medicina: in margine al recente documento" *La Civiltà Cattolica* 138,2 (1987) 247-261.

--------, "La 'nuova genetica': attualità, prospettive, problemi" in: Serra A, Santosuosso F, Bompiani A, Manni C, Cotta S, eds, **Medicina e Genetica Verso il Futuro**. L'Aquila-Roma: Japadre 1986, 5-23.

--------, "La diagnosi prenatale di malattie genetiche" *Medicina e Morale* 34,4 (1984) 433-448.

--------, "La realtà biologica del neo-concepito" *La Civiltà Cattolica* 126,3 (1975) 9-23.

--------, "La sperimentazione sull'embrione umano: una nuova esigenza della scienza e della medicina?" *Medicina e Morale* 43 (1993) 97-116.

--------, "Per un'analisi integrata dello 'status' dell'embrione umano. Alcuni dati della genetica e dell'embriologia" in: Biolo S, ed, **Nascita e Morte dell'Uomo**. Atti del 46 Convegno del Centro Studi Filosofici di Gallarate, Genova: Marietti 1993, 55-106.

--------, "Quando comincia un essre umano. In margine ad un recente documento" *Medicina e Morale* 37,3 (1987) 387-401.

--------, "Transcultural problems in the use of medical genetics in clinical practice" in: Srám RJ, Bulyzhenkov V, Prilipko L, Christen Y, eds, **Ethical Issues of Molecular Genetics in Psychiatry**. New York: Springer-Verlag 1991, 120-130.

Sgreccia E, "A proposito del 'pre-embrione' umano" *Medicina e Morale* 36,1 (1986) 5-17.

--------, "Ethical issues in prenatal diagnosis and fetal therapy" *Fetal Therapy* 4,suppl 1 (1989) 16-27.

--------, "La diagnosi prenatale" in: Congresso Internazionale di Teologia Morale (Roma, 7-12 aprile 1986), **Persona, Verità e Morale**. Roma: Città Nuova 1987, 315-331.

Simpson JL, Carson SA, "Preimplantation genetic diagnosis" *The New England Journal of Medicine* 327,13 (1992) 951-953.

Smith DJ, "Down's syndrome, amniocentesis, and abortion: prevention or elimination?" *Mental Retardation* 19,1 (1981) 8-11.

Smith PA, "The beginning of personhood: a thomistic perpective" *Laval Philosophique et Théologique* 39,2 (1983) 195-214.

Smurl JF, Weaver DD, Jarmas A, Padilla L-M, "Ethical considerations in medical genetics: the prenatal diagnosis of Hemophilia B" *American Journal of Medical Genetics* 17,4 (1984) 773-781.

Spagnolo AG, Di Pietro ML. "Feto a rischio per iperplasia surrenalica congenita: Quali i limiti etici della diagnosi e della terapia fetali?" *Medicina e Morale* 4 (1990) 759-778.

Spinsanti S, "La diagnostica prenatale" in: Goffi T, Piana G, eds, **Corso di Morale II: Diakonia (Etica della Persona)**. Brescia: Queriniana 1983, 212-216.

--------, "La normatività etica nel campo bio-medico" in: Goffi T, Piana G, eds, **Corso di Morale II: Diakonia (Etica della Persona)**. Brescia: Queriniana 1983, 127-175.

--------, "La tutela della vita" in: Goffi T, Piana G, eds, **Corso di Morale II: Diakonia (Etica della Persona)**. Brescia: Queriniana 1983, 198-219.

Steinbrook R, "In California, voluntary mass prenatal screening" *Hastings Center Report* 16,5 (1986) 5-7.

Still K, Kolatat T, et al, "Early third trimester selective feticide of a compromising twin" *Fetal Therapy* 4 (1989) 83-87.

Strasser M, "Mill and the right to remain uninformed" *Journal of Medicine and Philosophy* 11 (1986) 265-278.

Suarez A, "Hydatidiform moles and teratomas confirm the human identity of the preimplantation embryo" *Journal of Medicine and Philosophy* 15 (1990) 627-635.

Sullivan FA, "The authority of the magisterium on questions of natural moral law" in: Curran CE, McCormick RA, eds, **Readings in Moral Theology No. 6: Dissent in the Church**. Mahwah, New Jersey: Paulist 1988, 42-57.

Swint JM, Kaback MM, "Intervention against genetic disease: economic and ethical considerations" in: Agich GJ, Begley CE, eds, **The Price of Health**. Boston: D. Reidel 1986, 135-156.

Tauer CA, "Personhood and human embryos and fetuses" *Journal of Medicine and Philosophy* 10 (1985) 253-266.

--------, "The tradition of probabilism and the moral status of the early embryo" *Theological Studies* 45 (1984) 3-33.

Testa B, "La funzione del magistero ordinario nell'elaborazione teologica" *Anthropotes* 7 (1991) 67-82.

Tettamanzi D, "Problemi morali circa alcuni interventi sui feti/embrioni umani" *Medicina e Morale* 35,1 (1985) 23-43.

Theron S, "Consequentionalism and natural law" in: Congresso Internazionale di Teologia Morale (Roma, 7-12 aprile 1986), **Persona, Verità e Morale.** Roma: Città Nuova 1987, 177-193.

Thévenot X, "La compassion: une réponse au mal?" *Le Supplement* 172 (1990) 79-96.

--------, "Magistère et discernement moral" *Études* 362 (1985) 231-244.

Thévoz J-M, "Une recherche interdisciplinaire: la bioéthique" *Revue de Théologie et de Philosophie* 118 (1986) 67-79.

Tonti-Filippini N, "A critical note" *Linacre Quarterly* 56,3 (1989) 36-50.

Tormey JF, "Ethical considerations of prenatal genetic diagnosis" *Clinical Obstetrics and Gynecology* 19,4 (1976) 957-963.

Tymstra T, "Prenatal diagnosis, prenatal screening, and the rise of the tentative pregnancy" *International Journal of Technology Assessment in Health Care* 7,4 (1991) 509-516.

Vacek EV, "Proportionalism: one view of the debate" *Theological Studies* 46 (1985) 287-314.

Verp MS, Bombard AT, Simpson JK, Elias S, "Parental decision following prenatal diagnosis of fetal chromosome abnormality" *American Journal of Medical Genetics* 29,3 (1988) 613-622.

Verspieren P, "Prenatal diagnosis and selective abortion: an ethical issue" in: Malherbe J-F, ed, **Human Life: Its Beginnings and Development.** Paris: L'Harmattan 1988, 197-216.

--------, "Sur la pente de l'euthanasie" *Études* 360,1 (1984) 43-54.

--------, "Un droit à l'enfant?" *Études* 362,5 (1985) 623-628.

--------, ed, **Biologie, Médicine et Éthique,** *Les Dossiers de la Documentation Catholique*. Paris: Centurion 1987, especially 13-216.

Vidal M, "La 'razón eugenésica': exposición y valoración" *Moralia* 9 (1987) 327-340.

--------, "¿Existe el 'derecho a procrear'?" *Moralia* 9 (1987) 39-50.

--------, "Referencias al magisterio eclesiástico en la Instrucción 'Donum vitae'" *Moralia* 9 (1987) 265-281.

Walgrave JH, "Personalisme et anthropologie chrétienne" *Gregorianum* 65 (1984) 445-472.

Watkins D, "An alternative to termination of pregnancy" *The Practitioner* 233 (1989) 990-992.

Wertz DC, Fletcher JC, "Ethics and medical genetics in the United States: a national survey" *American Journal of Medical Genetics* 29,4 (1988) 815-827.

--------, Fletcher JC, "Fatal knowledge? Prenatal diagnosis and sexual selection" *Hastings Center Report* 19,3 (1989) 21-27.

--------, Sorenson JR, "Client reactions to genetic counseling: self-report of influence" *Clinical Genetics* 30,6 (1986) 494-502.

--------, Sorenson JR, Heeren TC, "Clients' interpretation of risks provided in genetic counseling" *American Journal of Human Genetics* 39,2 (1986) 253-264.

--------, Sorenson JR, Heeren TC, "Genetic counseling and reproductive uncertainty" *American Journal of Medical Genetics* 18,1 (1984) 79-88.

West R, "Ethical aspects of genetic disease and genetic counselling" *Journal of Medical Ethics* 14 (1988) 194-197.

Wolbert W, "La confusione tra parenesi ed etica normativa" *Rivista di Teologia Morale* 50 (1981) 227-236.687.

--------, "Parenesi ed etica normativa" *Rivista di Teologia Morale* 49 (1981) 11-39.

Yanguas JM, "Experimentación con embriones humanos" in: Congresso Internazionale di Teologia Morale (Roma, 7-12 aprile 1986), **Persona, Verità e Morale**. Roma: Città Nuova 1987, 109-121.

Zatti M, "Quando un 'pre-embrione' esiste, si tratta di un altro embrione" *Medicina e Morale* 5 (1991) 781-788.

[no author], "Ethical problems as prenatal diagnosis improves" *Obstetrics and Gynecology News* 19,12 (1984) 16.

III. BIO-MEDICAL LITERATURE

BOOKS

Berg K, ed, **Medical Genetics: Past, Present, Future**. New York: Alan R. Liss 1985.

--------, Tranoy KE, eds, **Research Ethics**. New York: Alan R. Liss 1983.

Chapman M, Grudzinskas G, Chard T, eds, **The Embryo. Normal and Abnormal Development and Growth**. London: Springer-Verlag 1991.

Cherry SH, **Understanding Pregnancy and Childbirth**. Indianapolis-New York: Bobbs-Merrill 1973.

Creasy RK, Resnik R, eds, **Maternal-Fetal Medicine: Principles and Practice**, 2nd ed. Philadelphia: Saunders 1989.

Elias S, Annas GJ, **Reproductive Genetics and the Law**. Chicago: Year Book Medical Publishers 1987.

Emery AEH, Rimoin DL, eds, **Principles and Practice of Medical Genetics**, 2nd ed. vols. I and II. New York: Churchill Livingstone 1990.

England MA, **Color Atlas of Life Before Birth: Normal Fetal Development**. Chicago: Year Book Medical Publishers 1990.

Evans MI, Dixler AO, Fletcher JC, Schulman JD, eds, **Fetal Diagnosis and Therapy: Science, Ethics and the Law**. Philadelphia: Lippincott 1989.

Gasser RF, **Atlas of Human Embryos**. Hagerstown, MD: Harper and Row 1975.

Haseltine FP, McClure ME, Goldberg EH, eds, **Genetic Markers of Sex Differentiation**. New York: Plenum 1987.

Johnson KE, **Human Developmental Anatomy**. New York: Wiley 1988.

Malherbe J-F, ed, **Human Life: its Beginnings and Development**. Paris: L'Harmattan 1988.

Mange AP, Mange EJ, **Genetics: Human Aspects**, 2nd ed. Sunderland, MA: Sinauer Associates 1990.

Moore KL, **The Developing Human: Clinically Oriented Embryology**, 4th ed. Philadelphia: Saunders 1988.

Nau H, Scott Jr WJ, eds, **Pharmacokinetics in Teratogenesis: Interspecies Comparison and Maternal/Embryonic-Fetal Drug Transfer**. Boca

Raton, FL: CRC 1987.

Nishimura H, ed, **Atlas of Human Prenatal Histology**, 1st ed. Tokyo-New York: Igaku-Shoin 1983.

Nora JJ, Fraser FC, **Medical Genetics: Principles and Practice**, 3rd ed. Philadelphia: Lea and Febiger 1989.

Romero R, Pilu G, Jeanty P, Ghidini A, Hobbins JC, **Prenatal Diagnosis of Congenital Anomalies**. Norwalk, CT: Appleton and Lange 1988.

Sadler TW, **Langman's Medical Embryology**, 5th ed. Baltimore: Williams and Wilkins 1985.

Sever JL, Brent RL, eds, **Teratogen Update: Environmentally Induced Birth Defect Risks**. New York: Liss 1986.

Shostak S, **Embryology: An Introduction to Developmental Biology**. New York: HarperCollins 1991.

Stedman's **Medical Dictionary**, 25th ed. Baltimore-Hong Kong-London-Sydney: Williams and Wilkins 1990.

Sutton HE, **An Introduction to Human Genetics**, 2nd ed. New York: Holt, Rinehart and Winston 1975.

Vogel F, Motulsky AG. **Human Genetics: Problems and Approaches**, 2nd ed. Berlin-Heidelberg: Springer-Verlag 1986.

Weaver RF, Hedrick PW, **Genetics**. Dubuque, IA: Brown 1989.

Whittle MJ, Connor JM, eds, **Prenatal Diagnosis in Obstetric Practice**. London: Blackwell 1989.

Wilson JG, **Environment and Birth Defects**. New York: Academic 1973.

--------, Fraser FC, eds, **Handbook of Teratology: Comparative, Maternal, and Epidemiologic Aspects**. New York: Plenum 1977.

Zuspan FP, Quilligan EJ, Iams JD, eds, **Manual of Obstetrics and Gynecology**, 2nd ed. St. Louis, MO: C.V. Mosby 1990.

ARTICLES

Abel EL, Sokol RJ, "Alcohol" in: Evans MI, Dixler AO, Fletcher JC, Schulman JD, eds, **Fetal Diagnosis and Therapy: Science, Ethics and the Law**. Philadelphia: Lippincott 1989, 140-149.

Adam C, Allen AC, Baskett TF, "Twin delivery: influence of the presentation and method of delivery on the second twin" *American Journal of Obstetrics and*

Gynecology 165 (1991) 23-27.

Anderson RL, Golbus MS, "Chemical teratogens" in: Evans MI, Dixler AO, Fletcher JC, Schulman JD, eds, **Fetal Diagnosis and Therapy: Science, Ethics and the Law**. Philadelphia: Lippincott 1989, 114-139.

Anderson WF, "Gene therapy" in: Evans MI, Dixler AO, Fletcher JC, Schulman JD, eds, **Fetal Diagnosis and Therapy: Science, Ethics and the Law**. Philadelphia: Lippincott 1989, 421-430.

Australian Research Commission, *Human Embryo Experimentation in Australia*, Senate Select Committee on Human Experimentation Bill, Australian Government Printing Office, 1985.

Balducci J, Rodis JF, Rosengren S, Vintzileos AM, Spivey G, Vosseller C, "Pregnancy outcome following first-trimester varicella infection" *Obstetrics and Gynecology* 79 (1992) 5-6.

Baumann P, Jovanovic V, Gellert G, Rauskolb R, "Risk of miscarriage after transcervical and transabdominal CVS in relation to bacterial colonization of the cervix" *Prenatal Diagnosis* 11 (1991) 551-557.

Beck F, Lloyd JB, "Comparative placental transfer" in: Wilson JG, Fraser FC, eds, **Handbook of Teratology: Comparative, Maternal, and Epidemiologic Aspects**. New York: Plenum 1977, 155-186.

Beeson JH, "Controversies surrounding antepartum Rh immune globulin prophylaxis" in: Evans MI, Dixler AO, Fletcher JC, Schulman JD, eds, **Fetal Diagnosis and Therapy: Science, Ethics and the Law**. Philadelphia: Lippincott 1989, 172-180.

Benacerraf BR, Gelman R, Frigoletto Jr. FD, "Sonographic identification of second-trimester fetuses with Down's syndrome" *New England Journal of Medicine* 317,22 (1987) 1371-1376.

Biddle FG, Fraser FC, "Maternal and cytoplasmic effects in experimental teratology" in: Wilson JG, Fraser FC, eds, **Handbook of Teratology: Comparative, Maternal, and Epidemiologic Aspects**. New York: Plenum 1977, 3-33.

Brent RL, "Radiation teratogenesis" in: Sever JL, Brent RL, eds, **Teratogen Update: Environmentally Induced Birth Defect Risks**. New York: Liss 1986, 145-163.

Bronshtein M, Mashiah N, Blumenfeld I, Blumenfeld Z, "Pseudoprognathism: an auxiliary ultrasonographic sign for transvaginal ultrasonographic diagnosis of cleft lip and palate in the early second trimester" *American Journal of Obstetrics and Gynecology* 165 (1991) 1314-1316.

Carr DH, "Detection and evaluation of pregnancy wastage" in: Wilson JG, Fraser

FC, eds, **Handbook of Teratology: Comparative, Maternal, and Epidemiologic Aspects**. New York: Plenum 1977, 189-213.

Charrow J, Nadler HL, "Prenatal diagnosis" in: Emery AEH, Rimoin DL, eds, **Principles and Practice of Medical Genetics**, 2nd ed. vol. II. New York: Churchill Livingstone 1990, 1458-1480.

Chervenak FA, Isaacson G, "Ultrasound detection of fetal anomalies" in: Evans MI, Dixler AO, Fletcher JC, Schulman JD, eds, **Fetal Diagnosis and Therapy: Science, Ethics and the Law**. Philadelphia: Lippincott 1989, 60-71.

Cohlan SQ, "Tetracycline staining of teeth" in: Sever JL, Brent RL, eds, **Teratogen Update: Environmentally Induced Birth Defect Risks**. New York: Liss 1986, 51-52.

Copel JA, Kleinman CS, "Diagnosis and management of fetal heart disease" in: Evans MI, Dixler AO, Fletcher JC, Schulman JD, eds, **Fetal Diagnosis and Therapy: Science, Ethics and the Law**. Philadelphia: Lippincott 1989, 412-421.

Copeland LJ, "Trophoblastic disease" in: Zuspan FP, Iams JD, eds, **Zuspan and Quilligan's Manual of Obstetrics and Gynecology**, 2nd ed. St. Louis, MO: Mosby 1990, 415-421.

Coutelle C, Williams C, Handyside A, Hardy K, Winston R, Williamson R, "Genetic analysis of DNA from single human oocytes: a model for preimplantation diagnosis of cystic fibrosis" *British Medical Journal* 299,6690 (1989) 22-24.

Crandall BF, Robinson L, Grau P, "Risks associated with an elevated maternal serum alpha-fetoprotein level" *American Journal of Obstetrics and Gynecology* 165 (1991) 581-586.

Cullen MT, Whetham J, Viscarello RR, Reece EA, Sanchez-Ramos L, Hobbins JC, "Transcervical endoscopic verification of congenital anomalies in the second trimester of pregnancy" *American Journal of Obstetrics and Gynecology* 165 (1991) 95-97.

D'Amelio R, Giorlandino C, Masala L, Garofalo M, Martinelli M, Anelli G, Zichella L, "Fetal echocardiography using transvaginal and transabdominal probes during the first period of pregnancy: a comparative study" *Prenatal Diagnosis* 11 (1991) 69-75.

De Paepe A, De Bie S, "Genetic counseling of a couple presenting respectively terminal transverse defects and congenital arthrogryposis" *Genetic Counseling* 2 (1991) 195-203.

Dekker GA, Sibai BM, "Early detection of preeclampsia" *American Journal of Obstetrics and Gynecology* 165 (1991) 160-172.

Dencker L, Danielsson BRG, "Transfer of drugs to the embryo and fetus after placentation" in: Nau H, Scott Jr. WJ, eds, **Pharmacokinetics in Teratogenesis: Interspecies Comparison and Maternal/Embryonic-Fetal Drug Transfer**. Boca Raton, FL: CRC 1987, 55-69.

Dolkart LA, Reimers FT, "Transvaginal fetal echocardiography in early pregnancy: normative data" *American Journal of Obstetrics and Gynecology* 165 (1991) 688-691.

Donnenfeld AE, Van de Woestijne J, Craparo F, Smith CS, Ludomirsky A, Weiner S, "The normal fetus of an acardiac twin pregnancy: perinatal management based on echocardiographic and sonographic evaluation" *Prenatal Diagnosis* 11 (1991) 235-244.

Doran TA, "Chorionic villus sampling as the primary diagnostic tool in prenatal diagnosis: should it replace genetic amniocentesis?" *Journal of Reproductive Medicine* 35,10 (1990) 935-940.

Drugan A, Timor-Tritsch IE, "Transvaginal ultrasonography" in: Evans MI, Dixler AO, Fletcher JC, Schulman JD, eds, **Fetal Diagnosis and Therapy: Science, Ethics and the Law**. Philadelphia: Lippincott 1989, 71-83.

Elias S, Gerbie AB, Simpson JL, Nadler HL, Sabbagha RE, Shkolnik A, "Genetic amniocentesis in twin gestations" *American Journal of Obstetrics and Gynecology* 138,2 (1980) 169-174.

Evans MI, Belsky RL, Greb A, Clementino N, Syner FN, "Alpha-fetoprotein: maternal serum and amniotic fluid analysis" in: Evans MI, Dixler AO, Fletcher JC, Schulman JD, eds, **Fetal Diagnosis and Therapy: Science, Ethics and the Law**. Philadelphia: Lippincott 1989, 44-60.

Evans MI, Bronsteen RA, "Multiple gestation" in: Evans MI, Dixler AO, Fletcher JC, Schulman JD, eds, **Fetal Diagnosis and Therapy: Science, Ethics and the Law**. Philadelphia: Lippincott 1989, 242-266.

Evans MI, Chrousos GP, Mann DW *et al*, "Pharmacologic suppression of the fetal adrenal gland *in utero*: attempted prevention of abnormal external masculinization in suspected congenital adrenal hyperplasia" *Journal of the American Medical Association* 253 (1985) 1015.

Evans MI, Quigg MH, Koppitch III FC, Schulman JD, "First trimester prenatal diagnosis" in: Evans MI, Dixler AO, Fletcher JC, Schulman JD, eds, **Fetal Diagnosis and Therapy: Science, Ethics and the Law**. Philadelphia: Lippincott 1989, 17-36.

Evans MI, Schulman JD, "Medical fetal therapy" in: Evans MI, Dixler AO, Fletcher JC, Schulman JD, eds, **Fetal Diagnosis and Therapy: Science, Ethics and the Law**. Philadelphia: Lippincott 1989, 403-412.

Fedele L, Dorta M, Brioschi D, Giudici MN, Candiani GB, "Magnetic resonance imaging in Mayer-Rokitansky-Küster-Hauser syndrome" *Obstetrics and Gynecology* 76 (1990) 593-596.

Ford N, "Letters: ethics, science, and embryos" *Tablet* February 3 (1990) 141-142.

Foulon W, Naessens A, Mahler T, De Waele M, De Catte L, De Meuter F, "Prenatal diagnosis of congenital toxoplasmosis" *Obstetrics and Gynecology* 76 (1990) 769-772.

Fowler MG, Kleinman JC, Kiely JL, Kessel SS, "Double jeopardy: twin infant mortality in the United States, 1983 and 1984" *American Journal of Obstetrics and Gynecology* 165 (1991) 15-22.

Fuccillo DA, "Congenital varicella" in: Sever JL, Brent RL, eds, **Teratogen Update: Environmentally Induced Birth Defect Risks**. New York: Liss 1986, 101-105.

Garden AS, Griffiths RD, Weindling AM, Martin PA, "Fast-scan magnetic resonance imaging in fetal visualization" *American Journal of Obstetrics and Gynecology* 164 (1991) 1190-1196.

Glass RH, "Sperm and egg transport, fertilization, and implantation" in: Creasy RK, Resnik R, eds, **Maternal-Fetal Medicine: Principles and Practice**, 2nd ed. Philadelphia: Saunders 1989, 108-115.

Goldman AS, Zackai EH, Yaffe SJ, "Fetal trimethadione syndrome" in: Sever JL, Brent RL, eds, **Teratogen Update: Environmentally Induced Birth Defect Risks**. New York: Liss 1986, 35-38.

Goldstein SR, "Embryonic ultrasonographic measurements: crown-rump length revisited" *American Journal of Obstetrics and Gynecology* 165 (1991) 497-501.

Goodfellow PN, Goodfellow PJ, Pym B, Banting G, Pritchard C, Darling SM, "Genes on the human Y chromosome" in: Haseltine FP, McClure ME, Goldberg EH, eds, **Genetic Markers of Sex Differentiation**. New York: Plenum 1987, 99-111.

Greenberg F, Del Junco D, Weyland B, Faucett WA, Schmidt D, Rose E, Alpert E, "The effect of gestational age on the detection rate of Down's syndrome by maternal serum alpha-fetoprotein screening" *American Journal of Obstetrics and Gynecology* 165 (1991) 1391-1393.

Grossman III JH, "Congenital syphilis" in: Sever JL, Brent RL, eds, **Teratogen Update: Environmentally Induced Birth Defect Risks**. New York: Liss 1986, 113-117.

Haddow JE, Holman MS, Palomaki GE, "Can gestational dates routinely derived from very early ultrasound be used to interpret maternal serum alpha-fetoprotein measurements?" *Prenatal Diagnosis* 12 (1992) 65-68.

Handyside AH, "Preimplantation diagnosis by DNA amplification" in: Chapman M, Grudzinskas G, Chard T, eds, **The Embryo. Normal and Abnormal Development and Growth.** London: Springer-Verlag 1991, 81-90.

--------, Kontogianni EH, Hardy K, Winston RML, "Pregnancies from biopsied human preimplantation embryos sexed by Y-specific DNA amplification" *Nature* 344,6268 (1990) 768-770.

--------, Lesko JG, Tarín JJ, Winston RML, Hughes MR, "Birth of a normal girl after *in vitro* fertilization and preimplantation diagnostic testing for cystic fibrosis" *New England Journal of Medicine* 327,13 (1992) 905-909.

--------, Penketh RJA, Winston RML, Pattinson JK, Delhanty JDA, Tuddenham EGD, "Biopsy of human preimplantation embryos and sexing by DNA amplification" *Lancet* 8634 (1989) 347-349.

Hanson JW, "Fetal hydantoin effects" in: Sever JL, Brent RL, eds, **Teratogen Update: Environmentally Induced Birth Defect Risks.** New York: Liss 1986, 29-33.

Hendren H, Lillehi C, "Pediatric surgery" *New England Journal of Medicine* 319,2 (1988) 89-96.

Herzog TJ, Angel OH, Darram MM, Evertson LR, "Use of magnetic resonance imaging in the diagnosis of cortical blindness in pregnancy" *Obstetrics and Gynecology* 76 (1990) 980-982.

Hogge WA, Golbus MS, "Surgical management of fetal malformations" in: Evans MI, Dixler AO, Fletcher JC, Schulman JD, eds, **Fetal Diagnosis and Therapy: Science, Ethics and the Law.** Philadelphia: Lippincott 1989, 395-403.

Huarte J, "Concepts fondamentaux d'embryologie" *L'Embryon: Un Homme: Actes du Congrès de Lausanne* 1986, Premier Congrès de la Société Suisse de Bioéthique 8 et 9 novembre 1986, Lausanne: Centre de documentation civique 1987.

Jauniaux E, Jurkovic D, Campbell S, Kurjak A, Hustin J, "Investigation of placental circulations by color Doppler ultrasonography" *American Journal of Obstetrics and Gynecology* 164 (1991) 486-488.

Kaaja R, Julkunen H, Ämmälä P, Teppo A-M, Kurki P, "Congenital heart block: successful prophylactic treatment with intravenous gamma globulin and corticosteroid therapy" *American Journal of Obstetrics and Gynecology* 165 (1991) 1333-1334.

Kamoun PP, Chadefaux B, "Eleventh week amniocentesis for prenatal diagnosis of some metabolic diseases" *Prenatal Diagnosis* 11 (1991) 691-696.

Kofinas AD, Simon NV, Sagel H, Lyttle E, Smith N, King K, "Treatment of fetal supraventricular tachycardia with flecainide acetate after digoxin failure" *American Journal of Obstetrics and Gynecology* 165 (1991) 630-631.

Korones SB, "Congenital rubella: An encapsulated review" in: Sever JL, Brent RL, eds, **Teratogen Update: Environmentally Induced Birth Defect Risks**. New York: Liss 1986, 77-80.

Krauer B, "Physiological changes and drug disposition during pregnancy" in: Nau H, Scott Jr. WJ, eds, **Pharmacokinetics in Teratogenesis: Interspecies Comparison and Maternal/Embryonic-Fetal Drug Transfer**. Boca Raton, FL: CRC 1987, 3-12.

Larsen Jr. JW, "Congenital toxoplasmosis" in: Sever JL, Brent RL, eds, **Teratogen Update: Environmentally Induced Birth Defect Risks**. New York: Liss 1986, 97-100.

--------, MacMillin MD, "Second and third trimester prenatal diagnosis" in: Evans MI, Dixler AO, Fletcher JC, Schulman JD, eds, **Fetal Diagnosis and Therapy: Science, Ethics and the Law**. Philadelphia: Lippincott 1989, 36-43.

Letovsky S, Berlyn MB, "CPROP: A rule-based program for constructing genetic maps" *Genommics* 12 (1992) 435-446.

Lin C-C, "Medical considerations in obstetric management" in: Evans MI, Dixler AO, Fletcher JC, Schulman JD, eds, **Fetal Diagnosis and Therapy: Science, Ethics and the Law**. Philadelphia: Lippincott 1989, 199-233.

Lurie IW, Lazjuk GI, Korotkova IA, Cherstvoy ED, "The cerebro-reno-digital syndromes: a new community" *Clinical Genetics* 39 (1991) 104-113.

Lynch L, Daffos F, Emanuel D, Giovangrandi Y, Meisel R, Forestier F, Cathomas G, Berkowitz RL, "Prenatal diagnosis of fetal cytomegalovirus infection" *American Journal of Obstetrics and Gynecology* 165 (1991) 714-718.

Martikainen MA, "Effects of intrauterine growth retardation and its subtypes on the development of the preterm infant" *Early Human Development* 28 (1992) 7-17.

McBride G, "Preimplantation genetic diagnosis" *British Medical Journal* 301,6757 (1990) 894-895.

McCormack MF, Mackenzie WE, Rushton DI, Newton JR, "Clinical and pathological factors in spontaneous abortion following chorionic villus sampling" *Prenatal Diagnosis* 11 (1991) 841-846.

McLaren A, "Prenatal diagnosis before implantation: opportunities and problems"

Prenatal Diagnosis 5 (1985) 85-90.

Miller JR, Lowry RB, "Birth defects registries and surveillance" in: Wilson JG, Fraser FC, eds, **Handbook of Teratology: Comparative, Maternal, and Epidemiologic Aspects**. New York: Plenum 1977, 227-242.

Miller RW, Mulvihill JJ, "Small head size after atomic irradiation" in: Sever JL, Brent RL, eds, **Teratogen Update: Environmentally Induced Birth Defect Risks**. New York: Liss 1986, 141-143.

Mills JL, "Malformations in infants of diabetic mothers" in: Sever JL, Brent RL, eds, **Teratogen Update: Environmentally Induced Birth Defect Risks**. New York: Liss 1986, 165-176.

Mulvihill JJ, "Fetal alcohol syndrome" in: Sever JL, Brent RL, eds, **Teratogen Update: Environmentally Induced Birth Defect Risks**. New York: Liss 1986, 13-18.

Muraskas JK, Carlson NJ, Halsey C, Frederiksen MC, Sabbagha RE, "Survival of a 280-g infant" *New England Journal of Medicine* 324,22 (1991) 1598-1599.

Narod S, "Counselling under genetic heterogeneity: A practical approach" *Clinical Genetics* 39 (1991) 125-131.

Newman CGH, "Clinical aspects of thalidomide embryopathy: a continuing preoccupation" in: Sever JL, Brent RL, eds, **Teratogen Update: Environmentally Induced Birth Defect Risks**. New York: Liss 1986, 1-12.

Petit P, Moerman P, Fryns JP, "The fetal phenotype of partial trisomy of the long arm of chromosome 4 (4q22-4qter)" *Genetic Counseling* 2 (1991) 163-165.

Pridjian G, Nugent CE, Barr M, "Twin gestation: influence of placentation on fetal growth" *American Journal of Obstetrics and Gynecology* 165 (1991) 1394-1401.

Read AP, Donnai D, "Preimplantation diagnosis with the polymerase chain reaction: scientifically possible, not widely available" *British Medical Journal* 299,6690 (1989) 3.

Rebello TM, Gray CTH, Rooney DR, Smith JH, Hackett GA, Loeffler FE, Horwell DH, Beard RW, Coleman DV, "Cytogenetic studies of amniotic fluid taken before the 15th week of pregnancy for earlier prenatal diagnosis: a report of 114 consecutive cases" *Prenatal Diagnosis* 11 (1991) 35-40.

Report of the Committee of Inquiry into Human Fertilisation and Embryology of the Department of Health and Social Security, Charman: Dame Mary Warnock DBE (London: Her Majesty's Stationery Office, 1984.

Reynolds DW, Stagno S, Alford CA, "Congenital cytomegalovirus infection" in: Sever JL, Brent RL, eds, **Teratogen Update: Environmentally Induced Birth Defect Risks**. New York: Liss 1986, 93-95.

Rhoads GG, Jackson LG, Schlesselman SE *et al*, "The safety and efficacy of chorionic villus sampling for early prenatal diagnosis of cytogenetic abnormalities" *New England Journal of Medicine* 320 (1989) 609-617.

Rogan WJ, "PCBs and cola colored babies: Japan, 1968, and Taiwan, 1979" in: Sever JL, Brent RL, eds, **Teratogen Update: Environmentally Induced Birth Defect Risks**. New York: Liss 1986, 127-130.

Romain DR, Chapman CJ, "Fragile site Xq27.3 in a family without mental retardation" *Clinical Genetics* 41 (1992) 33-35.

Rosa FW, "Penicillamine" in: Sever JL, Brent RL, eds, **Teratogen Update: Environmentally Induced Birth Defect Risks**. New York: Liss 1986, 71-75.

--------, Wilk AL, Kelsey FO, "Vitamin A congeners" in: Sever JL, Brent RL, eds, **Teratogen Update: Environmentally Induced Birth Defect Risks**. New York: Liss 1986, 61-70.

Sass H-M, "Brain life and brain death: a proposal for a normative agreement" *Journal of Medicine and philosophy* 14,1 (1989) 45-59.

Seeds JW, Cefalo RC, "Prenatal diagnosis: clinical considerations" in: Malherbe J-F, ed, **Human Life: Its Beginnings and Development**. Paris: L'Harmattan 1988, 117-124.

Semba R, Tanaka O, Tanimura T, "Digestive system" in: Nishimura H, ed, **Atlas of Human Prenatal Histology**, 1st ed. Tokyo-New York: Igaku-Shoin 1983, 171-240.

Seo K, McGregor JA, French JI, "Preterm birth is associated with increased risk of maternal and neonatal infection" *Obstetrics and Gynecology* 79 (1992) 75-80.

Serra A, "La diagnosi prenatale di malattie genetiche" *Medicina e Morale* 4 (1984) 433-448.

--------, Cagiano D, Neri G, Natale MT, Bova R, Maugiatti L, Bellati U, Garzetti GG, Serri FG, Noia G, Riccardi P, Colagrande C, Mirk P, Maresca G, "La diagnosi prenatale di malattie genetiche. Esperienze, prospettive, problemi" *Progresso Medico* 37 (1981) 1-18.

Shiota K, "Central nervous system" in: Nishimura H, ed, **Atlas of Human Prenatal Histology**, 1st ed. Tokyo-New York: Igaku-Shoin 1983, 19-48.

Silbergeld EK, Mattison DR, Bertin JE, "Occupational exposures and female reproduction" in: Evans MI, Dixler AO, Fletcher JC, Schulman JD, eds, **Fetal Diagnosis and Therapy: Science, Ethics and the Law**. Philadelphia: Lippincott 1989, 149-171.

Simpson JL, "Transmitting genetic disorders to offspring of mentally retarded individuals: principles underlying genetic counseling" in: Evans MI, Dixler AO, Fletcher JC, Schulman JD, eds, **Fetal Diagnosis and Therapy: Science, Ethics and the Law**. Philadelphia: Lippincott 1989, 94-101.

--------, Elias S, "Prenatal diagnosis of genetic disorders" in: Creasy RK, Resnik R, eds, **Maternal-Fetal Medicine: Principles and Practice**, 2nd ed. Philadelphia: Saunders 1989, 78-107.

Smidt-Jensen S, Philip J, "Comparison of transabdominal and transcervical CVS and amniocentesis: sampling success and risk" *Prenatal Diagnosis* 11 (1991) 529-537.

Smith R, "Rapid progress on preimplantation diagnosis" *British Medical Journal* 297,6641 (1988) 92.

South MA, Sever JL, "The congenital rubella syndrome" in: Sever JL, Brent RL, eds, **Teratogen Update: Environmentally Induced Birth Defect Risks**. New York: Liss 1986, 81-91.

Spielmann H, Vogel R, "Transfer of drugs into the embryo before and during implantation" in: Nau H, Scott Jr. WJ, eds, **Pharmacokinetics in Teratogenesis: Interspecies Comparison and Maternal/Embryonic-Fetal Drug Transfer**. Boca Raton, FL: CRC 1987, 45-53.

Suarez A, "Hydatidiform moles and teratomas confirm the human identity of the preimplantation embryo" *Journal of Medicine and Philosophy* 15,6 (1990) 627-635.

Sullivan FM, Smith SE, McElhatton PR, "Interpretation of animal experiments as illustrated by studies on caffeine" in: Nau H, Scott Jr. WJ, eds, **Pharmacokinetics in Teratogenesis: Interspecies Comparison and Maternal/Embryonic-Fetal Drug Transfer**. Boca Raton, FL: CRC 1987, 123-127.

Tabor BL, Soffici AR, Smith-Wallace T, Yonekura ML, "The effect of maternal cocaine use on the fetus: change in antepartum fetal heart rate tracings" *American Journal of Obstetrics and Gynecology* 165 (1991) 1278-1281.

Tanaka O, "Sense organs" in: Nishimura H, ed, **Atlas of Human Prenatal Histology**, 1st ed. Tokyo-New York: Igaku-Shoin 1983, 49-75.

Tanimura T, "Respiratory system" in: Nishimura H, ed, **Atlas of Human Prenatal Histology**, 1st ed. Tokyo-New York: Igaku-Shoin 1983, 241-

257.

--------, Shiota K, "Endocrine system" in: Nishimura H, ed, **Atlas of Human Prenatal Histology**, 1st ed. Tokyo-New York: Igaku-Shoin 1983, 259-291.

Timor-Tritsch IE, Monteagudo A, Warren WB, "Transvaginal ultrasonographic definition of the central nervous system in the first and early second trimesters" *American Journal of Obstetrics and Gynecology* 164 (1991) 497-503.

Tolmie JL, "Chromosomal disorders" in: Whittle MJ, Connor JM, eds, **Prenatal Diagnosis in Obstetric Practice**. Oxford: Blackwell 1989, 33-45.

Toncheva D, "Fragile sites and spontaneous abortions" *Genetic Counseling* 2 (1991) 205-210.

Treadwell MC, Bronsteen RA, Bottoms SF, "Prognostic factors and complication rates for cervical cerclage: a review of 482 cases" *American Journal of Obstetrics and Gynecology* 165 (1991) 555-558.

Van Lith JMM, "First-trimester screening for fetal chromosomal abnormalities. Preliminary results" *Prenatal Diagnosis* 11 (1991) 621-624.

Verlinsky Y, Rechitsky S, Evsikov S, White M, Cieslak J, Lifchez A, Valle J, Moise J, Strom CM, "Preconception and preimplantation diagnosis for cystic fibrosis" *Prenatal Diagnosis* 12 (1992) 103-110.

Warkany J, "Aminopterin and methotrexate: Folic acid deficiency" in: Sever JL, Brent RL, eds, **Teratogen Update: Environmentally Induced Birth Defect Risks**. New York: Liss 1986, 39-43.

--------, "Iodine deficiency" in: Sever JL, Brent RL, eds, **Teratogen Update: Environmentally Induced Birth Defect Risks**. New York: Liss 1986, 177-179.

--------, "Warfarin embryopathy" in: Sever JL, Brent RL, eds, **Teratogen Update: Environmentally Induced Birth Defect Risks**. New York: Liss 1986, 23-27.

Watson WJ, Katz VL, "Steroid therapy for hydrops associated with antibody-mediated congenital heart block" *American Journal of Obstetrics and Gynecology* 165 (1991) 553-554.

--------, Albright SG, Rao KW, Aylsworth AS, "Monozygotic twins discordant for partial trisomy 1" *Obstetrics and Gynecology* 76 (1990) 949-951.

Weiss B, Doherty RA, "Methylmercury poisoning" in: Sever JL, Brent RL, eds, **Teratogen Update: Environmentally Induced Birth Defect Risks**. New York: Liss 1986, 119-121.

Werler MM, Pober BR, Holmes LB, "Smoking and pregnancy" in: Sever JL, Brent RL, eds, **Teratogen Update: Environmentally Induced Birth Defect Risks.** New York: Liss 1986, 131-139.

West JD, "Sexing the preembryo" in: Chapman M, Grudzinskas G, Chard T, eds, **The Embryo. Normal and Abnormal Development and Growth.** London: Springer-Verlag 1991, 141-164.

--------, Gosden JR, Angell RR *et al*, "Sexing the human preembryo by DNA-DNA in situ hybridization" *Lancet* 1 (1987) 1345-1347.

Wolff DJ, Raffel LJ, Ferré MM, Schwartz S, "Prenatal ascertainment of an inherited dup(18p) associated with an apparently normal phenotype" *American Journal of Medical Genetics* 41 (1991) 319-321.

Yeoh SC, Sargent IL, Redman CWG, Wordsworth BP, Thein SL, "Detection of fetal cells in maternal blood" *Prenatal Diagnosis* 11 (1991) 117-123.

[no author], "Senate commences hearings on 'human life'" *Science* 212,4495 (1981) 648-649.